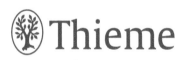

Neurosurgical Review

For Daily Clinical Use and Oral Board Preparation

Vasilios A. Zerris, MD, MPH, MSc, FAANS
Professor of Neurosurgery
European University Cyprus
Nicosia, Cyprus;
Chairman of Neurosurgery
Hygeia Hospital;
Chairman of Pediatric Neurosurgery
IASO Children's Hospital
Athens, Greece;
Diplomate of the American Board of Neurological Surgery
Woodbridge, Connecticut;
American Neurosurgical Associates
Athens, Greece

208 illustrations

Thieme
New York • Stuttgart • Delhi • Rio de Janeiro

Library of Congress Cataloging-in-Publication Data
is available from the publisher

Illustrations by Alexandros N. Vyziotis

Important note: Medicine is an ever-changing science undergoing continual development. Research and clinical experience are continually expanding our knowledge, in particular our knowledge of proper treatment and drug therapy. Insofar as this book mentions any dosage or application, readers may rest assured that the authors, editors, and publishers have made every effort to ensure that such references are in accordance with **the state of knowledge at the time of production of the book.**

Nevertheless, this does not involve, imply, or express any guarantee or responsibility on the part of the publishers in respect to any dosage instructions and forms of applications stated in the book. **Every user is requested to examine carefully** the manufacturers' leaflets accompanying each drug and to check, if necessary in consultation with a physician or specialist, whether the dosage schedules mentioned therein or the contraindications stated by the manufacturers differ from the statements made in the present book. Such examination is particularly important with drugs that are either rarely used or have been newly released on the market. Every dosage schedule or every form of application used is entirely at the user's own risk and responsibility. The authors and publishers request every user to report to the publishers any discrepancies or inaccuracies noticed. If errors in this work are found after publication, errata will be posted at www.thieme.com on the product description page.

Some of the product names, patents, and registered designs referred to in this book are in fact registered trademarks or proprietary names even though specific reference to this fact is not always made in the text. Therefore, the appearance of a name without designation as proprietary is not to be construed as a representation by the publisher that it is in the public domain.

© 2020. Thieme. All rights reserved.
Thieme Publishers New York
333 Seventh Avenue, New York, NY 10001 USA
+1 800 782 3488, customerservice@thieme.com

Thieme Publishers Stuttgart
Rüdigerstrasse 14, 70469 Stuttgart, Germany
+49 [0]711 8931 421, customerservice@thieme.de

Thieme Publishers Delhi
A-12, Second Floor, Sector-2, Noida-201301
Uttar Pradesh, India
+91 120 45 566 00, customerservice@thieme.in

Thieme Publishers Rio de Janeiro,
Thieme Publicações Ltda.
Edifício Rodolpho de Paoli, 25ª andar
Av. Nilo Peçanha, 50 – Sala 2508
Rio de Janeiro 20020-906, Brasil
+55 21 3172 2297

Cover design: Thieme Publishing Group
Cover image: Alexandros N. Vyziotis

Typesetting by DiTech Process Solutions, India

Printed in USA by King Printing Company, Inc.

ISBN 978-1-68420-021-4

Also available as an e-book:
eISBN 978-1-68420-022-1

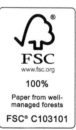

FSC
www.fsc.org
100%
Paper from well-managed forests
FSC® C103101

I dedicate this book to:

My wonderful parents, Athanasios and Anna. I owe everything to them. Their limitless love and kindness have been the foundation of my life. They are the most wonderful parents and people in the world.

My best friend Gerhard, who for 25 years has been not just my colleague, but above all, my brother in life.

To love. It's what gives life meaning.

Vasilios A. Zerris, MD, MPH, MSc, FAANS

Contents

Audios

Preface

The goal of this book is to present neurosurgical knowledge not in a time consuming long-winded text format, but rather digested in a high yield and easy to memorize format. Not to just present the data, but rather to "visualize" the knowledge. To convert vast complex neurosurgical information into a visual form that makes sense and is easy to recall. Several of the charts and tables also have associated audio files which are meant to further aid in creating the mental framework to easily comprehend and memorize the material.

Although the book is based primarily on notes taken while preparing for the ABNS oral board examination, it has been further enriched so that it serves as a handy and quick reference for daily clinical use by residents, fellows and practicing neurosurgeons throughout the world.

The New Oral Board Format and this Book

Recently the ABNS has changed the format of the oral boards and broken the examination down into three sections. The first session is general neurosurgery, the second section is based on the applicant's focused practice and the third session is based on the cases submitted by the applicant.

The main question is what material is included in the general session? Although an outline of included material is available on the ABNS website, the answer is likely twofold, meaning that there are two types of general sessions. The first is the general session that is taken by all neurosurgeons irrelevant of their sub-specialty focus. This session is meant to determine the applicant's ability to treat diseases that may show up when on-call or in the ER. The applicant is expected to be able to treat all neurosurgical emergencies and stabilize patients appropriately. The second type of general session is the one taken by applicants who select general neurosurgery as their focused practice and thus have two general neurosurgery sessions during their examination. This session is meant to determine the proficiency of applicants in diseases faced both on an emergent and on an elective basis by a community neurosurgeon.

For the purpose of this book, charts likely containing information relevant to the general neurosurgery session taken by all applicants, as well as the focused practice general neurosurgery session are marked with a G . Although we have tried to be inclusive with the choice of information for these sessions, we recommend that applicants strive for a thorough overview of the entire book.

Most of the cases presented at the end of the chapters are targeted towards material that may be tested in both general neurosurgery sessions.

Vasilios A. Zerris, MD, MPH, MSc, FAANS

Contributors

Gerhard M. Friehs, MD, FACGS
Professor of Neurosurgery
European University
Nicosia, Cyprus;
Scientific Director
IASO Children's Hospital
Athens, Greece;
Fellow of the American College of General Surgeons
Chicago, Illinois;
American Neurosurgical Associates
Athens, Greece

Steven W. Hwang, MD
Consulting Neurosurgeon
Pediatric Neurosurgery and Scoliosis
Shriners Hospital for Children
Philadelphia, Pennsylvania

Panagiotis Primikiris, MD, PhD
Staff Neurosurgeon
American Neurosurgical Associates
Athens, Greece

Alexandros N. Vyziotis, MD
Staff Neurosurgeon
American Neurosurgical Associates
Athens, Greece

Vasilios A. Zerris, MD, MPH, MSc, FAANS
Professor of Neurosurgery
European University Cyprus
Nicosia, Cyprus;
Chairman of Neurosurgery
Hygeia Hospital;
Chairman of Pediatric Neurosurgery
IASO Children's Hospital
Athens, Greece;
Diplomate of the American Board of
    Neurological Surgery
Woodbridge, Connecticut;
American Neurosurgical Associates
Athens, Greece

1 Peripheral Nerves

1.1 Diagnostic Approach for Peripheral Nerve Lesions (Table 1.1) G

History	1. Symptoms (sens., weakness, atrophy) 2. Mechanism of injury 3. Chronological progression of symptoms 4. Getting better/worse? 5. Inciting events?
Examination	1. Inspection (incl. postures) 2. Palpation (e.g., mass lesion, subluxation) 3. Motor examination 4. Sensory examination (fuzzy vs. discrete borders) 5. Reflexes (UMN vs. LMN) 6. Provocative tests (e.g. Tinel's sign) 7. Other: vascular examination, passive ROM (contractions)
Diagnostic studies	1. Electrophysiology (electromyogram [EMG], nerve conduction study [NCS]) 2. Imaging (US, CT, MRI)

1.2 Neuropathies

1.2.1 Nerve Pathologies Depending on Number and Location of Nerves Involved (Table 1.2a) G

	Dfn, features	Causes/specific syndromes
Mononeuropathy	One peripheral nerve involved	• Injury/iatrogenic • Compression/entrapment
Polyneuropathy	Diffuse lesions of many nerves involved: • Distal nerves > prox nerves involved • Motor + sensory (incl. pain) fibers involved	• Endocrinological diseases (DM, hypothyroidism) • Alcohol • Vitamin B12 deficiency • Heavy metals • Meds (e.g., chemotherapy) • Radiotherapy • Charcot–Marie–Tooth II (CMT II)
Mononeuritis multiplex	> 2 nerves involved in non-contiguous areas (simultaneous OR sequential)	• Autoimmune diseases (systemic lupus erythematosus [SLE], RA, sarcoid) • Vasculitis (polyarteritis nodosa)
Plexopathy	Brachial OR lumbosacral plexus involved	• Trauma • Brachial neuritis (Parsonage–Turner syndrome)

1.2.2 Other Classifications for Polyneuropathies (Table 1.2b) G

- Inherited vs. acquired
- Small fiber neuropathy (e.g., DM) vs. large fiber neuropathy (AKA sensory ataxic neuropathies)
- Neuropathies with predominantly motor deficits vs. with predominantly sensory deficits

1.2.3 Causes for Neuropathies (Table 1.2c) G

- Hereditary (CMT disorder)
- Traumatic (injuries, entrapment)
- Infection (Hansen's, AIDS, Guillain–Barré)
- Autoimmune (sarcoidosis, polymyalgia rheumatica)
- Ca (paraneoplastic, CTX, RTX)
- Metabolic (hypothyroidism, DM, uremic neuropathy, amyloid)
- Medicines, toxins (heavy metals), alcohol
- Vitamin B12 deficiency
- Pseudoneuropathy

1.2.4 Peripheral Neuropathy Versus Radiculopathy (Tab. 1.2d) G

	Radiculopathy	Neuropathy
Sensory distribution	Fuzzy	Discrete
Muscle atrophy	No (rare)	Yes

- Utilize patterns of innervation to differential diagnosis (DDx):
    - Sensory nerve distribution
    - Motor innervation

1.3 Peripheral Nerve Injuries G

1.3.1 Basics (Table 1.3a) G

Nerve anatomy	
Endoneurium	Surrounds myelinated OR unmyelinated axons
Perineurium	Surrounds fascicles
Mesoneurium (AKA interfascicular epineurium)	Separates fascicles
Epineurium	Surrounds nerve

1.3.2 Regeneration (Table 1.3b) G

- **Rate**   1 mm/d → 1 inch/mo
- **Signs**
  - Advancing Tinel's sign
  - Motor march phenomena
    (= motor reinnervation from
    prox. → dist.)

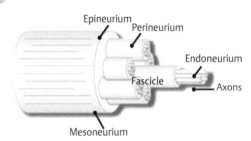

1.3.3 Mechs of Nerve Injury (Table 1.3c) G

- Trauma (compression–crush, concussive, laceration, stretch)
- Entrapment
- Ischemic
- Thermal, electrical, radiotherapy

1.3.4 Grading of Nerve Injuries (Table 1.3d) G

Seddon	Sunderland	Pathology dfn	Wallerian degeneration	NCS	Spontaneous recovery
Neuropraxia	I	Intact basement membrane (physiologic rather than anatomic transection/nerve in continuity)	NO (maybe just focal demyelinating injury)	No conduction across lesion Conduction prox. + dist. to lesion	Complete (in h/mo; ave: 6–8 wk)
	II	Complete interruption of axons—myelin sheaths with intact endoneurium			Good
Axonotmesis	III	Axons + endoneurium disrupted with intact perineurium	YES (dist. to injr)	Block distally	Variable (possibility of scarring)
	IV	Axons + endoneurium + perineurium disrupted with intact epineurium			Poor, neuroma formation
Neurotmesis	V	Complete transection (loss of continuity)	YES (dist. to injr)	Block distally	NO

Note: Pure grades of injury rarely exist; severity of most injury occurs along a continuum.

Epineurium
Perineurium
Endoneurium
Myelin
Axon

Conduction block

Axonal discontinuity

Axonal + endoneurium disruption

Perineurial rupture fascicle disruption

Nerve trunk discontinuity

— Wallerian degeneration

1.3.5 Peripheral Nerve Injury Grading Systems (Table 1.3e)

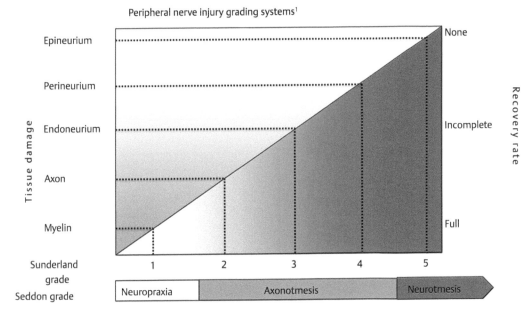

Peripheral nerve injury grading systems[1]

(Source: Adapted from Burnett et al.[1])

1.3.6 Management of Peripheral Nerve Injury (Table 1.3f) [G]

Evaluation (identify involved nerve, mech, degree of injury, time from injury)	• Hx • P/E (motor, sens, reflexes, autonomous nervous system involvement, trophic changes) • Electrophysiology • Imaging

Management	• Conservative (PT, splinting, pain meds)
	• Surgical repair:
	  – Options:
	    ◦ Neurolysis
	    ◦ Primary/secondary repair ± nerve graft
	    ◦ Nerve transfer
	  – Timing: rule of 3s

1.3.7 Timing of Nerve Exploration and Repair Rule of 3s (Table 1.3g) [G]

3 d/ASAP	Sharp clean lacerations
3 wk	• Blunt lacerations • Blast injuries
3 mo	Injury in continuity: stretch, compression, etc. (Mgt: follow nerve regeneration closely by clinical examinations ± EMG, NCS) → surgical exploration and repair if no recovery after 3 mo

1.3.8 Algorithm of Timing of Nerve Surgery[2,3] (Table 1.3h 🔊) G

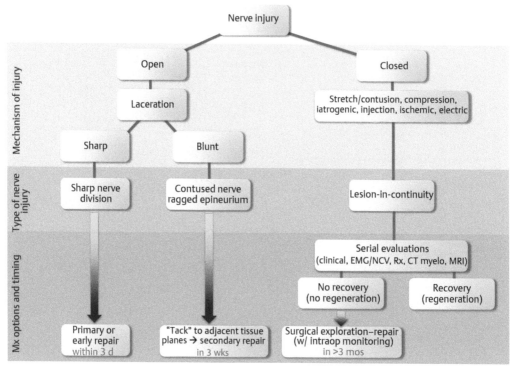

(Source: Adapted from Dubuisson and Kline[2] and Chung et al.[3])

1.3.9 Peripheral Nerve Repair: Surgical Pearls (Table 1.3i) G

- Trim back to healthy nerve (fascicular) tissue
- Tension-free neurorrhaphy + least possible microsutures
- Topographic specificity (= match surface landmarks)
- Magnification (microinstruments)
- Cover repair with fibrin glue
- No overriding fascicles
- Consider use of epineurial, grouped fascicular and fascicular repairs depending on circumstances
- Use max amount of graft (= maximal cross-sectional coverage of nerve stumps)

1.4 Brachial Plexus

1.4.1 Brachial Plexus Injuries (Table 1.4a) G

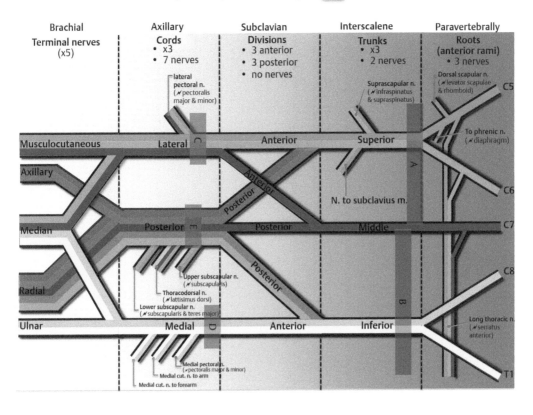

1.4.2 Brachial Plexus Injuries: Trunks (Table 1.4b) G

	Mech of injury	Motor deficits	Sensory deficits	UE posture	DDx
1. Upper trunk injury (C5, C6, ±C7); Erb–Duchenne palsy; common (A)	Forcible widening of shoulder–neck angle (shoulder pushed downward vs. head stabilized/pushed upward) • Motorcycle accidents • Falls • Parturition/obstetric	Weakness of muscles w/ C5, C6 ✗: • Infraspinatus • Supraspinatus • Deltoid • BB • Brachioradialis • Supinator (occ.)	Sens. loss in C5 + C6 dermatomes: • Lat. half of UA + forearm (FA) • Thumb (1st finger)	Bellhop's/waiter's tip position (see Table 1.10 • Arm hangs at side adducted–internally rotated • Elbow extension • Wrist–finger flexion	Versus C5, C6 nerve root injr: brachial plexus weakness involves more muscles: • +Rhomboids (✗ by dorsal scapular n.) • + Serratus anterior (✗ by long thoracic n.) • + Diaphragm (✗ by phrenic n.)

2. Lower brachial plexus injury (C8, T1, ±C7); Klumpke's palsy; rare (B)	• Forcible widening of chest wall–arm angle (traction of abducted arm)
	• Pancoast's syndrome due to chest tumor
	  – Pain along med. UA, FA
	  – Motor–sens. def.
	  – Horner's S.
		Weakness of muscles w/ C8, T1 ✗:
		• Hand grip
		• Finger spreading
		+ Horner s. (if T1 involved)
			Sens. loss in C5 + C6 dermatomes:
			• Med. FA+ hand
			• 5th finger
				Claw deformity:
				• FA supinations
				• Hyperextension of MCP joints
				• Flexion of IP joints	

1.4.3 Brachial Plexus Injuries: Cords (Table 1.4c)

	Motor deficits	Sensory deficits
1. **Lateral cord palsy** (C5, C6, C7; musculocutaneous n. palsy + lat. component of median n. palsy) (C)	a. Weakness of muscles w/ MCN ✗: • Weak elbow flex. (BB, brachialis, coracobrachialis) b. Weakness of muscles w/ lateral component of median n. ✗ (C5, C6, C7): • Pronator teres • Flexor carpi radialis (FCR) c. Weakness of clavicular head of pectoralis major (lat. pectoral n.)	a. Sens. loss of MCN n.: • Lat. FA (lat. antebrachial cut. n.) b. Sens. loss of lateral component of median n.: • Lat. Palm • Finger tips 1–3
2. **Medial cord palsy** (C8, T1; ulnar n. palsy + med. component of median n. palsy) (D)	a. Weakness of muscles w/ ulnar n. ✗: • Medial wrist flex. (FCU) • Distal IP joint flexion of fingers 4, 5 (flexor digitorum profundus [FDP]) • Finger 5 mvts (ADM, FDM, ODM) • Finger add–abd (interossei) b. Weakness of muscles w/ medial component of median n. ✗ (C8, T1): • Thumb mvts (opponens pollicis, FPB, APB) • Prox. IP joint ext. (lumbricals 1, 2) c. Weakness of sternal head of pectoralis major (med. pectoral n.)	a. Sens. loss of ulnar n.: • Med. hand • Fingers 4, 5 b. No cut. Innervation of med. component of median n. c. Sens. loss of br. from med. cord: • Med. UA (med. brachial cut. n.) • Med. FA (med. antebrachial cut. n.)
3. **Posterior cord palsy** (C5–C8, ±T1; radial n. palsy + axillary n. palsy) (E)	a. Weakness of muscles w/ radial n. ✗: • FA ext. (TB) • FA supination (supinator) • Wrist ext. (ECR longus–brevis, ECU) • Finger, thumb ext. (finger extensors) b. Weakness of muscles w/ axillary n. ✗: • Arm abd. (deltoid) c. Weakness of muscles w/ ✗ from br. of post. cord: • Arm add. + int. rotation (upper + lower subscapular n., thoracodorsal n.)	a. Sens. loss of radial n.: • Post. UA (post. brachial cut. n.) • Post. FA (post. antebrachial cut. n.) • Lower lat. UA (lower lat. brachial cut. n.) • Dorsolat. hand (superf. sens. radial n.) b. Sens. loss of axillary n.: • Upper lat. UA (upper lat. brachial cut. n.)

1.4.4 Dx of Preganglionic Injury (Nerve Root Avulsion) (Table 1.4d) G

Neuro def	• Prox upper roots:
	  – Phrenic palsy
	  – Serratus anterior/rhomboid paralysis (scapula alata = winged scapula)
	• Horner's syndrome (at T1 only)

EMG/NCS	• Denervation of posterior myotomes (segmental paraspinal muscles) • No motor action potentials (MAPs) • Normal sensory nerve action potentials (SNAPs) from clinically denervated skin • No somatosensory evoked potentials (SSEPs)
MRI/myelography	Intraspinal nerve root(let) Pseudomeningocele

1.4.5 Surgical Approach Based on Defining Clinical Level of Lesion (Table 1.4e) G

Approach		Location of injury
Anterior	Supraclavicular	Roots + trunks + proximal divisions
	Infraclavicular	Distal divisions + cords + terminal branches
	Combination of both	Potentially entire brachial plexus
Posterior	Posterior subscapularar	Roots + trunks + proximal divisions

Note: Indications for posterior subscapular approach (not commonly used): need for very proximal exposure to exiting roots, extensive scarring of anterior neck, and chest wall.

1.4.6 Supraclavicular Approach (Table 1.4f) G

1. Skin incision	• Starts: at jaw angle
	• Course:
	  1. Along posterior border of sternocleidomastoid (SCM)
	  2. At clavicle: turn laterally
	  3. Along superior border of clavicle
	• End: at midpoint of clavicle

2. Division of platysma muscle	

3. Exposure of posterior cervical triangle	• Caution: preserve spinal accessory nerve in superior edge of incision • Vessels crossing the operative field can be ligated • SCM: SCM is detached from clavicle → retracted medially • Omohyoid: cut + retract (tag edges for reapproximation)
4. Supraclavicular fat pad retraction	Dissect free supraclavicular fat pad → retract laterally → exposure of anterior scalene muscle
5. Identification proximal brachial plexus	1. Identify phrenic nerve on anterior surface of anterior scalene muscle 2. Follow phrenic nerve superiorly until it joins C5 spinal nerve 3. Identify C6 spinal nerve deep and slightly inferior to C5 (C5 + C6 form the superior trunk) 4. Identify C7 deep and inferior to C6 (C7 forms the middle trunk) 5. Identify the lower trunk deep and inferior to middle trunk 6. Identify C8, T1 spinal nerves (C8 + T1 form the lower trunk) 7. Trace trunks distally → identify divisions
6. Maneuver for better exposure of proximal brachial plexus	Anterior scalene muscle division resection with protection of phrenic nerve and internal jugular vein

1.4.7 Infraclavicular Approach (Table 1.4g)

1. Skin incision	• Starts: at midpoint of clavicle • Course: inferiorly along deltopectoral groove • End: anterior axillary crease
2. Cephalic vein resection	
3. Exposure of posterior cervical triangle	• Caution: preserve spinal accessory nerve in superior edge of incision • Vessels crossing the operative field can be ligated • SCM: SCM is detached from clavicle → retracted medially • Omohyoid: cut + retract (tag edges for reapproximation)
4. Pectoralis minor division	Division of pectoralis minor tendon insertion to coracoid process (leave muscle cuff for reapproximation)
5. Incision of clavipectoral fascia	
6. Identification of cords	1. Identify lateral cord → identify musculocutaneous nerve (from lateral cord) 2. Identify axillary artery inferomedial to lateral cord 3. Identify posterior cord posterior to axillary artery 4. Identify medial cord (+ its proximal sensory branches) inferomedial to axillary artery
7. Retraction of clavicle for exposure of divisions proximally	1. Detach pectoralis major from clavicle 2. Ligate suprascapular artery/vein 3. Resect subclavius muscle 4. Retract clavicle
8. Identification of brachial plexus terminal branches	1. Identify reverse Greek "Σ" formation of nerves (superior/lateral → inferior/medial: musculocutaneous, median, ulnar) 2. Identify radial and axillary nerves from posterior cord

1.4.8 Neurogenic Thoracic Outlet Syndrome (Table 1.4h)

Involved neural structures		C8, T1 +/ lower trunk irritated at scalene triangle
Causes		• Abnl fibrous band btw. ant. and mid. scalene m. • Elongated C7 transverse process/cervical rib
Sensory	Presentation	• Dull shoulder/axilla pain (not so concerning for pt)
	Examination	• Sens. loss: med. FA + med. hand • Roos' maneuver/elevated arm stress test: external arm rotation + abd. over head for 1–2 min → provocation • Tinel's sign: at supraclavicular area (not always)
Motor	Presentation	Progressive hand intrinsic weakness—atrophy (median n. > ulnar n. innerv. hand intrinsics)
Posture		Forward drooping shoulders

DDx		• R/O C8 radiculopathy:
		  – No neck/radicular pain
		  – C8 + T1 motor and sens. def. in thoracic outlet syndrome
		• R/O ulnar n. compression at elbow
		  – Weakness of both ABP (~by median n.) + ADM/FDI (~by ulnar n.) in thoracic outlet syndrome

Dx		C-spine XR: R/O C7 bony anomalies
Treatment (Tx)	Conservative	• Modification of activities • Physical therapy • Transcutaneous electrical nerve stimulation (TENS) • Pain meds (nonsteroidal anti-inflammatory diseases [NSAIDs], opiates, antiepileptics, antidepressants) • Nerve blocks
	Surgical	Surgical exploration + decompression via anterior supraclavicular approach (± transaxillary approach)

1.4.9 Parsonage–Turner Syndrome (Table 1.4i) [G]

Demographics		Males>, any age
Causes		• Unknown • Previous viral infection • Shoulder trauma/overuse • Surgery
Sensory	Presentation	• Sudden marked shoulder pain → pain radiation: – Down along UA – Up to the neck – To the scapula • Better with UA add. + FA flex. • Sens. loss: absent/minimal during acute phase
Motor	Presentation	• No weakness during acute phase → significant weakness occurs later after pain resolution • Most common muscles involved: – Deltoid – Supraspinatus, infraspinatus
DDx		MRI C-spine: R/O disk herniation
Dx		EMG/NCV (early and repeat in 6 weeks)
Management		a. Early stage (pain): – Pain meds (NSAIDs, opiates, antiepileptics, antidepressants) – Oral steroids (controversial) – TENS b. Later stage (weakness): – Physical therapy (strengthening exercises, range-of-motion exercises) – Electrical stimulation (controversial)
Prognosis		Self-limiting (wk) → near normal in 3 y

1.5 Entrapment Neuropathies

1.5.1 Median Nerve ([C5], C6, C7, C8, T1) Sites of Compression (Table 1.5a)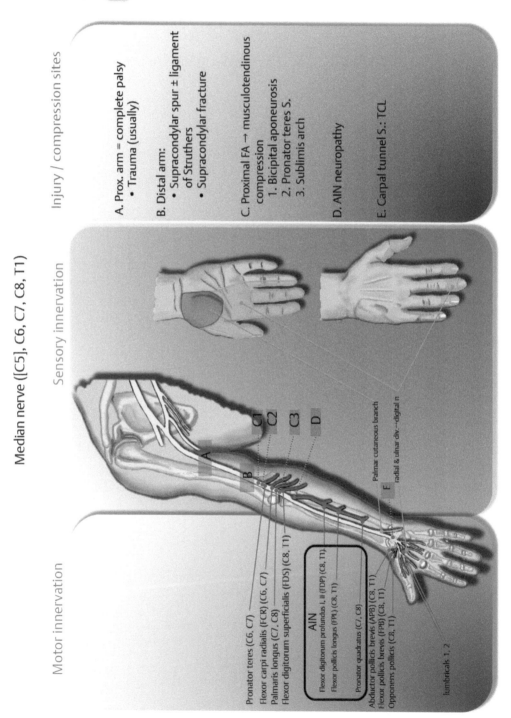

Median nerve ([C5], C6, C7, C8, T1)

Injury / compression sites

A. Prox. arm = complete palsy
- Trauma (usually)

B. Distal arm:
- Supracondylar spur ± ligament of Struthers
- Supracondylar fracture

C. Proximal FA → musculotendinous compression
 1. Bicipital aponeurosis
 2. Pronator teres S.
 3. Sublimis arch

D. AIN neuropathy

E. Carpal tunnel S.: TCL

Sensory innervation

Motor innervation

Pronator teres (C6, C7)
Flexor carpi radialis (FCR) (C6, C7)
Palmaris longus (C7, C8)
Flexor digitorum superficialis (FDS) (C8, T1)

AIN
Flexor digitorum profundus I, II (FDP) (C8, T1)
Flexor pollicis longus (FPL) (C8, T1)

Pronator quadratus (C7, C8)

Abductor pollicis brevis (APB) (C8, T1)
Flexor pollicis brevis (FPB) (C8, T1)
Opponens pollicis (C8, T1)

lumbricals 1, 2

C1
C2
C3
D

Palmar cutaneous branch
radial & ulnar div→digital n

A
B
E

1.5.2 Median Nerve Entrapment Sites: Motor and Sensory Deficits (Table 1.5b) G

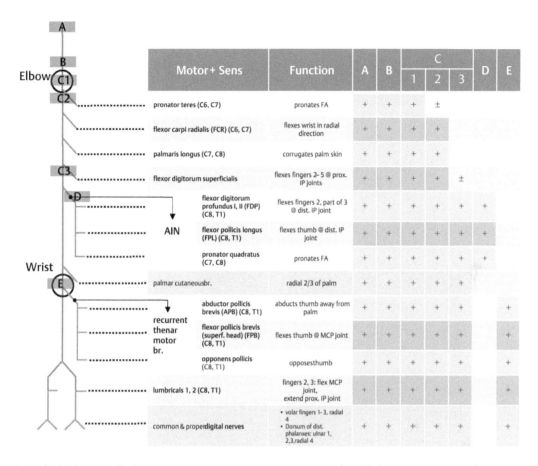

Motor+ Sens	Function	A	B	C 1	C 2	C 3	D	E
pronator teres (C6, C7)	pronates FA	+	+	+	±			
flexor carpi radialis (FCR) (C6, C7)	flexes wrist in radial direction	+	+	+	+			
palmaris longus (C7, C8)	corrugates palm skin	+	+	+	+			
flexor digitorum superficialis	flexes fingers 2–5 @ prox. IP joints	+	+	+	+	±		
flexor digitorum profundus I, II (FDP) (C8, T1)	flexes fingers 2, part of 3 @ dist. IP joint	+	+	+	+	+	+	
flexor pollicis longus (FPL) (C8, T1)	flexes thumb @ dist. IP joint	+	+	+	+	+	+	
pronator quadratus (C7, C8)	pronates FA	+	+	+	+	+	+	
palmar cutaneous br.	radial 2/3 of palm	+	+	+	+	+		
abductor pollicis brevis (APB) (C8, T1)	abducts thumb away from palm	+	+	+	+	+		+
flexor pollicis brevis (superf. head) (FPB) (C8, T1)	flexes thumb @ MCP joint	+	+	+	+	+		+
opponens pollicis (C8, T1)	opposes thumb	+	+	+	+	+		+
lumbricals 1, 2 (C8, T1)	fingers 2, 3: flex MCP joint, extend prox. IP joint	+	+	+	+	+		+
common & proper digital nerves	• volar fingers 1- 3, radial 4 • Dorsum of dist. phalanxes: ulnar 1, 2,3,radial 4	+	+	+	+	+		+

Legends: O Joint, ___ : mixed nerve, ___ : motor nerve, ___ : sensory nerve . In the table, boxes containing muscles are colored with blue shades and their deficits with gray shades. Boxes containing nerve br., which innervate skin as well as their deficit are colored green. Red boxes show possible entrapment sites.

1.5.3 Clinical Syndromes and Findings: Median Nerve Injury/Compression in Arm (Table 1.5c) G

Location of injury/compression	Causes	Motor	Sensation	Postures/signs	Dx	Pitfalls (mimicking/substitution)
Arm Proximal (A)	• Trauma (usually, + concomitant neurovascular injury) • Saturday night palsy: hanging arm over chair and fainting • Honeymooners palsy: arm under someone's neck • Pressure from crutch head	**Examination** Weakness[a]: • FA (pronator teres): no pronation • Wrist (FCR): weak flexion in ulnar direction • Thumb (ABP, OP): no opposition, no palmar abd • Second, third fingers: weakness of lumbricals	**Presentation** Numbness: • Radial two-thirds of palm • Volar surfaces of fingers 1–3 and radial half of 4 **Examination** Sensation loss: same distribution like numbness	Benedictine sign (orator's hand) 1. Pt makes fist 2. Finger flexion: • 1st: almost none • 2nd: partial • 3rd: weak • 4th, 5th: nl (see Table 1.10)		• Pronation: brachioradialis w/ gravity (↗ by radial n.) • Thumb opposition: FPB (deep head), add. pol. (both ↗ by ulnar n.) • Thumb abduction: FPB (deep head ↗ by ulnar n.), APL (↗ by radial n.)

Location of injury/ compression		Causes	Motor	Sensation	Postures/ signs	Dx	Pitfalls (mimicking/ substitution)
Arm	Distal (B)	**Entrapment** • Supracondylar spur: ≈ on med. humerus, 5 cm prox. to med. epicondyle (1%) + • Ligament of Struthers: lig. between supracondylar spur and med. epicondyle → median n. passes under this lig. (w/ brachial OR ulnar artery)	**Presentation** Insidious onset of FA, hand weakness **Examination** • Variable weakness ± wasting in any median n. innerv muscle • Pronator teres may be spared	**Presentation** Deep aching pain in prox. FA (occ. worsens w/ pronation–supination) Variable sensory loss **Examination** Tinel's sign: in dist med arm	OK sign: (see Table 1.5g, AIN neuropathy)	Dx of spur • XR • Palpation	
		Injury Supracondylar fractures: • Acute injury (esp. if displaced) • Delayed injury(callus formation)	Pseudo-anterior interosseous neuropathy[b] (often): Isolated AIN motor loss (partial median n. injr) + 1st, 2nd finger numbness (DDx vs. true AIN neuropathy)				

[a]Weakness of pronator teres implies injury above elbow.
[b]AIN exists as separate bundle in median n. before branching off.
Note: AIN fibers + sens fibers for first and second fingers placed post in median n. at dist arm.

1.5.4 Management for Injury of Median Nerve in Arm (A, B) (Table. 1.5d) G

Lesion type	Management options
Injury (A, B)	• Management options and timing follow general rules and rule of 3s for nerve injuries • Indications for surgery: progressive neurological deficit, intractable pain

1.5.5 Key Surgical Steps for Median Nerve Exposure in Arm (A, B) (Table 1.5e) G

1. Incision	1. Starts: from axillary fold 2. Courses: along the sulcus btw. BB and TB 3. Ends: 4 cm above med. epicondyle incision curves laterally
2. Anatomical structures encountered before median n.	1. Med. brachial cut. n.: beware—preserve prior to opening the brachialis fascia 2. Ulnar n.: the first nerve we might encounter is the ulnar n. (posteromed. vs. median n.) with the basilic vein
3. Median n. identification	• Dissect more lateral to ulnar n. to find the median n. • Median n. proximally courses laterally to brachial a. and then crosses medially

1.5.6 Clinical Syndromes and Findings: Median Nerve Entrapment in FA (Table 1.5f) [G]

Location of injury/ compression	Causes		Motor		Sensation	
FA	Entrapment	Musculo-tendinous compression (C)	(C1) Bicipital aponeurosis (very rare)	Presentation	Similar to compression due to ligament of Struthers	Presentation	Similar to compression due to ligament of Struthers: • Elbow pain radiating proximally and distally • Worse by resisted FA flexion
			(C2) Pronator teres syndrome: compression btw. two heads of pronator teres (unknown incidence)	Examination	• All muscles may be involved except for pronator teres • Weakness of flexion of 2nd, 3rd fingers (occasionally)	Presentation Examination	• Insidious onset of dull aching pain of proximal FA • Worse by repetitive pronation • Pronator teres tenderness • Hand sensation: nl • Tinel's sign: at antecubital fossa
			(C3) sublimis arch (arch of FDS)			Presentation	• Similar to pronator teres syndrome • Worse pain by FDS contraction

Note: AIN fibers + sens fibers for first and second fingers placed post in median n. at dist arm.

1.5.7 Clinical Syndromes and Findings: Median Nerve / AIN Injury/Compression in FA (Table 1.5g) [G]

Location of injury/compression	Causes	Motor	Sensation	Postures/signs	Dx	DDx
FA AIN (D)	• Unknown • Trauma/fracture • Parsonage–Turner S. • Anomalous muscle +/tendons	**Presentation** Weakness/clumsiness grasping objects with 1st and 2nd fingers **Examination** weakness: • FDP • PQ • FPL	**Presentation** **Examination** nl	• Progressive arm/FA pain followed by weakness • No numbness	OK sign: • nl: thumb and index fingertips touch together • In AIN palsy: volar surfaces of thumb and index touch together	• EMG/NCV • MRI: may show denervation of muscles innerv by AIN	• Cervical spine degenerative disease • Brachial plexopathy • Parsonage–Turner syndrome • Pseudo-AIN • Spontaneous painless rupture of FDS, FPL tendons in RA pts

Note: AIN fibers + sens fibers for first and second fingers placed post in median n. at dist arm.

1.5.8 Management for Entrapment of Median Nerve/AIN at Distal Arm/Elbow/Proximal FA (C, D) (Table 1.5h) G

Lesion type	Management options		
Entrapment (C, D)	Conservative	• NSAIDs • Activities modifications (avoidance of repetitive FA supination/pronation)	
	Surgery	Indications	No improvement > 8–12 wk
		Technique	Surgical exploration and decompression

1.5.9 Key Surgical Steps for Decompression of Median n./AIN at Distal Arm/Elbow/Proximal FA (C, D) (Table 1.5i) G

1. Landmarks	Mark biceps tendon
2. Incision	1. Starts: 2–3 cm above med. epicondyle over the medial IM septum 2. Courses: curves lateral just med. to BB tendon 3. Ends: continues into FA btw. FDS and brachioradialis
3. Median n. identification	Find median n. proximally btw. biceps and IM septum →follow into FA
4. Division of three points of compression	a. Lacertus aponeurosis (oblique) b. Deep head of pronator teres c. Arch of FDS (sublimis arch) d. Also divide any other constricting fibrous bands/collateral vessels

Note: There is a still controversy regarding conservative vs. surgical management of AIN entrapment.

1.5.10 Clinical Syndromes and Findings: Median Nerve Entrapment in Carpal Tunnel (Table 1.5j) Ⓖ

Compression site	Causes	Motor	Sensation	Postures/ signs	Dx
Hand (E)	Entrapment	Carpal tunnel syndrome (compression by transverse carpal lig.)	Systemic diseases: – Hypothyroidism, acromegaly, DM – Chronic renal dialysis – RA – Obesity – Vitamin B6 deficiency – Alcoholism • Pregnancy • Trauma • Space occupying lesions • Genetic • Anatomical variations • Repetitive wrist movements	Presentation • Hand clumsiness • Weak grip strength Examination • Thenar muscle wasting • Weakness: – Thumb opp (OP) – Thumb abduction (APB) – Thumb flexion (FPB)	Presentation • Aching pain and paresthesias in radial half of palm, fingers 1–3 • Insidious onset • Pain wakes pt up at night • Relief: by shaking hand away; strike Examination • Fingers 1–3, half of 4: – Hypesthesia/hyperesthesia – ↓Vibratory sensation • Thenar eminence: nl • Tinel's sign: at wrist	• Phalen's test: forceful wrist flexion →↑ paresthesias • Reverse Phalen's test: wrist extension → paresthesias	• NCS: a. Sensory studies (earliest, most sensitive): – ↑Latency at carpal tunnel > 3.7 ms – ↓Amplitude OR absent b. Motor studies (APB): ↑latency at carpal tunnel > 4 ms EMG: DDx vs.: 1. Other median n. entrapment sites 2. Brachial plexus lesions 3. C6, C7 radiculopathies

Note: AIN fibers + sens fibers for first and second fingers placed post in median n. at dist arm.

1.5.11 Management for Entrapment of Median Nerve at Carpal Tunnel (E) (Table 1.5k) G

Lesion type	Management options		
Carpal tunnel syndrome (E)	Conservative	• NSAIDs, steroids • Steroid injections • Splint • Tx of underlying systematic diseases	
	Surgery	Indications	• Failure of conservative measures • Progressive OR nonimproving sensory loss • Muscle atrophy/weakness • EMG findings of axonal loss
		Technique	Surgical exploration and division of transverse carpal ligament (TCL)
		Outcomes	• Excellent results for most pts (pain/paresthesias relieved, motor improvement) • Surgical decompression is better for symptom relief vs. conservative Tx • Factors in favor of good outcome: symptoms <3y, no muscle atrophy/weakness, no OR low degree of demyelination/axonal loss

1.5.12 Key Surgical Steps for Median Nerve Decompression at the Carpal Tunnel (E) (Table 1.5l) G

1. Incision	1. Starts: at distal wrist crease 2. Courses: along ulnar side of palmar crease pointing to ulnar edge of middle finger up to 4 cm (ulnar to palmaris longus tendon) 3. Ends: at point where incision intersects Kaplan's line (= line parallel to distal border of extended thumb)
2. Division of layers	1. Subcutaneous fat 2. Palmar fascia 3. Thenar—hypothenar muscles (occ.) cover TCL in midline 4. TCL

3. TCL division	1. Incise midpoint of TCL w/ scalpel → should put you on ulnar side of nerve
	2. Dissect median nerve off TCL w/ fine scissors
	3. Extents of incision:
	  a. Distal: until you find palmar fat pad
	  b. Proximal: ≈ 2 cm prox. to wrist crease until the deep FA fascia is found

4. Preservation of median n. branches	• Recurrent motor branch • Palmar cutaneous branch

Recur. motor branch	• Origin:
	  – 50% past the transverse ligament
	  – 30% subligamentous
	  – 20% transligamentous
	• Location: at intersection of Kaplan line–radial border of third finger
	• Must be preserved

1.6 Ulnar Nerve

1.6.1 Ulnar Nerve (C7, C8, T1) (Table 1.6a)   G

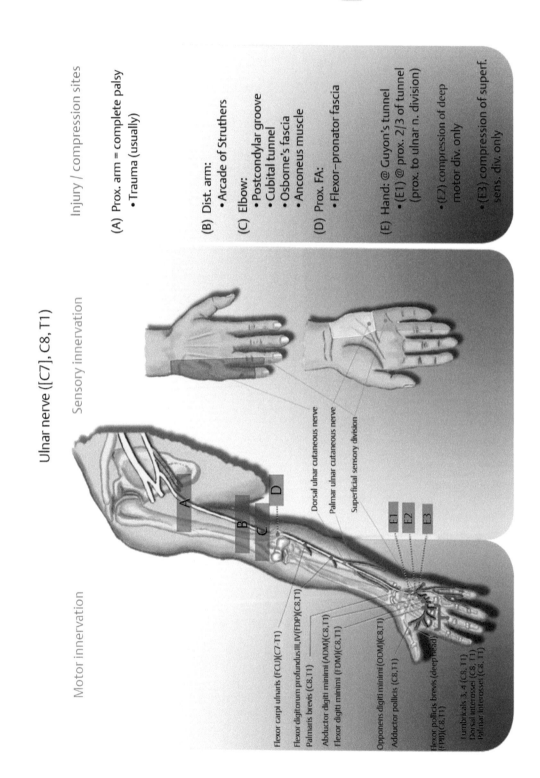

Injury / compression sites

(A) Prox. arm = complete palsy
 • Trauma (usually)

(B) Dist. arm:
 • Arcade of Struthers

(C) Elbow:
 • Postcondylar groove
 • Cubital tunnel
 • Osborne's fascia
 • Anconeus muscle

(D) Prox. FA:
 • Flexor–pronator fascia

(E) Hand: @ Guyon's tunnel
 • (E1) @ prox. 2/3 of tunnel (prox. to ulnar n. division)
 • (E2) compression of deep motor div. only
 • (E3) compression of superf. sens. div. only

Ulnar nerve ([C7], C8, T1)

Sensory innervation

Motor innervation

Dorsal ulnar cutaneous nerve
Palmar ulnar cutaneous nerve
Superficial sensory division

Flexor carpi ulnaris (FCU)(C7-T1)
Flexor digitorum profundus III,IV(FDP)(C8,T1)
Palmaris brevis (C8,T1)
Abductor digiti minimi (ADM)(C8,T1)
Flexor digiti minimi (FDM)(C8,T1)
Opponens digiti minimi (ODM)(C8,T1)
Adductor pollicis (C8,T1)
Flexor pollicis brevis (deep head) (FPB)(C8,T1)
Lumbricals 3, 4 (C8, T1)
Dorsal interossei (C8, T1)
Palmar interossei (C8, T1)

1.6.2 Ulnar Nerve Entrapment Sites: Motor and Sensory Deficits (Table 1.6b) G

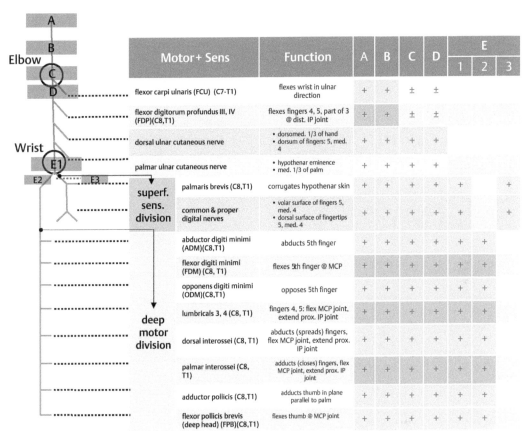

Motor+ Sens	Function	A	B	C	D	E 1	E 2	E 3
flexor carpi ulnaris (FCU) (C7-T1)	flexes wrist in ulnar direction	+	+	±	±			
flexor digitorum profundus III, IV (FDP)(C8,T1)	flexes fingers 4, 5, part of 3 @ dist. IP joint	+	+	±	±			
dorsal ulnar cutaneous nerve	• dorsomed. 1/3 of hand • dorsum of fingers: 5, med. 4	+	+	+	+			
palmar ulnar cutaneous nerve	• hypothenar eminence • med. 1/3 of palm	+	+	+	+			
superf. sens. division palmaris brevis (C8,T1)	corrugates hypothenar skin	+	+	+	+	+		+
common & proper digital nerves	• volar surface of fingers 5, med. 4 • dorsal surface of fingertips 5, med. 4	+	+	+	+	+		+
abductor digiti minimi (ADM)(C8,T1)	abducts 5th finger	+	+	+	+	+	+	
flexor digiti minimi (FDM) (C8, T1)	flexes 5th finger @ MCP	+	+	+	+	+	+	
opponens digiti minimi (ODM)(C8,T1)	opposes 5th finger	+	+	+	+	+	+	
deep motor division lumbricals 3, 4 (C8, T1)	fingers 4, 5: flex MCP joint, extend prox. IP joint	+	+	+	+	+	+	
dorsal interossei (C8, T1)	abducts (spreads) fingers, flex MCP joint, extend prox. IP joint	+	+	+	+	+	+	
palmar interossei (C8, T1)	adducts (closes) fingers, flex MCP joint, extend prox. IP joint	+	+	+	+	+	+	
adductor pollicis (C8,T1)	adducts thumb in plane parallel to palm	+	+	+	+	+	+	
flexor pollicis brevis (deep head) (FPB)(C8,T1)	flexes thumb @ MCP joint	+	+	+	+	+	+	

Legends: **O** joint, —— : mixed nerve, —— : motor nerve, ···· : sensory nerve. In the table, boxes containing muscles are colored with blue shades and their deficits with gray shades. Boxes containing nerve br., which innervate skin, as well as their deficits are colored with green shades. The only one orange box implies that this division is mixed. Red boxes show possible entrapment/injury sites.

1.6.3 Clinical Syndromes and Findings: Ulnar Nerve Injury/Compression in Arm (Table 1.6c) | G

Location of injury/compression	Causes	Motor	Sensation	Postures/signs
Arm **Complete palsy (A)**	• Trauma (usu.) (GSW, lacerations, blunt injury) • Compression (by crutch, Saturday night palsy)	**Examination** • Weakness: – Weak wrist flexion in radial direction only (FCU paralysis vs. intact FCR) – No dist. IP joint flexion of the fourth and fifth fingers (partial FDP weakness) – Hand intrinsic muscle weakness (residual muscle function from median n. ~) • Muscle wasting: – Hypothenar eminence – Dorsal interosseous muscles – Thenar eminence (due to adductor pollicis)	**Examination** Loss of sensation: • Hypothenar eminence (~ by palm. ulnar cut. br.) • Volar surface of fingers 5, med. half of 4 (~ by superf. sens. div.) • Dorsomed. one-third of hand + dorsum of finger 5, med. half of 4 (~ by dors. ulnar cut. n.) If sens. loss >2 cm prox. to wrist →suspect higher level of injury (med. cord/C8, T1 roots)	**Examination** • Ulnar claw hand: – Test: pt opens hand → fingers 4, 5: MCP joint hyperextension (unopposed EDC function) + partial flex. of both IP joints (resid. tone of FDP) – Due to Loss of function: third and fourth lumbricals, interossei; FDM • Wartenburg's sign: – Definition: on finger abduction more abducted fifth finger (unopposed action of EDM, EDC) – Due to Loss of function: third palmar interosseous • Froment's sign: – Test: pull apart a piece of paper held btw. volar surface of each straightened thumb+closed fist → thumb IP joint flexes (FPL) – Due to Loss of function: adductor pollicis
Arcade of Struthers (B) (50%, arcade of fascia from IM septum to su-perf. surface of med. head of TB over ulnar n.)	• Causes secondary compression by tethering the relocated ulnar n. after nerve transposition w/o transection of arcade of Struthers			

1.6.4 Management for Injury of Ulnar Nerve in Arm (A) (Table 1.6d)   G

Lesion type	Management options
Injury (A)	• Management options and timing follow general rules and rule of 3's for nerve injuries • Outcome of ulnar nerve repair is worse vs. median / radial nerve repair

1.6.5 Key Surgical Steps for Ulnar Nerve Exposure in Arm (A) (Table 1.6e)   G

1. Incision	1. Starts: from prox. axillary fold over pectoralis major tendon 2. Course: along the sulcus btw. BB and TB 3. Ends: distally btw. med. epicondyle and olecranon
2. Anatomical structures to protect	Med. brachial cut. n.: beware—preserve prior to opening the brachialis fascia
3. Ulnar nerve identification	Ulnar n. is located posteromedially to median n. next to basilic vein
4. Further steps	1. Incise IM septum (ulnar n. pierces septum 8 cm prox. to medial epicondyle) 2. Identify ulnar n. within triceps epimysium

1.6.6 Clinical Syndromes and Findings: Ulnar Nerve Injury/Compression in Elbow (Table 1.6f) G

Compression/injury site	Causes	Motor	Sensation	Postures/signs	Dx	DDx
Elbow (C): • Olecranon notch • Most common	• Postocondylar groove (most common compression site) • Cubital tunnel S. (btw. two heads of FCU) • Arcuate lig. btw. two heads of FCU (AKA Osborne's fascia) • Tardive ulnar palsy (cubitus valgus deformity due to elbow fracture) • Anconeus muscle • Iatrogenic (due to operative positioning)	Presentation Clumsiness, due to hand intrinsic muscle weakness (↘ by ulnar n.)	Presentation • Sensory changes in fingers 4, 5: – Hyper/hypesthesia, paresthesias – Intermittent – (Worse by prolonged FA flex) – Wakes up pt at night (less common vs. CTS) • Numbness • Pain (in post-condylar region → radiating down medial FA to hand)	• Ulnar claw hand • Wartenberg's sign • Froment's sign (see Table 1.6c and Table 1.10)	• NCS: a. Sensory studies (more sensitive): – ↑latency at elbow b. Motor studies (FDI): – motor conduction at elbow <50 m/sec – ↓CMAP – EMG: denervation	DDx vs. C8/T1 /lower trunk lesions (+ abnl muscles ↘ by median n.)

Compression/injury site	Causes	Motor	Sensation	Postures/signs	Dx	DDx
		Examination • Tests for hand intrinsic muscle weakness: – Rapid thumb–fingertip touching – Synchronous digit flex–ext – Power grip testing • FCU, FDP weakness: rare in cubital tunnel S. • Muscle atrophy: – Hypothenar – FDI	Examination • Light touch: maybe abnl • Vibration sense: may be abnl • Two-point discrimination: maybe abnl • Provocative maneuvers: FA flex for 1 min. • R/O snapping/dislocation of ulnar n. by palp. during elbow flex. • Tinel's sign: at postcondylar groove			

1.6.7 Clinical Syndromes and Findings: Ulnar Nerve Injury/ Compression in FA (Table 1.6g) G

Location of injury/ compression	Causes		Motor	Sensation
FA	Entrapment	Flexor–pronator fascia (D): • Very rare • Thickened flexor–pronator fascia • Compression in prox–mid FA, where ulnar n. passes btw. FCU and flexor-pronator mass • Worse by rep. FA pronation–wrist flex.	Like (C)	Like (C)
	Injury	Compression/transection of dorsal ulnar cutaneous nerve • Ulnar fracture • Lacerations • Blunt trauma	Presentation Examination	Numbness/ hypesthesia in dorsomed. one-third of hand Tinel's sign (maybe) at medial ulna (≈5 cm prox. to wrist)

1.6.8 Management for Injury of Ulnar Nerve Injury/Compression in Elbow/FA (B, C, D) (Table 1.6h) G

Lesion type	Management options		
Injury (C)	Management options and timing follow general rules and rule of 3's for nerve injuries		
Entrapment (B, C, D)	Conservative	• Indications: mild sens. symptoms only • Management: avoid repetitive elbow flexion, leaning on flexed	
	Surgical	Indications	• Severe persistent sens. symptoms worsening quality of life • Weakness/muscle atrophy
		Techniques	• In situ decompression • Nerve transposition
		Outcome	• Improvement in ≈70–80% (esp. pain, sensory symptoms) • Not as successful as carpal tunnel decompression • Factors for poor outcome: duration of symptoms, hand intrinsic muscle weakness, age, systemic peripheral nerve disorders

1.6.9 Key Surgical Steps for Ulnar Nerve Decompression in Elbow/ FA (B, C, D) (Table 1.6i) G

1. Incision	1. Starts: 5 cm prox. to medial epicondyle (in sulcus btw. brachialis and triceps m.) 2. Curves: in btw medial epicondyle–olecranon 3. Ends: 4–5 cm distally to med. epicondyle in FA (btw. FCU and FDP)
2. Skin–subQ tissue division	
3. Anatomical structures to protect	Medial antebrachial cutaneous n.: beware of and preserve
4. Ulnar n. tracing	Trace nerve and decompress (prox → distally): 1. Arcade of Struthers 2. Postcondylar humeral groove 3. Cubital tunnel w/ arcuate lig. (AKA Osborne's fascia) ± anconeus m. (rare) 4. Flexor–pronator fascia

Note: At elbow, ulnar n. lies in cubital tunnel. At prox. FA, ulnar n. courses btw. FCU and FDP in the epimysium of the latter.

1.6.10 Clinical Syndromes and Findings: Ulnar Nerve Injury/Compression at Guyon's Tunnel (Table 1.6j) G

Compression/injury site	Causes	Motor	Sensation	Postures/signs
Hand (at Guyon's tunnel; E); (rare) **Zone 1 (E1):** compression before ulnar n. div. in prox. two-thirds of tunnel	• Fracture • Ganglion cyst	Presentation • Clumsiness due to intrinsic hand muscle weakness • Hand grip weakness	Presentation Numbness/tingling on volar surfaces of fingers 5 + med. half of 4 Examination • Sens. loss on volar surfaces of fingers 5 + med. half of 4 • ±↓light touch • ±↓vibration sense • ±↑distance in two-point discrimination (more advanced cases) • Tinel's sign at Guyon's tunnel • ±Phalen's/reverse Phalen's positive test	• Ulnar claw hand (quite severe due to intact FCU) • Wartenberg's • Froment's (see Table 1.6c and Table 1.10)
Zone 2 (E2): compression of deep motor br. only →no sens. loss	• Ganglion cyst	Presentation • Clumsiness due to intrinsic hand muscle weakness • Hand grip weakness (like zone 1)	Normal	Palmaris brevis sign (+): if this muscle contracts, the prox. superf. sens. div. is intact
Zone 3 (least common) (E3): compression of superf. sens. div. only → intact motor function except for palmaris brevis	• Distal ulnar a. thrombosis/aneurysm (Dx: Doppler)	Normal	Examination Test volar surface of finger 5 for sensation (same sens. examination as zone 1)	Palmaris brevis sign (–) (maybe)

1.6.11 Management for Ulnar Nerve Compression/Injury at Guyon's Tunnel (E) (Table 1.6k) G

Lesion type	Management options		
Injury	Management options and timing follow general rules and rule of 3s for nerve injuries		
Entrapment (E)	Conservative	• Indications: mild–moderate sens. symptoms only • Management: wrist splint, activity modification	
	Surgery	Indications	Severe persistent sens. symptoms worsening QOL Weakness/muscle atrophy Failure of conservative measures
		Technique	Ulnar n. decompression throughout Guyon's tunnel
		Outcome	Factors for better outcome: shorter duration + less degree of severity of symptoms See also Table 1.6l: Common causes of failure of ulnar n. decompression at Guyon's tunnel

1.6.12 Key Surgical Steps for Ulnar Nerve Decompression in Guyon's Tunnel (E) (Table 1.6l) G

1. Incision (Z-shaped)	1. Starts: 4 cm prox. to the wrist (at ulnar aspect of FA over FCU tendon) 2. Courses: btw. pisiform–hamate bones 3. Ends: 4 cm distally to the wrist toward midline
2. Skin–subQ tissue division	
3. Anatomical structures to protect	Palmar ulnar cutaneous n.: beware of and preserve
4. Ulnar n. exposure	Dissect FCU tendon → retract medially → exposure of ulnar n. + ulnar a. (radially to n.)
5. Tracing of ulnar n.	Trace nerve and decompress by dividing (prox → distal): 1. Palmar carpal ligament 2. Palmaris brevis muscle fibers 3. Hypothenar fat–fibrous tissues–muscles ! If concomitant carpal tunnel → incise TCL (= floor of Guyon's tunnel) !! Always trace both deep motor and superf. sens. branches and visualize entire tunnel !! Always locate deep motor br. near free edge of hypothenar muscles → trace it around the hamate + release it from tendinous bands

Note: R/O—treat common causes of failure of ulnar n. decompression at Guyon's tunnel: double crush phenomenon (compression at 2 sites), concomitant carpal tunnel S., other causes (tumor, aneurysm, nonhealing hook of hamate/pisiform fractures).

1.7 Radial Nerve

1.7.1 Radial nerve (C5, C6, C7, C8, [T1]) (Table 1.7a) G

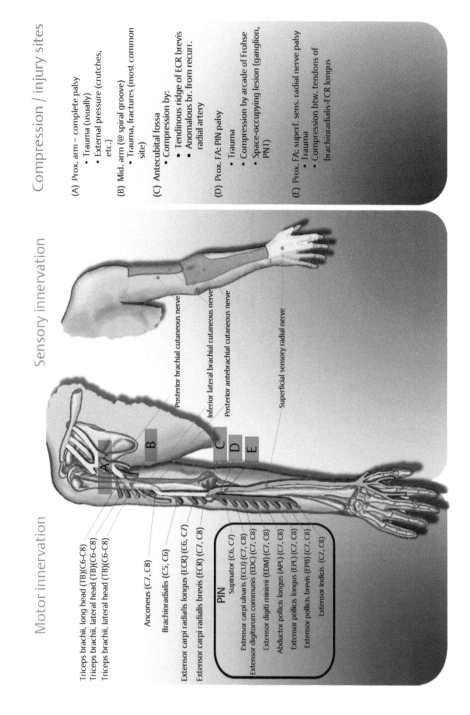

Compression / injury sites

(A) Prox. arm = complete palsy
- Trauma (usually)
- External pressure (crutches, etc.)

(B) Mid. arm (@ spiral groove)
- Trauma, fractures (most common site)

(C) Antecubital fossa
- Compression by:
  - Tendinous ridge of ECR brevis
  - Anomalous br. from recurr. radial artery

(D) Prox. FA: PIN palsy
- Trauma
- Compression by arcade of Frohse
- Space-occupying lesion (ganglion, PNT)

(E) Prox. FA: superf. sens. radial nerve palsy
- Trauma
- Compression btw. tendons of brachioradialis-ECR longus

Sensory innervation

Posterior brachial cutaneous nerve

Inferior lateral brachial cutaneous nerve

Posterior antebrachial cutaneous nerve

Superficial sensory radial nerve

Motor innervation

Triceps brachii, long head (TB)(C6-C8)
Triceps brachii, lateral head (TB)(C6-C8)
Triceps brachii, lateral head (TB)(C6-C8)

Anconeus (C7, C8)

Brachioradialis (C5, C6)

Extensor carpi radialis longus (ECR) (C6, C7)

Extensor carpi radialis brevis (ECR) (C7, C8)

PIN
Supinator (C6, C7)
Extensor carpi ulnaris (ECU) (C7, C8)
Extensor digitorum communis (EDC) (C7, C8)
Extensor digiti minimi (EDM) (C7, C8)
Abductor pollicis longus (APl) (C7, C8)
Extensor pollicis longus (EPl) (C7, C8)
Extensor pollicis brevis (EPb) (C7, C8)
Extensor indicis (C7, C8)

1.7.2 Radial nerve entrapment sites: motor and sensory deficits (Table 1.7b) G

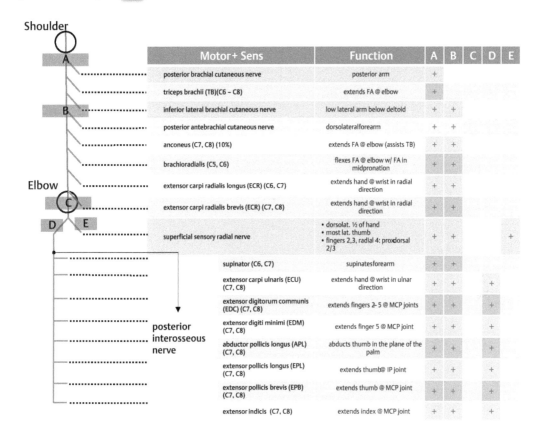

Motor + Sens	Function	A	B	C	D	E
posterior brachial cutaneous nerve	posterior arm	+				
triceps brachii (TB)(C6 – C8)	extends FA @ elbow	+				
inferior lateral brachial cutaneous nerve	low lateral arm below deltoid	+	+			
posterior antebrachial cutaneous nerve	dorsolateral forearm	+	+			
anconeus (C7, C8) (10%)	extends FA @ elbow (assists TB)	+	+			
brachioradialis (C5, C6)	flexes FA @ elbow w/ FA in midpronation	+	+			
extensor carpi radialis longus (ECR) (C6, C7)	extends hand @ wrist in radial direction	+	+			
extensor carpi radialis brevis (ECR) (C7, C8)	extends hand @ wrist in radial direction	+	+			
superficial sensory radial nerve	• dorsolat. ½ of hand • most lat. thumb • fingers 2,3, radial 4: proxdorsal 2/3	+	+			+
supinator (C6, C7)	supinates forearm	+	+			
extensor carpi ulnaris (ECU) (C7, C8)	extends hand @ wrist in ulnar direction	+	+		+	
extensor digitorum communis (EDC) (C7, C8)	extends fingers 2–5 @ MCP joints	+	+		+	
extensor digiti minimi (EDM) (C7, C8)	extends finger 5 @ MCP joint	+	+		+	
abductor pollicis longus (APL) (C7, C8)	abducts thumb in the plane of the palm	+	+		+	
extensor pollicis longus (EPL) (C7, C8)	extends thumb @ IP joint	+	+		+	
extensor pollicis brevis (EPB) (C7, C8)	extends thumb @ MCP joint	+	+		+	
extensor indicis (C7, C8)	extends index @ MCP joint	+	+		+	

posterior interosseous nerve

Legends: O Joint, — : mixed nerve, — : motor nerve, ⋯ : sensory nerve. In the table, boxes containing muscles are colored with blue shades and their deficits with gray shades. Boxes containing nerve br., which innervate skin, as well as their deficits are colored with green shades. Red boxes show possible entrapment/injury sites.

1.7.3 Clinical Syndromes and Findings: Radial Nerve Compression/Injury in Arm (Table 1.7c) G

Compression/injury site	Causes	Motor	Sensation	Postures/signs	DDx	Pitfalls (mimicking/substitution)
		Examination	Examination			
Proximal arm (A) (complete palsy w/ injury at axilla)	• Trauma • Iatrogenic (im deltoid injection) • Pressure (crutches, Saturday night, honeymooner's; see median n.)	Weakness: • TB →no elbow ext. • Brachioradialis → • Weak elbow flex • ECU, ECR → wrist drop • Supinator → weak supination • EDC, EDM, extensor indici →no finger extension (2–5) at MCP joints • APL, EPL, EPB → no thumb extension	Sens. loss: • Postbrachialcut. n. → post arm • Postantebrachial cut. n. → post. FA • Inf lat brachial cut. n. → lower anterolat arm • Superf br. of radial n. + dors. digital n. → dorsolat hand	Wrist and finger drop: • Semiflexed fingers • Thumb metacarpal bone volar to palm (see Table 1.10)	• Radial nerve injr at spiral groove – No TB weakness – No post. arm sens. loss • Posterior cord injury: – + Deltoid weakness (↗by axillary n.) – + Latissimus dorsi weakness (↗by thoracodorsal n.) • C7 palsy: – Numbness only in Volar – dorsal 3rd • Digit – + Weak C7 muscles with median n. ↗	Mimicking of finger extension at MCP due to tenodesis occurs with: • Wrist flexion (esp. w/ sclerosis) • Partial finger flexion →hand intrinsics may extend MCP joint

Compression/injury site	Causes	Motor	Sensation	Postures/signs	DDx	Pitfalls (mimicking/substitution)
Mid arm (B) (injury at spiral groove = most common trauma site)	• Trauma(-direct contusion, midhumeral fracture) • Iatrogenic (im deltoid injection)	Examination Weakness: • Brachioradialis • All muscles dist. to elbow	Examination Sens. loss: • Post. antebra-chial cut. n. → post. FA • Inf lat brachial cut. n. → lower anterolat arm		Radial n. injr. at axilla: • + TB palsy • + Post. arm sens. loss (posterior brachial cut. n.)	

1.7.4 Management for Radial Nerve Injury in Arm

Key surgical steps for radial nerve exposure (posterior cord–axilla) (anterior approach) (A) (Table 1.7d) G

1. Incision	2 cm below clavicle into deltopectoral groove
2. Pectoral groove exposure	1. Open pectoral groove 2. Ligate cephalic vein 3. Cut–reflect pectoralis minor
3. Identification of key anatomical structures	Identify lateral cord + axillary artery
4. Dissection of median + musculocutaneous n.	Dissect median + musculocutaneous n. → so you can retract lateral cord medially w/o traction injury
5. Identification of posterior cord	Identification of posterior cord behind axillary artery → divides into radial n. + axillary n.
6. Identification of radial nerve	Identification of radial nerve as it exits in triangular space (btw. medial and long head of triceps and teres major)

Note: Outcome of radial nerve repair in midhumeral level: good, but not complete recovery of wrist + finger extension

Key Surgical Steps for Radial Nerve Exposure in Arm Beyond Axilla (Posterior Approach) (B) (Table 1.7e)   G

1. Incision	Incision line connecting acromion and midolecranon
2. Identification of distal triceps tendon	Find characteristic flame—like distal triceps tendon → follow prox. to identify groove btw. long and lateral head of triceps
3. Identification of radial n. proximally	Follow groove proximally until you run into the teres major → find radial nerve exit from triangular space
4. Trace radial nerve distally	1. Follow radial nerve distally till you find nerve branches to triceps 2. Nerve then goes into spiral groove 3. Nerve then pierces lateral IM septum → comes to anterior compartment (flexors)
5. Separate anterior incision	To follow radial nerve further (distally to its piercing the IM septum) a separate anterior incision is required

Note: ! Options and timing of management for radial nerve injuries at the arm follow general rules and rule of 3s for nerve injuries.

!! Most radial nerve injuries due to midhumeral fractures are neurapraxic → high probability of spontaneous recovery.

1.7.5 Clinical Syndromes and Findings: Radial Nerve Compression/Injury at Antecubital Fossa/FA (Table 1.7f) G

Location of injury/compression		Causes	Motor	Sensation	Postures	DDx
Ante-cubital fossa (C)	PIN entrap-ment — **Radial tunnel[a] syndrome (controversial, clinical Dx w/o confirmatory tests)**	Compression sites: • Anterior margin of elbow joint/radial head • Tendinous ridge on ECR brevis m. • Anomalous br. from recurr. radial artery/vein	Normal	Presentation	• Pain at radial tunnel • Dull ache, deep in muscles • Worse during resisted third finger ext. w/ full elbow extension + FA supination • Sensation: nl	• PIN compression at supinator • Tennis elbow (= lateral epicondylitis) – Much more common – Sharp localized pain at lateral epicondyle – Worsening w/passive hand pronation + flexion
	Supinator syndrome (controversial)	Arcade of Frohse: compression at ant. margin of pocket formed by superf. + deep head of supinator m. through which PIN passes (fibrous in 30%)	Presentation: Sudden/progressive finger extension weakness Examination: Spared TB, brachioradialis, supinator function	Presentation: Pain at supinator m. Examination: Normal		• Parsonage–Turner S. – R/O subtle palsies of other UE n. • Rupture of extensor tendons

(Continued) ▲

Location of injury/compression	Causes	Motor	Sensation	Postures	DDx
FA (D) PIN injury/compression – Posterior interosseous nerve palsy	• Trauma • Compression at supinator • DM • SOL (lipoma, PNT, ganglion) • Idiopathic (Parsonage–Turner S.)	Examination • Wrist ext. weakness in ulnar direction (ECU function loss vs. spared ECR longus, brevis function usu.) → no wrist drop • Finger ext. weakness at MCP joints • Spared brachioradialis function (always)	Presentation Dull ache in prox. FA ext. muscles near radial head Examination Normal	• Radial deviation of wrist drop • Finger drop	

Radial tunnel: submuscular course of radial n. btw. lateral IM septum and supinator (covered by brachioradialis, ECR brevis, and longus muscles).

1.7.6 Clinical Syndromes and Findings: Radial Nerve Compression/Injury at FA (Table 1.7g) G

Compression/injury site	Causes	Motor	Sensation		Dx	DDx
FA	Superf. radial n. palsy (AKA Wartenberg's syndrome/cheiralgia paresthetica) (E)	• Trauma • Iatrogenic (venipuncture, surgery for de Quervain's tenosynovitis) • Tight watches • Pinching btw. brachioradials and ECR longus tendons	Normal	Presentation	Pain, numbness, hyperesthesia on dorsolat. hand	NCS	De Quervain's tenosynovitis of thumb's extensor tendon: • No sens. loss
				Examination	• Worse w/ forced FA pronation + ulnar wrist deviation • Tinel's sign		

Note: Paramount for PIN palsy: nl sens + spared brachioradialis.
Pseudoulnar claw hand (weakness begins from 5, 4 fingers).

1.7.7 Management for Entrapment of Radial Nerve/PIN at Elbow/FA (C, D) (Table 1.7h) G

Lesion type	Management options	
PIN entrapment (radial tunnel syndrome, supinator syndrome) (C, D)	Conservative	• Rest OR immobilization (w/ wrist dorsiflexion splint) • Activity/occupation/hobbies modification (avoidance of repetitive elbow extension, FA supination/pronation w/ wrist extension)
	Surgical	Indications	• Failure of conservative measures after several mo • R/O other treatable causes (lateral epicondylitis)
		Technique	Surgical exploration–decompression (see Table 1.7i)
		Outcome	Good results in 65–70% of patients
PIN injury (D)	Management options and timing follow general rules and rule of 3s for nerve injuries	

1.7.8 Approaches for radial nerve decompression in radial tunnel syndrome and PIN decompression (C, D) (Table 1.7i) 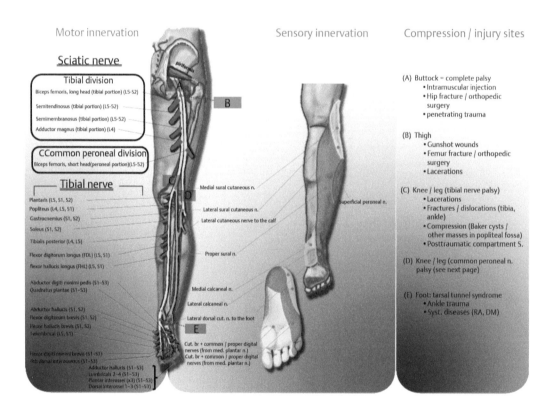 G

Approaches	1. Anterior proximal (incision btw. brachioradialis and brachialis) 2. Posterior proximal (incision btw. brachioradialis and ECRL)
Sites for exploration–decompression	Release of following structures: 1. Radial recurrent vessels (before supinator) 2. Arcade of Frohse (leading edge of supinator) ± complete section of superf. supinator head 3. Extensor carpi radialis brevis

Note: R/O lateral epicondylitis before Dx of radial tunnel syndrome.

1.8 Sciatic Nerve (L4, L5, S1, S2, S3) and Tibial Nerve (L4, L5, S1, S2, S3) (Table 1.8a) G

1.8.1 Common Peroneal Nerve (L4, L5, S1, S2) (Table 1.8b) G

Compression / injury sites

(D) Knee / leg (common peroneal n. palsy:
- Trauma (stretch / contusion injury, fracture)
- Ganglion cysts (tibiofibular joint)
- Compression:
  - Of common peroneal @ fibular tunnel
  - Of deep peroneal n. under fibrous edge of EDL
- Strawberry picker's palsy (squatting)
- Posttraumatic compartment S.

Sensory innervation

Motor innervation

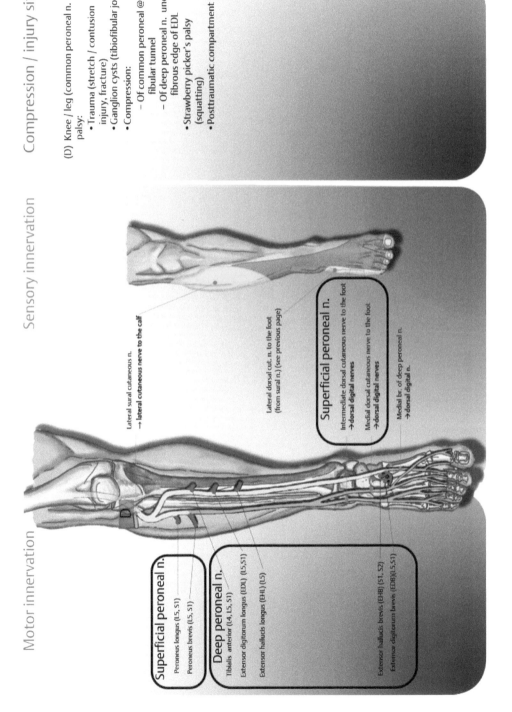

Lateral sural cutaneous n.
→ lateral cutaneous nerve to the calf

Lateral dorsal cut. n. to the foot (from sural n.) (see previous page)

Superficial peroneal n.
Intermediate dorsal cutaneous nerve to the foot
→dorsal digital nerves
Medial dorsal cutaneous nerve to the foot
→dorsal digital nerves

Medial br. of deep peroneal n.
→dorsal digital n.

Superficial peroneal n.
Peroneus longus (L5, S1)
Peroneus brevis (L5, S1)

Deep peroneal n.
Tibialis anterior (L4, L5, S1)
Extensor digitorum longus (EDL) (L5, S1)
Extensor hallucis longus (EHL) (L5)

Extensor hallucis brevis (EHB) (S1, S2)
Extensor digitorum brevis (EDB)(L5, S1)

1.8.2 Sciatic Nerve (Table 1.8c)

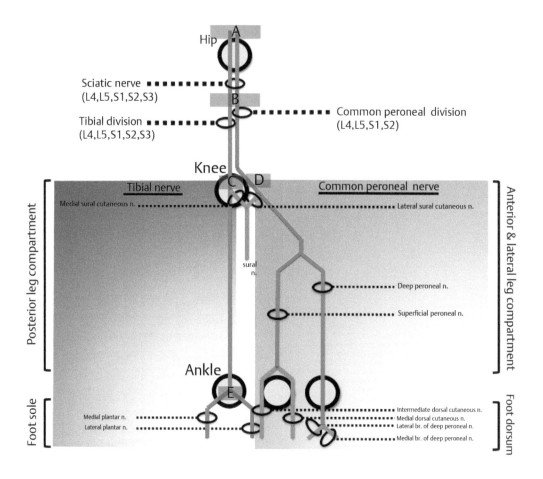

1.8.3 Sciatic Nerve Entrapment Sites: Motor and Sensory Deficits (Table 1.8d–f) G

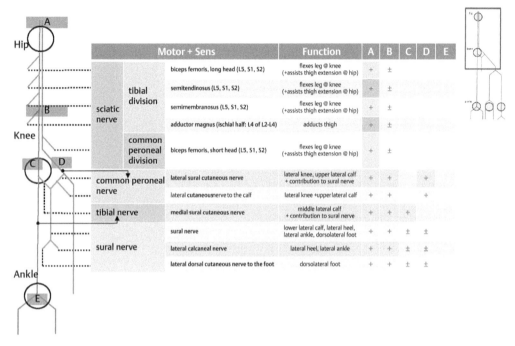

Motor + Sens			Function	A	B	C	D	E
sciatic nerve	tibial division	biceps femoris, long head (L5, S1, S2)	flexes leg @ knee (+assists thigh extension @ hip)	+	±			
		semitendinosus (L5, S1, S2)	flexes leg @ knee (+assists thigh extension @ hip)	+	±			
		semimembranosus (L5, S1, S2)	flexes leg @ knee (+assists thigh extension @ hip)	+	±			
		adductor magnus (ischial half: L4 of L2-L4)	adducts thigh	+	±			
	common peroneal division	biceps femoris, short head (L5, S1, S2)	flexes leg @ knee (+assists thigh extension @ hip)	+	±			
common peroneal nerve		lateral sural cutaneous nerve	lateral knee, upper lateral calf + contribution to sural nerve	+	+		+	
		lateral cutaneous nerve to the calf	lateral knee +upper lateral calf	+	+		+	
tibial nerve		medial sural cutaneous nerve	middle lateral calf + contribution to sural nerve	+	+	±		
		sural nerve	lower lateral calf, lateral heel, lateral ankle, dorsolateral foot	+	+	±	±	
sural nerve		lateral calcaneal nerve	lateral heel, lateral ankle	+	+	±	±	
		lateral dorsal cutaneous nerve to the foot	dorsolateral foot	+	+	±	±	

Legends: O Joint, ▭ : mixed nerve, ▭ : motor nerve, ▭ : sensory nerve. In the table, boxes containing muscles are colored with blue shades and their deficits with gray shades. Boxes containing nerve br., which innervate skin, as well as their deficits are colored with green shades. Boxes containing mixed nerves are colored with orange shades. Red boxes show possible entrapment/injury sites. The same color coding applies for the following two tables as well.

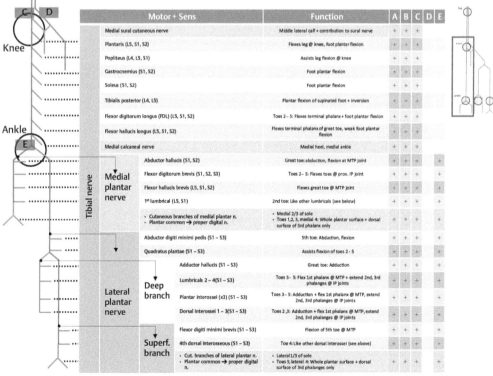

Motor + Sens			Function	A	B	C	D	E
Tibial nerve		Medial sural cutaneous nerve	Middle lateral calf + contribution to sural nerve	+	+	+		
		Plantaris (L5, S1, S2)	Flexes leg @ knee, foot plantar flexion	+	+	+		
		Popliteus (L4, L5, S1)	Assists leg flexion @ knee	+	+	+		
		Gastrocnemius (S1, S2)	Foot plantar flexion	+	+	+		
		Soleus (S1, S2)	Foot plantar flexion	+	+	+		
		Tibialis posterior (L4, L5)	Plantar flexion of supinated foot + inversion	+	+	+		
		Flexor digitorum longus (FDL) (L5, S1, S2)	Toes 2– 5: Flexes terminal phalanx + foot plantar flexion	+	+	+		
		Flexor hallucis longus (L5, S1, S2)	Flexes terminal phalanx of great toe, weak foot plantar flexion	+	+	+		
		Medial calcaneal nerve	Medial heel, medial ankle	+	+	+		
	Medial plantar nerve	Abductor hallucis (S1, S2)	Great toe: abduction, flexion at MTP joint	+	+	+	+	
		Flexor digitorum brevis (S1, S2, S3)	Toes 2– 5: Flexes toes @ prox. IP joint	+	+	+	+	
		Flexor hallucis brevis (L5, S1, S2)	Flexes great toe @ MTP joint	+	+	+	+	
		1st lumbrical (L5, S1)	2nd toe: Like other lumbricals (see below)	+	+	+	+	
		• Cutaneous branches of medial plantar n. • Plantar common → proper digital n.	• Medial 2/3 of sole • Toes 1,2, 3, medial 4: Whole plantar surface + dorsal surface of 3rd phalanx only	+	+	+	+	
	Lateral plantar nerve	Abductor digiti minimi pedis (S1 – S3)	5th toe: Abduction, flexion	+	+	+	+	
		Quadratus plantae (S1 – S3)	Assists flexion of toes 2 - 5	+	+	+	+	
	Deep branch	Adductor hallucis (S1 – S3)	Great toe: Adduction	+	+	+	+	
		Lumbricals 2 – 4 (S1 – S3)	Toes 3– 5: Flex 1st phalanx @ MTP + extend 2nd, 3rd phalanges @ IP joints	+	+	+	+	
		Plantar interossei (x3) (S1 – S3)	Toes 3– 5: Adduction + flex 1st phalanx @ MTP, extend 2nd, 3rd phalanges @ IP joints	+	+	+	+	
		Dorsal interossei 1 – 3 (S1 – S3)	Toes 2,3: Adduction + flex 1st phalanx @ MTP, extend 2nd, 3rd phalanges @ IP joints	+	+	+	+	
	Superf. branch	Flexor digiti minimi brevis (S1 – S3)	Flexion of 5th toe @ MTP	+	+	+	+	
		4th dorsal interosseous (S1 – S3)	Toe 4: Like other dorsal interossei (see above)	+	+	+	+	
		• Cut. branches of lateral plantar n. • Plantar common → proper digital n.	• Lateral 1/3 of sole • Toes 5, lateral 4: Whole plantar surface + dorsal surface of 3rd phalanges only	+	+	+	+	

(Continued) ▶   **45**

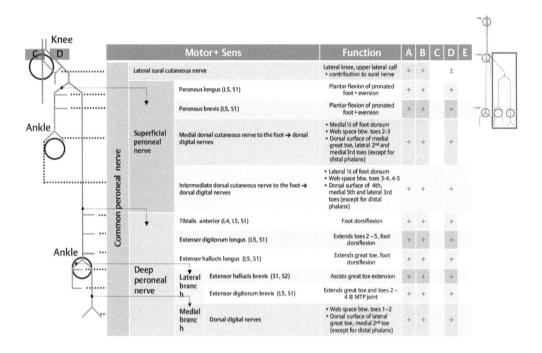

Motor+ Sens		Function	A	B	C	D	E
	Lateral sural cutaneous nerve	Lateral knee, upper lateral calf + contribution to sural nerve	+	+		±	
Superficial peroneal nerve	Peroneus longus (L5, S1)	Plantar flexion of pronated foot + eversion	+	+		+	
	Peroneus brevis (L5, S1)	Plantar flexion of pronated foot + eversion	+	+		+	
	Medial dorsal cutaneous nerve to the foot → dorsal digital nerves	• Medial ½ of foot dorsum • Web space btw. toes 2-3 • Dorsal surface of medial great toe, lateral 2nd and medial 3rd toes (except for distal phalanx)	+	+		+	
	Intermediate dorsal cutaneous nerve to the foot → dorsal digital nerves	• Lateral ½ of foot dorsum • Web space btw. toes 3-4, 4-5 • Dorsal surface of 4th, medial 5th and lateral 3rd toes (except for distal phalanx)	+	+		+	
Deep peroneal nerve	Tibialis anterior (L4, L5, S1)	Foot dorsiflexion	+	+		+	
	Extensor digitorum longus (L5, S1)	Extends toes 2 – 5, foot dorsiflexion	+	+		+	
	Extensor hallucis longus (L5, S1)	Extends great toe, foot dorsiflexion	+	+		+	
Lateral branch	Extensor hallucis brevis (S1, S2)	Assists great toe extension	+	+		+	
	Extensor digitorum brevis (L5, S1)	Extends great toe and toes 2 – 4 @ MTP joint	+	+		+	
Medial branch	Dorsal digital nerves	• Web space btw. toes 1–2 • Dorsal surface of lateral great toe, medial 2nd toe (except for distal phalanx)	+	+		+	

1.8.4 Clinical Syndromes and Findings: Sciatic Nerve Compression/Injury at Buttock (Table 1.8g) [G]

Compression/injury site	Causes	Motor	Sensation	DDx	Dx
Buttock (A) (complete sciatic palsy)	• Injection: presentation: – Sciatica – Motor–sens def (mild > severe) • Hip fracture, orthopaedic surgery (sciatic n. posterior to hip joint) • Penetrating trauma (uncommon due to deep location of n.)	Examination • Weakness: – Knee flexion (uncommon due to very proximal origin of nerve branches) – All ankle mvts – All foot mvts	Examination • Sensation loss: • Lateral lower leg • Nearly all foot except for med. malleolus (~saphenous n.)	• S1 radiculopathy includes: – + gluteal nerve palsy • Sacral plexus lesions include: – + gluteal nerve palsy – + pudendal n. deficits – + post. cut. n. to the thigh deficit	• Required tests for DDx: – EMG/NCS – Imaging
	• Piriformis syndrome (definition: compression of sciatic n. by piriformis m. at its exit from pelvis) (controversial) – Neurogenic (w/ objective clin. findings) – Non-neurogenic (w/o objective clin. findings)	Normal	Presentation Pain: • At buttock • Sciatic n. distribution • Worse: when sitting on hard surfaces Examination Provocative maneuvers: • Resisting thigh abduction at knee (piriformis contracts) • Resisting hip internal rotation (piriformis is stretched)	• L-spine disk herniation (MRI for DDx) • Pelvic tumors (pelvic MRI)	• EMG/NCS: usu. nl • Dx of exclusion (usu. something else) • MRI

Note: Sensation loss of foot w/ sciatic injury at buttock is very dangerous for foot injury.

1.8.5 Clinical Syndromes and Findings: Sciatic Nerve Compression/Injury at Thigh (Table 1.8h) G

Compression/ injury site	Causes	Motor		Sensation
Thigh (B) a. Complete palsy (both divisions) b. Partial palsy (one OR mainly one division, peroneal is more susceptible vs. tibial)	• GSW • Lacerations • Femur fracture/ orthop. surgery	Examination	Weakness: • All muscles except for hamstrings (knee flexion) • For partial palsies involved muscles depend on the mainly affected div.	Sensation loss: (depends on the division affected, i.e., one OR both): • Lateral lower leg • Nearly all foot except for med. malleolus (⁄ saphenous n.)

1.8.6 Management for Compression/Injury of Sciatic Nerve at Buttock/Thigh (A, B) (Table 1.8i) G

Lesion type	Management options		
Injury	Management options and timing follow general rules and rule of 3's for nerve injuries		
Piriformis syndrome (entrapment at buttock)	Conservative	• Pain meds (NSAIDs, meds for neuropathic pain) • Physical therapy (massage) • Ultrasound • Trigger point injections	
	Surgical	Indications	R/O all other causes of sciatica + failure of conservative options for > 4–6 mo **(Do everything to avoid surgery, due to generally not good surgical outcome)**
		Techniques	1. Piriformis division 2. Coagulation of compressive veins 3. ± Neurolysis

Note: There are more chances for tibial division injuries than peroneal division ones to recover function after nerve repair.

1.8.7 Key Surgical Steps for Sciatic Nerve Exposure at Buttock (A) (Table 1.8j) [G]

1. Incision	Curved incision: 1. Starts: posterior inferior iliac spine 2. Courses: around buttock cc → along gluteal crease 3. Ends: midline of posterior thigh
2. Divide gluteus maximus	Divide gluteus maximus (near greater epitrochanter) → retract medially (leave cuff for reapproximation)
3. Identification of sciatic nerve	Identify–trace sciatic nerve proximally up to sciatic notch
4. Division of piriformis	Improves access to sciatic notch
5. Preserve structures	Protect: • Posterior femoral cutaneous nerve • Inferior gluteal artery + nerve • Sciatic branches to hamstring muscles

Note: !! It is recommended to **divide sciatic nerve to its peroneal and tibial divisions** for separate evaluation of nerve action potentials (NAPs) and better repair of the lesion.

!!! Injury of the peroneal division is more unlikely to recover even after treatment.

1.8.8 Key Surgical Steps for Sciatic Nerve Exposure at Thigh (B) (Table 1.8k)

1. Incision	Straight midline incision along posterior thigh (btw. hamstrings)
2. Identify long head of biceps femoris muscle	Identify long head of biceps femoris muscle just inferior to gluteus maximus
3. Identification of sciatic nerve proximally	Identify sciatic nerve in fat pad lateral and deep to long head of biceps femoris
4. Trace sciatic nerve distally	1. Follow sciatic nerve distally under long head of biceps femoris (this muscle crosses over sciatic nerve from medially to laterally) 2. Split biceps femoris and semitendinosus/semi-membranosus → find sciatic nerve distally
5. Preserve structures	Protect: • Posterior femoral cutaneous nerve • Sciatic branches to hamstring muscles

Note: The above approaches can be combined for longer exposure.

1.8.9 Clinical Syndromes and Findings: Common Peroneal n. and Tibial n. Compression/Injury at Knee/Leg (Table 1.8I) G

Compression/injury site		Causes	Motor		Sensation		DDx
Knee/leg	Tibial n. palsy (C)	• Lacerations • Tibial fracture • Ankle fracture/ dislocations • Baker's cysts/ other masses in popliteal fossa • Posttraumatic compartment S.	Examination	Weakness: • Plantar flex. (gastrocnemius, soleus) → lesion level at OR proximal to popliteal fossa • Foot inversion (tibialis posterior) → if spared, lesion level at deep post. compartment of midleg • Toes flexion (FDL, FHL, FDB, FHB) → if FDL, FHL spared, lesion level at lower one-third of leg OR dist. to tarsal tunnel • Foot intrinsic muscles	Examination	Sens. loss • Sole • Med. heel • ± tibial n. contribution to sural n.	

Compression/injury site	Causes	Motor	Sensation	DDx

Common peroneal n. (CPN) palsy (D) (most common LE n. injury)	• Stretch/contusion injury
	• Fracture
	• Ganglion cysts(tibiofibular joint)
	• Compression of common peroneal at fibular tunnel (= tunnel btw. fibrous edge of peroneus longus and fibular head)
	• Compression of deep peroneal n. under fibrous edge of EDL
	• Strawberry picker's palsy (squatting position for long periods) ◊ b/l common peroneal palsy
	• Posttraumatic compartment S.
		Examination
		Weakness:
		• Foot dorsiflexion (tibialis anterior)
		• Foot eversion (peroneus longus +brevis)
		• Toe extension (EDL, EHL, EHB)
			Presentation
			• Pain + numbness radiating from fibular head down along the lateral leg over the foot dorsum
			• Lateral cutaneous n. of calf may be spared (origin prox. to fibular tunnel)
			
			Examination
			• Tinel's sign at fibular head)
			• Sensation loss:
			  – Lower lateral leg
			  – Dorsal + lateral foot
			  – ± CPN contribution to sural n.
				• L5 radiculopathy:
				  – Hx of back pain
				  – Much more common!
				  – EMG/NCS: tibialis posterior is involved (~by L5 via tibial n.)
				• Injury of peroneal division of sciatic nerve above knee:
				  – EMG: denervation of short head of biceps (see Table 1.8m)

1.8.10 DDx of Foot Drop (Table 1.8m ◀ᴗ) G

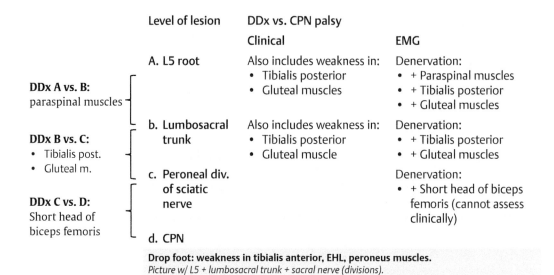

	Level of lesion	DDx vs. CPN palsy	
		Clinical	EMG
DDx A vs. B: paraspinal muscles	A. L5 root	Also includes weakness in: • Tibialis posterior • Gluteal muscles	Denervation: • + Paraspinal muscles • + Tibialis posterior • + Gluteal muscles
DDx B vs. C: • Tibialis post. • Gluteal m.	b. Lumbosacral trunk	Also includes weakness in: • Tibialis posterior • Gluteal muscle	Denervation: • + Tibialis posterior • + Gluteal muscles
DDx C vs. D: Short head of biceps femoris	c. Peroneal div. of sciatic nerve		Denervation: • + Short head of biceps femoris (cannot assess clinically)
	d. CPN		

Drop foot: weakness in tibialis anterior, EHL, peroneus muscles.
Picture w/ L5 + lumbosacral trunk + sacral nerve (divisions).

1.8.11 Management for Compression/Injury of CPN at Knee/ Leg (D) (Table 1.8n) G

Lesion type	Management options		
Injury	Management options and timing follow general rules and rule of 3s for nerve injuries		
Entrapment/ compression	Conservative(usually)	• Pain meds (NSAIDs, antiepileptics, antidepressants) • Ankle support (orthosis, boots) • Physical therapy (strengthening) • Avoidance of external pressure	
	Surgical	Indications	Failure of conservative options for >3–4 mo
		Techniques	• For entrapment: neurolysis ± partial osteotomy of fibular head • For intraneural cyst: cyst drainage + transection of feeding articular br.

1.8.12 Key Surgical Steps for CPN Exposure at Knee/Leg (D) (Table 1.80) G

1. Landmarks	a. Fibular head b. Biceps femoris tendon c. Midline of popliteal fossa
2. Incision	1. Starts: just superior of popliteal fossa 2. Courses: along midline of popliteal fossa → curves slowly laterally to cross the fossa obliquely → posteroinferior to fibular head 3. Ends: peroneus longus
3. Identify CPN	Identify CPN in fat pad medial to biceps femoris tendon (do not confuse CPN with biceps femoris tendon!)
4. Trace CPN distally	1. Over lateral head of gastrocnemius 2. Over fibular head
5. Peroneus longus incision	Trace nerve up to peroneus longus → divide its fascia + muscle fibers → until you find it splitting into superficial + deep peroneal branches
6. Identify deep peroneal n.	Identify deep branch piercing the IM septum on its way to the anterior compartment
7. ± Fibular head partial osteotomy	Rongeur posterior part of fibular head (less angulated course of deep peroneal nerve)

Caution: Not to injure the nerve during incision.
Generally good results of both CPN repair after injury and of CPN decompression in case of entrapment/compression.

1.8.13 Clinical Syndromes and Findings: Compression of Tibial and CPN at Foot (Table 1.8p) G

Compression/injury site	Causes	Motor		Sensation		DDx	Dx
Foot		Examination		Presentation		• Peripheral neuropathy:	
Tarsal tunnel syndrome (E) (uncommon) (definition: medial + lateral plantar n., which are br. from tibial n., are compressed under flexor retinaculum)	• Ankle trauma • Syst. diseases (RA, DM)		Weakness of foot intrinsic muscles (uncommon)		Sole pain (at metatarsals), numbness ± paresthesias Worse w/ walking, standing Better w/ rest, elevation	– + Sens. loss outside tibial n. – + Absent Achilles tendon reflex – EMG/NCS	
				Examination	• Pinprick, vibration, two-point discrimination: abnl (possibly) • Tinel's sign: posterior to med. malleolus → may radiate down into the foot • Valleix phenomenon: percussion posterior to med. malleolus → may radiate up along tibial n.	• Mass lesion (lipoma, ganglion cysts, etc.) (50%) – MRI • S1 radiculopathy – R/O with EMG/NCS • Musculoskeletal causes • EMG/NCS	

Compression/injury site	Causes	Motor	Sensation	DDx	Dx
Anterior tarsal tunnel syndrome (very rare) (definition: compression of distal deep peroneal n. under one/both extensor retinaculum on foot dorsum)	• Tight shoes • Local trauma	Examination — Weakness (± wasting) of EDB	Presentation — • Dull ache on foot dorsum • Numbness at first web space (possibly) Examination — Tinel's sign		
Morton neuroma (definition: chronic irritation of common plantar n. due to repetitive pinching btw. third, fourth metatarsal heads and deep transverse metatarsal lig.)			Presentation — • Pain btw. third and fourth metatarsals → radiation to 3, 4 toes • Worse w/ walking • Better w/ rest, elevation Examination — • Provocation: squeeze metatarsals → pain into 3, 4 toes • Tinel's sign		U/S

1.8.14 Management for Compression/Injury of Tibial Nerve and its Branches (Table 1.8q) G

Lesion type	Management options			Outcome
Injury	Management options and timing follow general rules and rule of 3s for nerve injuries			Repair of tibial nerve lacerations usually have a very good result
Tarsal tunnel syndrome (E)	Conservative (usually)	• Pain meds (NSAIDs, antiepileptics, antidepressants) • Appropriate shoes • Physical therapy • Immobilization		
	Surgical	Indications	• Failure of conservative options • Mass lesion	Good result in around 65 – 70%
		Techniques	Surgical exploration and nerve decompression	
Morton neuroma	Conservative	• Appropriate shoes (no heels, no narrow shoes) • Injections (local anesthetics + steroids)		
	Surgical	Indications	Failure of conservative options	
		Approaches	Neuroma resection though: • Plantar approach (easier, better exposure vs. incision on dorsal surface) • Dorsal approach (difficult, limited exposure vs. avoidance of incision on plantar surface)	Success rate: 75%

1.8.15 Key Surgical Steps for Exposure of Tibial Nerve and its Branches at Knee/Leg/Foot

Key surgical steps for tibial nerve exposure at popliteal fossa (C) (Table 1.8r) G

Positioning	Prone
1. Incision	1. Starts: midline of thigh just superior of popliteal fossa 2. Courses: runs medially to cross the fossa obliquely 3. Ends: down the leg medial to midline
2. Identify tibial nerve	Identify tibial nerve btw. two heads of gastrocnemius
3. Protect vasculature	Protect popliteal artery/vein and saphenous vein (An artery follows tibial nerve all the way to the foot, proximally called popliteal and distally posterior tibial)

Key surgical steps for tibial nerve exposure at leg (C) (Table 1.8s)

Positioning	Supine
1. Incision	At medial leg along medial surface of tibia
2. Identify tibial nerve	Identify tibial nerve btw. flexor digitorum longus and soleus muscle
3. Protect structures	Protect posterior tibial artery/vein and saphenous nerve

Key surgical steps for decompression in tarsal tunnel syndrome (E) (Table 1.8t)

Positioning	Supine
1. Incision	1. Center: curves around posterior aspect of medial malleolus 2. Proximal extent: 5 cm proximally into the leg 3. Distal extent: 5 cm distally along the medial border of the sole
2. Identify tibial nerve	Identify tibial nerve anterior to flexor digitorum longus tendon coursing under the flexor retinaculum (along with posterior tibial artery/vein)
3. Trace–unroof tibial nerve and its branches	1. Divide flexor retinaculum ligament 2. May have to cut muscle fibers of abductor hallucis muscle to expose nerve 3. Find and decompress the three tibial nerve branches (mediolateral plantar nerve + medial calcaneal br.)

1.9 Meralgia Paresthetica (Table 1.9) G

Definition	Irritation of lateral femoral cutaneous nerve (idiopathic/rep. minor trauma)	
Predisposition		• Obesity/extreme weight loss • Ascites • Pregnancy
Sensory	Presentation	• Pain • Numbness • Paresthesias } on anterolat. thigh • +/hyperesthesias • Worse w/ standing • Better w/ sitting/hip flex.
	Examination	• Sens. changes/hyperesthesia on lat. thigh • Tenderness along lat. inguinal lig. • Provocative mnvr: hip ext. • Tinel's sign: no (usu.)
Motor	Presentation	NO symptoms
	Examination	Nl
DDx		• Intra-abdominal masses/pathology • L2 radiculopathy: pain/sens. changes more over anteromedial thigh ± psoas weakness • Lumbar plexus lesion } more extensive sens. • Femoral n. entrapment } changes ± weakness • Peripheral neuropathy/DM
Dx		• Nerve block (many false negatives) • EMG/NCS (may help) • CT/MRI L-spine, pelvis, hip
Tx	Conservative	• Risk factor modification (body weight loss, looser belts/pants) • Pain meds (NSAIDs, tricyclic) • Injections (corticosteroid + local anesthetic)
	Surgical	• Compressive pathology → decompression • No compressive pathology → neurectomy

1.10 Postures (Table 1.10)   G

Location of lesion	Posture	Examination/ posture description	Nonfunctioning muscles involved in posture	Non opposed muscles involved in posture
Upper trunk injury (Duchenne–Erb's palsy)	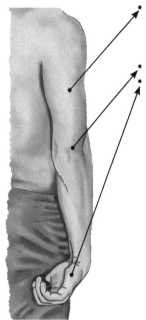 Bellhop's/waiter's tip position	• Arm hangs at side adducted, internally rotated • Elbow extension • Wrist–finger flexion	Muscles w/ C5, C6 ↗: • Infraspinatus • Supraspinatus • Deltoid • Biceps • Brachioradialis • Supinator (occ.)	
Median n. injury (complete injury at proximal arm)	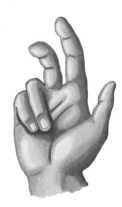 Benedictine sign (orator's hand)	1. Ask pt to make a fist 2. Ginger flexion: • 1st: almost none • 2nd: partial • 3rd: weak • 4th, 5th: nl	• Flexor digitorum profundus: flexes fingers 2, part of 3 at dist. IP joint • Lumbricals 1, 2: flex MCP joint, extend prox. IP joint (fingers 2, 3)	Extensor digitorum: MCP joint of fingers 2, 3 remain extended

(Continued) ▶

Location of lesion	Posture	Examination/ posture description	Nonfunction- ing muscles involved in posture	Non opposed muscles involved in posture
AIN injury	nl abnl OK sign	• nl: thumb and index fingertips touch together • In AIN palsy: volar surfaces of thumb and index touch together	• Flexor digitorum profundus: flexes fingers 2, part of 3 at dist. IP joint • Flexor pollicis longus: flexes thumb at dist. IP joint	
Radial n. injury (com- plete injury at proximal arm)	Wrist and finger drop	• Semiflexed fingers • Thumb me- tacarpal bone volar to palm	• Wrist exten- sors (ECR, ECU) • Finger exten- sors (EDC)	

Location of lesion	Posture	Examination/ posture description	Nonfunction-ing muscles involved in posture	Non opposed muscles involved in posture

Ulnar nerve injury at:
• Proximal arm
• Elbow
• Hand (Guyon's tunnel)
	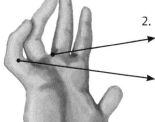
	
	Claw hand
		1. Ask pt to open hand
		2. Fingers 4, 5:
		  • MCP joint hyperexten-sion
		  • Partial flex. of both IP joints
			• 3rd, 4th lumbricals + all interossei: flex MCP joint, extend prox. IP joint
			• Flexor digiti minimi: flexes fifth finger at MCP
				• Extensor digitorum communis (unoppo-sed): MCP joint hype-rextension
				• Residu-al tone of flexor digitorum profundus: partial flex. of both IP joints

	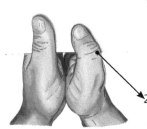 Froment's sign	1. Pull apart a piece of paper held btw. volar surface of each straightened thumb–closed fist 2. Thumb IP joint flexes (flexor pollicis longus)	• Adductor pol-licis: adducts thumb in plane parallel to palm	• Flexor pollicis longus: substitutes by flexing IP joint of thumb
	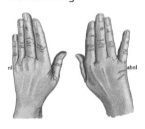 Wartenberg's sign	1. Ask pt to adduct all fingers 2. Fifth finger is more abducted	• Third palmar interosseous: adducts fifth finger	Unopposed action of: • Extensor digiti minimi • Extensor digitorum communis

61

1.11 Peripheral Nerve Tumors

1.11.1 Classification of Peripheral Nerve Tumors (Table 1.11a)   G

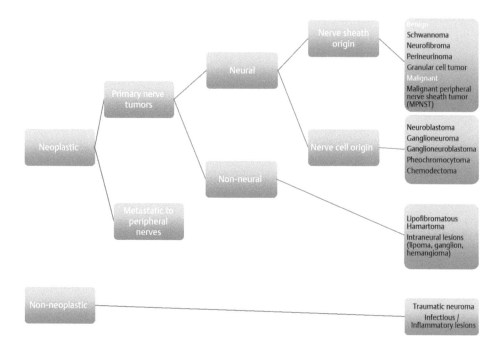

1.11.2 Peripheral Nerve Tumors (Table 1.11b)   G

Presentation	• Mass • Sens (pain, paresthesia, hyper/hypoalgesia) • Motor • ANS dysfunction

Physical examination	• Tumor features:
	  – Location, margins, relations to adjacent structures
	  – Size
	  – Consistency
	  – Tumor mobility vs. direction of nerves
	  – Auscultation
	  – Tinel's sign
	• Look for neurocutaneous stigmata (phakomatosis)
	• Neuro examination (motor, sens, reflexes)

1.11.3 Schwannomas versus Neurofibromas (Table 1.11c) G

	Schwannomas	Neurofibromas
Origin/pathology	Cells that resemble Schwann cells in ultrastructure Types: • Cellular • Plexiform • Melanotic	Cells: Schwann cell precursors, axons, fibroblasts, mast cells, perineural cells Types: • Solitary (90%) • Plexiform and multiple
Frequency	Most common PNT in the adult	Most common PNT in younger adults (average age: 20–30)
Associated syndromes	NF2	NF1 (plexiform and multiple types)
Macro features	• Smooth • Well encapsulated • Firm	
Growth pattern vs. peripheral nerves of origin	Grow eccentrically to the nerve	Encompass nerve fibers
MRI features	Ovoid enhance T1: iso, T2: ↑	Fusiform, multinodular enhance T1: iso, T2: ↑
Surgery	Surgical cure <5% recurrence Weakness post-op (4/5): 9%	Slight weakness post-op: 22–34%
Malignancy	(Almost) no risk	5–10% for plexiform and multiple types

1.11.4 Management (Table 1.11d) G

Observation	• Indications: – Small – Asymptomatic
Surgical removal	• Indications: – Large or enlarging lesions – Symptomatic – Uncertain pathology – Painful • Surgical pearls: – Use of IOP electrical stimulation and evoked EMGs – Magnification for fascicular dissection

1.11.5 Malignant Peripheral Nerve Sheath Tumor (MPNST) (Table 1.11e)

Causes	• Spontaneous • RTX (15 y later) • NF1 association (most often)
Symptoms/signs	• Rapidly enlarging mass, usu very painful • Motor loss early and often progressive (which is rare for benign nerve tumor) • Often non mobile, feels fixed
Imaging features	• Heterogeneous • Necrosis • Invasion of surrounding compartments **None is diagnostic**
Operative features	Firm, indurated, no good planes
Outcomes	Still relatively poor w/ 5yS = 30–50%

1.12 Abbreviations

- ≈: approximately
- (+): positive
- +: plus
- #: fracture
- /: or
- +/: and/or
- Ø: none
- 5yS: 5-year survival
- Abd: abduct, abduction
- Abnl: abnormal
- Add.: adduct, adduction
- ADM: adductor digiti minimi
- AKA: also known as
- APL: abductor pollicis longus
- ANS: autonomic nervous system
- Ant.: anterior
- Anterolat.: anterolateral
- Anteromed: anteromedial
- APL: abductor pollicis longus
- Art.: artery
- BB: biceps brachii
- Br.: branch
- Btw.: between
- CMAP: compound muscle action potential

- CMT: Charcot–Marie–Tooth
- CTS: carpal tunnel syndrome
- C-spine: cervical spine
- CTX: chemotherapy
- Cut.: cutaneous
- Def: deficit
- Dfn: definition
- Dist: distal
- Div.: division
- DM: diabetes melitus
- Dors.: dorsal
- Dorsolat.: dorsolateral
- Dorsomed.: dorsomedial
- D/T: due to
- ECR: extensor carpi radialis
- ECU: extensor carpi ulnaris
- EDB: extensor digitorum brevis
- EDC: extensor digitorum communis
- EDL: extensor digitorum longus
- EDM: extensor digiti minimi
- EHB: extensor hallucis brevis

- EHL: extensor hallucis longus
- EPB: extensor pollicis brevis
- EPL: extensor pollicis longus
- Ext: extension, extensors, extend
- Ext rot: external rotation
- Flex: flexion
- FDB: flexor digitorum brevis
- FDI: first dorsal interosseous
- FDL: flexor digitorum longus
- FDM: flexor digiti minimi
- FHB: flexor hallucis brevis
- FDI: first dorsal interosseous
- FDL: flexor digitorum longus
- FDM: flexor digiti minimi
- FHB: flexor hallucis brevis
- FHL: flexor hallucis longus
- FPI: first palmar interosseous
- GSW: gunshot wound
- Hx: history
- Immob: immobilize
- Incl.: including
- Inj.: injection
- Injr: injury

(Continued) ▶

- Innerv, ✗: innervation, innervated
- Int: internal
- I: incidence
- im: intramuscular
- IM: intermuscular
- IP: interphalangeal
- LE: lower extremity
- Lig.: ligament
- LMN: lower motor neuron
- Lvl: level
- L-spine: lumbar spine
- m.: muscle
- MCN: musculocutaneous nerve
- MCP: metacarpal phalangeal
- Mnvr: maneuver
- Mech.: mechanism
- Mid.: middle
- MTP: metatarsophalangeal
- Mvt(s): movement(s)
- n.: nerve

- Occ: occasionally
- ODM: opponens digiti minimi
- Opp: opposition
- Orhop: orthopaedic
- p: possibility
- Palm.: palmar
- Palp.: palpation
- PIN: posterior interosseous nerve
- PNT: peripheral nerve tumor
- Poll.: pollicis
- Posteromed: posteromedial
- Pron: pronation
- Prox: proximal
- Pr ter: pronator teres
- Pt: patient
- PT: physiotherapy
- QOL: quality of life
- RA: rheumatoid arthritis
- recurr.: recurrent
- Rep.: repetitive

- Resid.: residual
- Resp: respectively
- R/O: rule out
- ROM: range of motion
- Rot: rotation
- RTX: radiotherapy
- S.: syndrome
- sens.: sensory
- SOL: space occupying lesion
- Spont: spontaneous
- subQ: subcutaneous
- Substit.: substitute
- Superf.: superficial
- t: time
- TB: triceps brachii
- T-spine: thoracic spine
- UA: upper arm
- UE: upper extremity
- UMN: upper motor neuron
- Usu: usually
- w/: with
- XR: X-ray

1.13 Cases

1.13.1 Brachial Plexus Stab Wound

Chief complaint/History of present illness	• A 26 y/o male is brought to the emergency room (ER) after being involved in an altercation during which he was stabbed with a sharp knife in the region above his left clavicle.
	• The patient is cleared by the trauma, vascular, and orthopaedics team.
	• You are asked to examine the patient because of upper extremity weakness.
Physical examination	On examination the patient is found to have Bellhop's/waiter's tip position.

(Continued) ▶

Imaging

CT, CTA and MRI are negative with the exception of soft tissue injury in the region of the stab wound.

1. **What is your diagnosis?**
   Based on the upper extremity posture (Bellhop's/Porter's tip position) the patient must have suffered an injury of the upper trunk of the brachial plexus. (See Table 1.4b and Table 1.10).

2. **What motor and sensory deficits do you expect to see in this patient?**
   - Muscles with C5/C6 innervation are involved:
     - Infraspinatus, supraspinatus (external arm rotation).
     - Deltoid (arm abduction).
     - Biceps, brachioradialis (elbow flexion).
     - Occasionally supinator is also involved (forearm supination).
   - Sensory loss in C5 + C6 dermatomes:
     - Lateral half of arm and forearm.
     - Thumb.

3. **What is your management plan?**
   Stab wound injury of the brachial plexus is an open injury that causes sharp nerve division. Thus, the nerve repair should be performed within 3 days from injury. (See Table 1.3g and Table 1.3h).

4. **Describe your surgical approach.**
   (See Table 1.4f).

5. **How fast do you expect the patient to improve his motor function?**
   After brachial plexus repair 12 to 18 months are required to determine the extent of motor recovery.

6. **The patient presents 6 weeks postoperatively with burning sensation in the lateral half of his upper arm and forearm. On examination, he has skin discoloration, loss of hair, and severe allodynia to light touch. What is your diagnosis and management?**
   Patient suffers from complex regional pain syndrome. (See Table 7.1e).

1.13.2 Ulnar Neuropathy

Chief complaint/History of present illness	• A 55 y/o professional tennis player presents to your office. Over the past 6 months he has been experiencing significant paresthesias and numbness along the fourth and fifth digit of his right hand that wakes him up at night.
Physical examination	• Weakness of abduction and adduction primarily of the fourth digit. • Decreased light touch along the fourth and fifth digits. • His neurological examination is completely normal.

1. **What is the most likely diagnosis?**
   The combination of weakness of abduction and adduction primarily of the fourth digit with hypesthesia along the fourth and fifth fingers should raise suspicion for ulnar neuropathy. (See Table 1.6b).

2. **How would you differentiate an ulnar nerve lesion from a C8/T1 radiculopathy or thoracic outlet syndrome?**
   - C8/T1 radiculopathy and neurogenic thoracic outlet syndrome (TOS) are also accompanied by sensation disturbances of upper extremity proximally to the wrist along the medial arm and medial forearm.
   - C8/T1 radiculopathy may be accompanied by neck pain whereas neurogenic TOS may also present with dull shoulder and axilla pain.
   - Neurogenic TOS may present with weakness of both median nerve innervated muscles (e.g., abductor pollicis brevis [APB]) and ulnar nerve-mediated muscles (e.g., abductor digiti minimi [ADM]).
   - Electromyography and nerve conduction studies (EMG/NCS) may further assist in differential diagnosis. (see Table 1.4h and Table 1.6f)

3. **What are the expected neurophysiological findings with ulnar nerve compression at the elbow?**
   (See Table 1.6f).

4. **List the potential anatomical structures causing ulnar nerve compression at the elbow.**
   Postcondylar groove, cubital tunnel, Osborne's fascia, anconeus muscle. (See also Table 1.6f).

5. **Describe the surgical procedure for ulnar nerve decompression at the elbow.**
   (See Table 1.6i).

6. **Postoperatively, the patient complains of numbness in the medial forearm. What are your concerns?**
   Medial antebrachial cutaneous nerve may have been injured during the procedure. (See Table 1.6i).

1.13.3 Carpal Tunnel Syndrome

Chief complaint/History of present illness	• A 45 y/o right-handed secretary presents with numbness and tingling in the right thumb, index and middle finger. • She also describes episodes of pain in the same fingers especially at night, which wake her up and are relieved by shaking her hand. • She also reports weak grip strength. • Her medical history is remarkable for diabetes mellitus.
Physical examination	• Mild loss of sensation to light touch in the right thumb, index and middle finger. • Mild right thenar atrophy. • Mild weakness of the APB and the opponens pollicis. • Tinel's sign is positive at wrist. • Phalen's test is positive.

1. Which are the clinical signs/tests that can support diagnosis of carpal tunnel syndrome? How are they elicited?
   Tinel's sign, Phalen's test, reverse Phalen's test. (See Table 1.5j).

2. What is the most probable clinical diagnosis?
   Median nerve entrapment at carpal tunnel.

3. What are the expected neurophysiological findings with ulnar nerve compression at the elbow?
   NCS and EMG. (See Table 1.5j).

4. What is the differential diagnosis? What further diagnostic tests are you going to order to rule out other possible diagnoses?
   • Other median nerve entrapment sites, brachial plexus lesions, C6/C7 radiculopathies
   • EMG/nerve conduction velocity test (NCV), magnetic resonance imaging (MRI) C-spine. (See Table 1.5j).

5. What are the possible entrapment sites of median nerve? (See Table 1.5a and Table 1.5b)

6. What are the motor and sensory deficits when median nerve is compressed at carpal tunnel? (See Table 1.5b).

7. What are the conservative management measures?
   (See Table 1.5k).

8. What are the indications for surgical decompression of median nerve at the carpal tunnel? (See Table 1.5k).

9. Describe the key surgical steps of surgical decompression of median nerve at the carpal tunnel.
   (See Table 1.5l).

10. What are the variations of the recurrent motor branch in relation to the transverse carpal ligament?
    (See Table 1.5l).

References

1. Burnett MG, Zager EL. Pathophysiology of peripheral nerve injury: a brief review. Neurosurg Focus. 2004; 16(5):E1
2. Dubuisson A, Kline DG. Indications for peripheral nerve and brachial plexus surgery. Neurol Clin. 1992; 10(4):935–951
3. Chung KC, Yang LJ-S, McGillicuddy JE. Practical Management of Pediatric and Adult Brachial Plexus Palsies. Edinburgh: Elsevier; 2012

Suggested Readings

Stephen M. Russel. Examination of Peripheral Nerve Injuries: An Anatomical Approach. New York, NY: Thieme; 2006
Midha R, Zager EL. Surgery of Peripheral Nerve: A Case Based Approach. New York, NY: Thieme; 2008
Manniker AH. Operative Exposures in Peripheral Nerve Surgery. New York, NY: Thieme; 2005

2 Spine and Spinal Cord

2.1 Key Myotomes and Dermatomes and Their Main Function (Table 2.1) ⟨G⟩

	Motor	Sensory	Remarks
C2	None	*Greater occipital nerve:* occiput sensation	
C4	Diaphragm	Clavicle	C3–C5 keep the diaphragm alive
C5	*Deltoid:* arm abduction	Lateral arm	
C6	*Biceps and brachioradialis:* forearm flexion	Thumb	Biceps tendon reflex Radioperiosteal reflex
C7	*Triceps:* forearm extension	Fingers 2 and 3	Triceps tendon reflex
C8	*Finger flexors:* grip strength	Fingers 4 and 5	
T1	*Hand intrinsics:* finger abduction	Inside of arm and forearm	
T4	Intercostals	Nipples	
T10	Upper abdominal muscles	Umbilicus	Abdominal cutaneous reflex
T12	Lower abdominal muscles	Belt line	Abdominal cutaneous reflex
L1	Adductors	Groin	
L2	Iliopsoas, adductors	Inside thigh	Cremasteric reflex
L3	Adductors, quadriceps	Anterior thigh	
L4	Quadriceps	Anterior thigh and shin	Patellar tendon reflex
L5	Foot extensors	Lateral thigh and calf to big toe	

CAUTION:
a. *L5 radiculopathy:* weakness of foot extension (anterior tibialis) + foot inversion (posterior tibialis) + internal rotation of flexed hip (gluteus medius)
b. *Peroneal nerve palsy:* ONLY foot extensor weakness; the other muscles are spared

	Motor	Sensory	Remarks
S1	Gastrocnemius	Posterolateral calf to little toe	Achilles tendon reflex
S2	Toe flexors	Posterior thigh	
S3, S4	Bowel and bladder function	Perianal	Bulbocavernosus reflex

2.2 Spine Injuries

2.2.1 Management of Cervical Spine Fractures (Table 2.2a) G

Always Rule Out Vertebral Artery Injury

Fracture	Radiographic appearance	Description	Treatment
Occipital condyle fracture		**POTENTIALLY UNSTABLE** **Anderson and Montesano classification:** a. *Type I:* comminuted from impact (axial loading) b. *Type II:* extension of linear basilar skull fracture c. *Type III:* • avulsion of bone fragment (rotation, lateral bending) • considered *unstable* • CT is diagnostic test of choice • supplemental MRI to assess ligaments	• Simple unilateral type I or II: collar • Bilateral or type III: halo • Fracture with ligamentous injury/instability or severe type III: occipitocervical fusion

Atlanto-occipital dislocation (AOD)		**UNSTABLE**
		• CT is test of choice especially in children
		• Highest sensitivity test is the **condyle–C1 interval (CC1):**
		  a. Adults: < 1.4 mm
		  b. Pediatrics: < 2.5 mm
		• **On X-ray or CT**, the following may also be used:
		  1. *Basion–axial interval (BAI):*
		    a. *Adults:* ≤ 12 mm
		    b. *Pediatrics:* 0–12 mm but never negative
		  2. *Basion–dental interval (BDI):*
		    a. *Adults:* ≤ 12 mm
		    b. Pediatrics: variable because of odontoid ossification stage
		  3. *Powers ratio/Dublin method:* have low sensitivity - would avoid using.
		  4. *Posterior axial line (PAL):* posterior margin of C2 body
		• Upper cervical **prevertebral soft tissue swelling** should prompt CT to rule out AOD
			• **Always surgical:** occipitocervical fusion, any technique
			• **DO NOT USE TRACTION** (10% risk of neurological deterioration)

Fracture	Radiographic appearance	Description	Treatment
C1 ring fracture (AKA Jefferson's fracture)	**Type 1** **Type 2** **Type 3**	**POTENTIALLY UNSTABLE** a. **Type 1:** single posterior arch fracture b. **Type 2:** anterior and posterior ring fractures. Four-point fracture is classic Jefferson's. c. **Type 3:** lateral mass fracture **Stability** (rule of Spence) depends to a large extent on whether transverse ligament is intact. This can be indirectly assessed by whether the combined overhang of the lateral masses of C1 on C2 is more or less than 7 mm → More than 7 mm implies a disrupted transverse ligament. Obtain MRI to assess.	a. **Type 1:** collar b. **Type 2:** • Intact transverse ligament → halo • Disrupted transverse ligament → surgery (C1/C2 fusion or occipitocervical fusion) c. **Type 3:** halo
Atlantoaxial rotatory deformity	 **Type 1** **Type 2**	Grading is based on degree of atlantodental interval (ADI) in the presence of rotation **POTENTIALLY STABLE** **Type 1:** • Anterior subluxation of C1 on C2 • Both joints affected • Symmetric lateral mass subluxation • Pivot point is dens • Fixed rotation • Transverse ligament intact • Normal ADI **POTENTIALLY UNSTABLE** **Type 2:** • Anterior subluxation of C1 on C2 • Only one joint affected • Pivot point is intact joint • Transverse ligament disrupted • ADI < 5 mm	• If transverse ligament is intact or suffers from bony avulsion, attempt **reduction** through traction followed by **halo vest** immobilization, • **Surgery** if: a. irreducible or b. reduction is not maintained following termination of halo treatment c. transverse ligament disrupted

(Continued) ▶

Fracture	Radiographic appearance	Description	Treatment
	Type 3	**POTENTIALLY UNSTABLE** **Type 3:** • Anterior subluxation of C1 on C2 • Both joints affected • Asymmetric lateral mass subluxation • Asymmetric pivot around dens • Transverse ligament disrupted • ADI > 5 mm	
	Type 4	**POTENTIALLY UNSTABLE** **Type 4:** Posterior displacement of C1 on C2	
Insuffi-ciency of transverse ligament	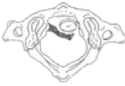	a. **ADI 3–5 mm:** partial transverse ligament disruption b. **ADI 5–8 mm:** complete transverse ligament disruption with low risk of neurological injury c. **ADI > 10 mm:** complete ligamentous disruption with high risk of neurological injury	1. May attempt **halo immobilization treatment**, if ADI ≤ 5 mm secondary to: • purely ligamentous injury or • atlantodental instability due to bone evulsion of tubercle where transverse ligament attaches on C1 2. **C1/C2 fusion**, if ADI > 5 mm OR because of purely ligamentous injury

Fracture	Radiographic appearance	Description	Treatment
Odontoid fracture	Type 1	**STABLE** **Type 1:** oblique avulsion fracture through odontoid tip	Rigid collar (nearly 100% success rate)

	Type 2	**POTENTIALLY UNSTABLE**
		Type 2: fracture through the base of the odontoid Stability depends primarily on whether transverse ligament is intact
			1. **Halo immobilization**
			2. Consider **surgery** instead of halo if:
			   • ≥ 50 years old
			   • posterior fracture displacement
			   • any fracture displacement > 6 mm
			   • angulation > 10°
			   • fracture comminution
			Surgical options:
			a. odontoid screw may be used in acute phase
			b. C1/C2 transarticular or C1/C2 Harms fusion in acute phase or for pseudoarthrosis
			3. Consider **cervical collar** with goal of "stable non-union" for elderly patients who cannot tolerate surgery or halo

(Continued) ▶

Fracture	Radiographic appearance	Description	Treatment
Cont'd	Type 3 	**STABLE** **Type 3:** Fracture extends into C2 body cancellous bone and may involve C1/C2 joint uni- or bilaterally	1. Collar (90% success rate) or 2. Halo

Os odontoideum		**POTENTIALLY UNSTABLE**
		Significant translation of os anterior or posterior to C2 peg may indicate instability
			1. **Observation** in case of no symptoms or neurological signs and no instability
			2. **Surgery** in case of symptoms or neurological signs or instability:
			  a. *reducible neurologic compression* (via traction etc): reduce and then C1/C2 fusion
			  b. *irreducible ANTERIOR neurologic compression:* ventral decompression (transoral, endoscopic transnasal) followed by fusion stabilization for instability
			  c. *irreducible POSTERIOR neurologic compression:* posterior decompression (laminectomy) followed by fusion stabilization for instability

Fracture	Radiographic appearance	Description	Treatment
Traumatic spondylolisthesis of C2 AKA Hangman's fracture	Type 1	**STABLE** **Type 1:** vertical pars fracture of axis: • Displacement of C2 on C3 < 3 mm • No angulation	Collar or halo
	Type 2	**UNSTABLE** **Type 2:** like type 1 PLUS disruption of C2/C3 disk and posterior longitudinal ligament (PLL): • Displacement of C2 on C3 > 3 mm • Possible angulation. Mostly displacement rather than angulation	Traction followed by halo
	Type 2a	**UNSTABLE** **Type 2a:** oblique pars fracture: • Displacement of C2 on C3 < 3 mm • Significant angulation > 11 degrees	Reduce via hyperextension and place in situ compression halo **CAUTION:** avoid traction → may worsen angulation
	Type 3	**UNSTABLE** **Type 3:** like type 2 PLUS bilateral facet disruption and possible ALL ligament disruption: • Displacement of C2 on C3 > 3 mm • Significant angulation > 11 degrees	1. **Open reduction** 2. Followed by **C2/C3 fusion** with lag screws across fracture line

(*Continued*) ▶

Fracture	Radiographic appearance	Description	Treatment
Cervical wedge compression fracture		a. **STABLE**, if posterior elements are intact (simple) b. **UNSTABLE**, if posterior elements are disrupted (complex)	a. **Simple compression:** collar b. **Complex compression:** consider treatment with halo or directly proceed with surgical stabilization
Cervical teardrop fracture		**UNSTABLE** Usually **associated with:** • Anterior inferior bone fragment • Posterior displacement of vertebral body into spinal canal • Kyphosis (flexion angulation of the spine) • Posterior ligamentous disruption May be confused with avulsion fracture. Always obtain CT	1. **Surgical fusion** anterior or posterior 2. **± decompression** anterior or posterior as needed

Cervical subluxation, locked or jumped facet joints		**UNSTABLE**
		a. **Unilateral:**
		  • Usually < 50% subluxation
		  • *Clinically:*
		    – 25% intact
		    – 35% root deficit
		    – 25% incomplete spinal cord injury
		    – 15% quadriplegia
		b. **Bilateral:**
		  • Usually > 50% subluxation
		  • *Clinically:*
		    – 75% quadriplegia
		    – 15% incomplete spinal cord injury
		    – 10% intact
		Imaging:
		a. *Sagittal CT* shows facet dislocation ("bow-tie" sign)
		b. *Axial CT* shows "naked" facet sign
			CAUTION: If possible, obtain MRI prior to reduction to rule out disk herniation
			a. **For patients with neurological deficit,** attempt closed reduction with traction followed by surgical stabilization (anterior cervical discectomy and fusion [ACDF] or posterior fusion or both)
			b. **For patients without neurological deficit,** you may proceed with open reduction and arthrodesis:
			• preferred method is by drilling off facet to allow for reduction, followed by posterior instrumented fusion.
			• ACDF with divergent distraction pin placement has also been described as an alternate method for reduction and fusion

Fracture	Radiographic appearance	Description	Treatment
Facet separation fracture		**POTENTIALLY UNSTABLE** Fracture through ipsilateral lamina and pedicle. Floating facet	1. Consider **halo immobilization,** if there is: • minimal displacement of facet fracture fragments • with no other ligamentous injury and • no neurologic deficit 2. Otherwise, proceed with **surgery.** *Surgical options:* a. *Posterior instrumented fusion* from level above to level below without placement of screw into fractured facet. If needed, decompress affected nerve root b. *ACDF* may also be considered
Comminuted facet fracture		**POTENTIALLY UNSTABLE** • Multiple fractures of pedicle and within facet. • May cause angulation in coronal plane	
Split fracture		**POTENTIALLY UNSTABLE** • Unilateral lateral mass fracture. • Fracture line is vertical	
Traumatic spondylolysis		**POTENTIALLY UNSTABLE** • Bilateral horizontal pars interarticularis fracture • Separates anterior from posterior spinal elements	
Cervical distraction–extension injuries	Type 2	**UNSTABLE** **Type 1:** • Fracture through vertebral body or disk space • Posterior elements intact • Usually presents only with lordotic angulation **Type 2:** • Similar to type 1 but posterior elements are disrupted • Usually presents with lordotic angulation and retrolisthesis	**Type 1:** a. *With fracture through bone:* Halo vest b. *With fracture through disc space:* ACDF **Type 2:** A 360-degree circumferential fusion PLUS decompression as needed
Spinous process fracture AKA "clay shoveler's fracture		**STABLE**	**No specific treatment is necessary:** • Pain relief • Collar for comfort

General Comments on Spine and Spinal Cord Injury (Table 2.2b)

Methylprednisolone: in the 2013 updated guidelines for the management of acute cervical spine and spinal cord injury, the use of methylprednisolone is NOT RECOMMENDED.

Timing of surgery:

a. *Complete spinal cord injury:*
- surgery as soon as the patient is medically stable (after spinal shock)
- *Goal of surgery:* spinal stabilization to allow for sitting position and early rehabilitation

b. *Incomplete spinal cord injury:*
- early decompression and stabilization
- *Goal of surgery:* functional recovery (spinal cord decompression)

Cervical Spine Closed Reduction Protocol (Table 2.2c)

- Rule out skull fractures
- *Always* place pins with patient's eyes closed
- Closed reduction is **contraindicated** if MRI shows disk herniation
- If flexion or extension is necessary during traction, consider external auditory meatus as neutral point

Protocol:

1. **Start weight:** cervical level × 3 in lb
2. Obtain X-ray
3. **Increase weight** by 5–10 lb every 10–15 min until reduced → **Maximum weight in pounds:** 5–10 lb × cervical level
4. Check X-ray after every weight increase
5. Once reduction is achieved, **leave the patient in traction** with 5–10 lb until definitive treatment (surgery or halo vest)

Add muscle relaxants, narcotics, or general anesthesia (*must use somatosensory evoked potentials [SSEP]/motor evoked potential [MEP]*)

Stop closed reduction if:
- Level is reduced
- Occipitocervical instability develops (condyle–C1 lateral mass distance > 5 mm)
- Any disc space height > 10 mm (= overdistraction)
- Neurological or SSEP/MEP deterioration

How to Clear a Cervical Spine (Table 2.2d 🔊)

a. **Asymptomatic patient**	Patients **DO NOT NEED radiographic cervical spine evaluation** if: • Awake • Asymptomatic without neck pain or tenderness • Without injury detracting from accurate evaluation • Have not received CNS depressant medication or pharmacotherapy for pain • Able to complete functional range of motion evaluation

b. **Symptomatic patient**	**Remember:** you MUST rule out BOTH bone injury and ligamentous injury!
	1. **Bone injury** is best ruled out by CT: only if negative, proceed to rule out ligamentous injury
	2. **Ligamentous injury** is best ruled out by:
	  • *MRI with short tau inversion recovery (STIR) images* within 48 h after injury OR
	  • *flexion/extension X-rays* once the patient no longer has symptoms or limiting pain

c. **Obtunded or unreliable patient**	1. Rule out bone injury with CT: only if negative, proceed to rule out ligamentous injury 2. Rule out ligamentous injury with MRI with STIR images within 48 h after injury 3. If MRI is not available, you may consider manual flexion/extension X-rays under fluoroscopic guidance

2.2.2 Management of Thoracic and Lumbar Spine Fractures (Table 2.3) G

Three-column model (DENIS)	1. **Anterior column:**
	  • Anterior longitudinal ligament (ALL)
	  • Anterior 50% of vertebral body and disc
	
	2. **Middle column:**
	  • Posterior 50% of vertebral body and disk
	  • Posterior longitudinal ligament (PLL)
	
	3. **Posterior column:**
	  • Pedicles
	  • Posterior bones (laminae, facet joints, spinous processes)
	  • Ligaments (ligamentum flavum, interspinous, supraspinous)
	  • Facet joint capsule
	
	Potentially unstable if:
	• ≥ 2 columns are involved
	• Fracture below T8 and middle column involved
	• Any of the following:
	  – loss of height > 50%
	  – canal compromise > 50%
	  – kyphosis > 20°

Fracture	Radiographic appearance	Description	Treatment
Transverse process fracture Acute traumatic pars interarticularis (uni- or bilateral) fracture without nerve root compression Laminar fracture Spinous process fracture		STABLE	No specific treatment necessary. May chose to brace.

Compression fracture		STABLE
		 Involves anterior column only.
			1. Thoracic lumbar sacral orthosis (TLSO) brace
			 2. Consider **vertebroplasty,** if after TLSO brace for 3 mo:
			   a. the patient continues to have pain
			   b. without anatomical progression
			   c. with continued high signal on STIR MRI imaging
			 3. Consider **kyphoplasty or surgical fusion,** if after TLSO brace for 3 mo the patient presents with anatomical progression (ie. progressive kyphosis or loss of height)

Fracture	Radiographic appearance	Description	Treatment
Burst fracture		**POTENTIALLY UNSTABLE** Fractures above T8 are more stable because of rib cage support 1. Involves anterior and middle column 2. Most commonly involves superior endplate 3. Less commonly involves inferior endplate or both endplates	**A. In neurologically intact patients:** 1. *TLSO brace*, if there is no evidence of posterior element disruption: • Kyphosis < 15° • no spinous process or facet splaying • no high signal in posterior elements on STIR MRI) 2. *Surgical stabilization* is recommended, if there is involvement of posterior elements: • Kyphosis > 15° • Spinous process or facet splaying • High signal in posterior elements on STIR MRI **B. In neurologically compromised patients** *Surgical decompression and stabilization must be performed.* i. *In thoracic region:* anterior compression should be treated with anterior approach ii. *In lumbar spine:* anterior compression may be reduced with the use of a down-angled curette or via transpedicular approach *If posterior stabilization is performed:* • 2 levels above + 2 levels below fracture is minimum requirement
"Seat belt" fracture AKA Chance fracture		**UNSTABLE** 1. Distraction of middle and posterior columns 2. No or mild compression of anterior column	**A. In neurologically intact patients** with bone injury *WITHOUT significant ligamentous injury*: place in and reduce with hyperextension cast **B. In neurologically compromised patients** or those with bone injury ALONG *WITH significant ligamentous injury*: proceed with surgical stabilization and decompression if needed
Fracture dislocation		**UNSTABLE** **Failure of all three columns:** bone or ligament disruption with displacement	Posterior surgical stabilization with anterior or posterior decompression (corpectomy) if needed

2.2.3 Management of Sacral Spine Fractures (Table 2.4)

Disease	Radiographic appearance	Description	Treatment
Zone 1		1. Fracture **through ala only** 2. No involvement of sacral foramina or sacral canal 3. May cause L5 nerve root injury	
Zone 2		1. Fracture **through sacral foramina** 2. No involvement of sacral canal 3. May cause unilateral L5, S1, S2 nerve root injuries 4. Usually normal bladder function	1. Consider **nonoperative management** for: • nondisplaced fractures • without symptomatic neurological compromise 2. **Iliosacral screw stabilization with decompression** (as needed) for: • significant fracture displacement OR • those with neurologic compromise. **REMEMBER:** Concurrent orthopaedic management required to assess pelvis
Zone 3: vertical		1. Fracture longitudinally **along sacral canal** 2. Usually **associated with:** • pelvic ring fracture • bladder dysfunction • saddle hypesthesia	
Zone 3: transverse		1. Fracture **transverses entire sacrum** horizontally 2. Usually direct trauma to sacrum 3. **Usually associated with:** • bladder and bowel dysfunction • saddle hypesthesia	

2.2.4 Penetrating Spine Injuries (Table 2.5)

Indications for surgery	• Military weapon: debridement • Copper bullet: remove • Lead bullet in joint or disc space or bursa • Migrating bullet • Bullet that traversed gastrointestinal (GI) or respiratory tract: debridement for infection reduction • Cerebrospinal fluid (CSF) leak • Spinal instability

2.3 Management of Degenerative Cervical Spine Disease (Table 2.6) G

Condition	Imaging	Causes, diagnostic tests and other	Treatment
Cervical radiculopathy without myelopathy		1. Disc herniation 2. Foraminal stenosis	1. **Nonsurgical treatment**, if primarily sensory symptoms with no or minimal weakness *Treatment options:* • Oral anti-inflammatory medications • Neuropathic pain medications • Traction • Cervical epidural steroid injections 2. Consider **surgical treatment**, if: • 6 weeks of conservative measures are ineffective or • patient initially presents with significant weakness **Surgical options** for radiculopathy due to foraminal stenosis or disk herniation without significant midline component: • *Posterior laminoforaminotomy/ diskectomy* (preferred due to motion segment preservation and lack of need for implant) • *Anterior cervical discectomy with instrumented fusion or disk replacement* is the other option

(Continued) ▶

Condition	Imaging	Causes, diagnostic tests and other	Treatment

Cervical myelopathy		1. Central disc herniation
		2. Anterior compression due to spondylotic changes
		3. Posterior element compression (ligamentous hypertrophy or spondylotic changes)
		
		For diagnostic verification of myelopathy, **preoperative SSEP** may be considered
			Myelopathy = surgery!
			Predictors of poor prognosis:
			  a. Older age
			  b. Symptoms duration > 1 – 2 y
			  c. Poor preoperative status
			  d. Spinal cord signal ($\downarrow$ T1 and $\uparrow$ T2)
			  e. Spinal cord atrophy
			
			Surgical options depending on compressive pathology:
			1. *Disc herniation:*
			  a. *Disc herniation 1–3 levels* → anterior decompression and stabilization
			  b. *Disc herniation > 3 levels with preserved lordosis* → posterior decompression ± instrumented fusion
			2. *Anterior spondylotic compression:*
			  a. Consider *corpectomy with anterior fusion*. Consider augmenting anterior fusion with posterior instrumented fusion, if corpectomy involves ≥ 2 vertebral bodies.
			  b. Consider *posterior decompression ± instrumented fusion* in patients with preserved lordosis
			3. *Posterior element compression:* posterior decompression ± instrumented fusion
			• **CAUTION:** *posterior decompression without fusion* carries an increased risk of instability and kyphosis. Posterior instrumented fusion or laminoplasty may be used in order to reduce this risk.
			• **CAUTION:** *C5 palsy* in 5% of posterior decompressive surgeries. Consider steroid tapper. Prognosis is good (may take several months to improve).

Condition	Imaging	Causes, diagnostic tests and other	Treatment
Ossified PLL (OPLL)		**More common:** 1. Asian population 2. Males 3. Age > 50 y	1. **Asymptomatic patients:** observation 2. **Patients with radicular symptoms ONLY:** treat with laminoforaminotomy 3. **Patients with myelopathy ± radicular symptoms.** a. *Neutral or lordotic cervical spine:* preferred approach is posterior indirect decompression ± instrumented fusion b. *Kyphotic cervical spine:* i. anterior decompression with epidural dissection using microscope ii. If > 2 level corpectomy is performed, augment anterior fusion with posterior instrumented fusion **REMEMBER:** It is preferable to avoid anterior approaches because of the increased risk of CSF leak and anterior spinal artery injury *(Continued)* ▶

Condition	Imaging	Causes, diagnostic tests and other	Treatment

Cervical kyphosis		**Common causes:**
		a. Degenerative
		b. Iatrogenic (post-laminectomy)
			A. **Cord compression due to kyphosis ONLY:**
			  i. *If kyphosis is reducible:*
			    1. Reduce with traction, followed by
			    2. Posterior instrumented fusion
			  ii. *If kyphosis cannot be reduced:*
			    a. *Ankylosed posterior elements:*
			      1. Posterior release/facetectomy
			      2. ± Anterior release (ACD/ corpectomy/fusion), if facetectomy does not provide enough lordosis
			      3. + Posterior instrumented fusion
			    b. *Non-ankylosed posterior elements:*
			      i. Anterior release (ACD/corpectomy/fusion) to create lordosis
			      ii. ± Posterior instrumented fusion
			
			B. **Cord compression due to kyphosis PLUS significant anterior compressive pathology (osteophytes, etc.):**
			Careful with closed reduction!!
			  i. *If kyphosis is reducible:*
			    1. Start with anterior decompression (ACD/corpectomy/fusion),
			    2. ± Posterior instrumented fusion in reduced lordosed position
			  ii. *If kyphosis cannot be reduced:*
			    a. Ankylosed posterior elements:
			      1. Start with anterior decompression (ACD/corpectomy/fusion), because anterior compression is significant
			      2. Posterior release/facetectomy
			      3. Plus posterior instrumented fusion
			    b. Non-ankylosed posterior elements:
			      1. Start with anterior decompression (ACD/corpectomy/fusion)
			      2. ± Posterior instrumented fusion

Condition	Anatomy	Causes, diagnostic tests and other	Treatment
Central cord syndrome	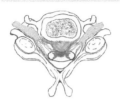	**Typical presentation:** 1. Motor deficit is greater in upper extremities than in lower 2. ± Sensory deficit below injury 3. ± Bowel and bladder dysfunction	A. **In the absence of compression/ instability:** patient may be treated conservatively B. **If compression and instability are present:** i. *Patient with deteriorating neurological status:* urgent surgery is recommended → anterior or posterior approach ± fusion (depending on the pathology and instability) ii. *Patient with a stable or improving neurological deficit:* elective surgery is recommended → anterior or posterior approach ± fusion (depending on pathology and instability)
Rheumatoid arthritis	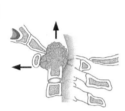	1. Erosion of odontoid and pannus formation behind C2 2. Basilar invagination secondary to erosive destruction of lateral masses C1	A. **Asymptomatic patients:** there are no guidelines for prophylactic surgery B. **Symptomatic patients:** i. *Compression due to basilar invagination only:* 1. attempt to reduce patients with traction 2. a. *If reducible* → proceed with occipitocervical (OC) fusion b. *If irreducible* → consider transoral decompression followed by OC fusion ii. *Compression due to pannus formation only:* transoral decompression → followed by C1/C2 fusion or OC fusion. There is evidence that in some cases OC fusion alone leads to involution of pannus iii. *If both are present:* traction + transoral decompression + OC fusion

2.4 Other Spine or Spinal Cord Conditions (Table 2.7)

Condition	Causes, presentation, diagnostic tests and other	Treatment

Syringomyelia	**Causes**
	a. *Primary:* idiopathic
	b. *Secondary:*
	  • Chiari malformation
	  • Postinfectious
	  • Neoplastic
	  • Postsurgical
	  • Posttraumatic
		a. **Asymptomatic**
		Observation with neurological and radiographic follow-up
		b. **Symptomatic**
		  1. *First treat primary CSF flow abnormality* if possible (i.e., decompression for Chiari)
		  2. *If there is no resolution or no primary CSF flow abnormality*, then consider shunt:
		    • Syringo-subarachnoid or
		    • syringo-peritoneal/pleural, etc.

Spinal epidural lipomatosis	• Hypertrophy of epidural fat tissue • Thoracic and lumbar spine **Common causes:** • Prolonged steroid use (chronic obstructive pulmonary disease [COPD]) • Cushing's disease • Obesity • Hypothyroidism **Presentation:** usually presents with radicular symptoms ± back pain. **Diagnostic tests:** obtain EMG to verify radiculopathies	**Treatment:** • Correct cause, if possible (stop steroid use) • Laminectomy for persistent symptoms **Outcome:** usually good
Spinal epidural hematoma	• Usually thoracic spine **Common causes:** • Anticoagulation • Nonsteroidal anti-inflammatory drugs (NSAIDs) • Trauma (lumbar puncture, spinal anesthesia) • Idiopathic	**Treatment:** • Reverse anticoagulation • Surgical evacuation

2.5 Spinal Infections (Table 2.8) G

Condition	Causes, presentation and other	Diagnostic tests	Treatment
Spinal epidural abscess	**Most common organism:** Staphylococcus aureus followed by Streptococcus **Risk factors:** • Immune compromise • Diabetes • IV drug abuse • Renal failure • Alcoholism **Typical symptoms:** • Back pain • + fever • + sweats/chills • ± neurological deficit (usually develops within 3–4 d from when back pain starts) !! Even small abscesses can have fulminant course with rapid neurological deterioration	**Imaging:** Contrast-enhanced MRI	**A. Nonsurgical treatment:** 1. Isolate microorganism 2. Treat with appropriate antibiotics **CAUTION:** Extremely close observation and treatment with antibiotics alone may be an option if the patient is asymptomatic and abscess is very small. Patients may decompensate very rapidly **B. Surgical treatment:** Generally spinal epidural abscess *is a surgical disease*

Diskitis and vertebral osteomyelitis	**Disk space INVOLVED:**
	a. Typically involves only one disk *(diskitis)* or
	b. disk and adjacent vertebral bodies *(osteomyelitis)*
	
	Most common organism: S. aureus followed by Escherichia coli
	
	Risk factors and symptoms are similar to epidural abscess
		1. Contrast-enhanced MRI
		2. **CT and flexion–extension (Flex/Ex) films** for assessment of stability
		3. If infection is occult, **technetium-99 three-phase scan or gallium-67 scan**
			A. Nonsurgical treatment:
			• **Indications:**
			  a. Positive culture obtained (blood culture, CT-guided biopsy)
			  b. No neurological deficits
			  c. No spinal instability
			  d. Limited disease that responds to antibiotic treatment
			  e. No or minimal spinal epidural abscess component
			• **Treatment:** IV antibiotics for 6 wk PLUS 6 wk oral antibiotics + bracing
			B. Surgical treatment: if any of the above nonsurgical indications are not present, in addition to antibiotic treatment, also consider:
			1. Surgical debridement
			2. + instrumentation, if necessary (not contraindicated)

(Continued) ▶

Condition	Causes, presentation and other	Diagnostic tests	Treatment
Tuberculosis of the spine AKA Pott's disease	**Disk space SPARING** Almost never in cervical or sacral spine **Presentation:** usually associated with back pain of a long chronicity	1. **Imaging:** a. MRI b. CT c. Flex/Ex films 2. **Culture:** has to be maintained for 3 mo before it is considered negative	A. **Nonsurgical treatment** Antibiotics + bracing IF: a. No neurological deficit b. No deformity or instability B. **Surgical treatment** if any of the above nonsurgical indications are not present, consider: 1. Extensive debridement 2. + stabilization 3. + antibiotics

2.6 Management of Degenerative Thoracic and Lumbar Spine Disease (Table 2.9) G

Disease	Anatomy	Presentation, diagnostic tests and other	Treatment
Thoracic disk herniation	Laminectomy Transpedicular Costotransversectomy Lateral extracavitary	ALWAYS obtain CT to see if lesion is calcified	**Surgical approaches:** 1. Transpedicular 2. Costotransversectomy 3. Lateral extracavitary approach 4. Transthoracic 5. Laminectomy alone is usually NOT a good option **Ventral approaches:** a. *T1–T3:* approach through median sternotomy b. *T3–T5:* right thoracotomy (left side is difficult due to aorta) c. *T6–T10:* left or right thoracotomy d. *T11–L2:* lateral thoracoabdominal approach with detachment of diaphragm right or left (left preferred to avoid liver) **REMEMBER: For approaches near the lung:** • Always double lumen intubation • Neurovascular bundle runs underneath rib on rostral aspect Vein (superior) Artery Nerve (inferior) **REMEMBER:** • The more midline the lesion, the more lateral the exposure • For each targeted disk space, expose rib numbered after INFERIOR vertebral body (eg. for T6/T7 disk space → expose rib 7)

Disease	Anatomy	Presentation, diagnostic tests and other	Treatment
Ankylosing spondylitis		a. Squared vertebral bodies b. "Bamboo" spine c. Sacroiliitis d. HLA-B27 (human leukocyte antigen B27)	**Treat back pain with:** 1. NSAIDs 2. Sulfasalazine 3. Immune-modulating medications **CAUTION:** • In case of surgery perform *awake intubation* (rigid cervical spine) • If *instrumented fusion* is required: 1. use long segment fusion with multiple points of fixation 2. consider anterior/posterior instrumentation **REMEMBER:** Because of rigidity of spine, minor trauma can lead to severe injury (usually fracture dislocation)
Lumbar spinal stenosis		**CAUTION:** ALWAYS rule out vascular claudication	A. **Nonsurgical treatment includes:** 1. NSAIDs 2. Neuropathic medications 3. Physical therapy 4. Epidural steroid injections B. **Surgical treatment:** • *Indications:* a. if nonsurgical treatments fail b. if the patient presents with significant or progressive associated neurological deficits (including weakness or bowel/bladder problems) • *Surgical tips:* a. Always address *foraminal stenosis* in addition to central stenosis b. Preserve the *pars interarticularis* to avoid instability c. Consider adding *fusion* to decompression if preoperative listhesis is present
Spondy-lolisthesis	Grading system for spondylolisthesis (expressed as % of vertebral body anteroposterior (AP) diameter): a. *Grade 1:* 1–24% b. *Grade 2:* 25–49% c. *Grade 3:* 50–74% d. *Grade 4:* 75–99% e. *Grade 5:* 100% and higher, spondyloptosis		

(Continued) ▶

Disease	Anatomy	Presentation, diagnostic tests and other	Treatment
Degenerative spondylo- listhesis = posterior elements are intact		a. Usually presents after age 40 y b. More common in women c. Most commonly **L4/L5** d. Usually causes **central stenosis** e. **Symptoms are** usually because of associated stenosis	A. **Nonsurgical treatment:** similar to spinal stenosis B. **Surgical treatment:** decompression PLUS fusion has better long-term outcomes than simple decompression

Isthmic spon- dylolisthesis = posterior elements are disrupted posterior elements		a. Usually at **L5/S1**
		b. Rarely causes central stenosis
		c. Causes primarily **foraminal stenosis**
		d. **Common symptoms** include back pain and L5 radiculopathy
			A. **Nonsurgical treatment:**
			1. *Back pain:* If patient presents with back pain, obtain CT, Flex/ Ex films and bone scan:
			  a. *Fracture is acute,* if bone scan is "hot" and CT does not show corticated fracture line → start with TLSO brace for 3 mo for fracture healing
			  b. *Fracture is old,* if bone scan is "cold" → treat symptomatically with NSAIDs and possibly injections into fracture line
			2. *Radiculopathy:*
			  a. NSAIDs
			  b. Epidural injections
			
			B. **Surgical treatment**
			• *Indications:*
			  a. Patients failing to respond to nonsurgical therapy
			  b. Visible rapid anatomical progression of disease
			• *Goal of surgery* is stabilization and decompression of neural elements if radicular symptoms exist
			• *Surgical plan:*
			  a. *Grades 1 & 2:* it is usually not necessary to reduce. Simple posterior instrumented fusion ± decompression
			  b. *Grade ≥ 3:* reduction is suggested, usually via the anterior approach with interbody device followed by posterior decompression + instrumented fusion.

Disease	Anatomy	Presentation, diagnostic tests and other	Treatment
Lumbar disk herniation, lumbar radiculopathy	a. **Midline/lateral gutter disks** affect transversing root. (e.g., L4/L5 disks → L5 radiculopathy b. **Far lateral/foraminal disks** affect exiting root. (e.g., L4/L5 disks → L4 radiculopathy CAUTION: Location of disk herniation must coincide with neurological symptoms, so beware of mimickers (meralgia paresthetica, peroneal nerve compression, etc.)	**Most common location:** L4/ L5 and L5/S1 (95% of all lumbar disk herniations)	A. **Nonsurgical treatment:** 1. Short-term bed rest 2. NSAIDs ± oral opioids 3. ± Physical or chiropractic therapy 4. Epidural steroid injections B. **Surgical treatment** • *Indications:* a. Cauda equina syndrome (emergent) b. Progressive motor deficits c. Inability to control pain d. Nonresolution of symptoms after 6 wk of nonsurgical treatment • *Surgical technique:* a. *Microdiscectomy ± laminectomy.* Use pedicle as anatomic point for localization of disk fragment on imaging and for intraoperative identification!! b. *Fusion* NOT recommended as routine treatment following primary disk excision but it is considered for recurrent disk herniations
Cauda equina syndrome	a. Urinary retention → check for postvoid residual b. Urinary and/or fecal incontinence c. Diminished anal sphincter tone d. Sexual dysfunction e. Saddle hypesthesia f. Significant weakness in more than one nerve root distribution g. Severe radicular pain (REMEMBER: absence of pain may indicate severe nerve damage and worse prognosis)		**Surgery as soon as possible!!** • *Surgical technique:* Depending on pathology, wide decompression with laminectomy is recommended • *Timing of surgery:* There is evidence that surgical intervention within 48 h of symptom onset carries a better prognosis • *Prognostic factors:* a. *Better prognosis* if on initial presentation patient has only motor and sensory deficits (including saddle anesthesia) b. *Worse prognosis* if urinary retention is present

(Continued) ▶

Disease	Description	Treatment

Low back pain	**Modic changes types in MRI:**
	a. *Type 1:* bone marrow edema adjacent to disk space:
	• T1 ↓
	• T2 ↑
	b. *Type 2:* replacement of bone marrow by fat:
	↑ on T1 and T2
	c. *Type 3:* reactive osteosclerosis:
	• T1 ↓
	• T2 ↑
	
	Rule out pathologic causes such as:
	a. Fracture
	b. Instability
	c. Metastasis/tumor
	d. Infection
		A. **Nonsurgical treatment:**
		1. Short-term bed rest
		2. Limit heavy lifting
		3. Physical therapy
		4. *Analgesics:*
		  a. NSAIDs are preferred
		  b. addition of opioids or muscle relaxers not better than adding placebo
		5. *Interventional pain treatments* including:
		  a. epidural steroid injections
		  b. medial branch blocks/ablations
		
		B. **Surgical treatment:**
		In the absence of pathologic causes, fusion for back pain may be considered for selected patients even without stenosis or listhesis *when symptoms are:*
		a. Lasting more than 2 y.
		b. Refractory to conservative treatment.
		c. Associated with one- or two-level degenerative disk disease

2.7 Spinal Instrumentation Placement (Table 2.10) [G]

The surgical procedures described in this chart are based on standard trajectories and the main author's instrumentation placement technique.

Disease	Anatomy	Surgical technique
Occipital plate placement		1. **Study pre-op MRI/CT** to identify thickness of occipital bone. Midline occipital bone is thickest. 2. **First, place screws in cervical spine** and then choose and place occipital plate. This way, it lines up with the cervical screws for easy rod placement 3. **Place occipital plate as close to external occipital protuberance as possible** but not above it since that increases the risk of injury to the transverse sinus and leads to prominence of the plate under the skin 4. **Drill pilot holes** in stepwise fashion until inner cortex is breached for bicortical screw purchase 5. **Tap holes and place screws** **Complication management** a. *If there is CSF return*, place bone wax in hole and then place screw b. *If there is venous bleeding* due to occipital sinus violation, tamponade by placing screw (which is shorter than tapped depth)

Disease	Anatomy	Surgical technique
C1 lateral mass screw	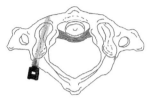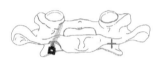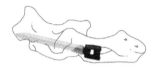	<ul><li>**Study pre-op MRI/MRA/CTA** to determine course of vertebral artery and location of carotid in relation to anterior border of C1</li><li>**Entry point:** midpoint of lateral mass.<ul><li>*To identify*, follow inferior border of lateral aspect of C1 lamina with subperiosteal dissection down to the lateral mass. Use micro Penfield 4 to identify medial and lateral border of C1 lateral mass.</li><li>*Significant bleeding of venous plexus* may be encountered around C2 nerve root → Control bleeding with morselized thrombin-soaked gelatin sponge.</li><li>*C2 nerve root can be sacrificed* if needed.</li></ul></li><li>**Trajectory:** *Target* on lateral fluoroscopy is the anterior C1 tubercle:<ul><li>*Medial* 15°</li><li>*Superior* 20°</li></ul></li><li>**Depth:** VERY LONG ≥ 30 mm<ul><li>Needs to be proud dorsally to be able to connect to C2 screw</li><li>*Beware* of location of carotid artery anterior to C1</li></ul></li></ul>
C2 isthmus screw	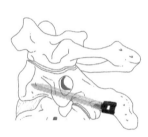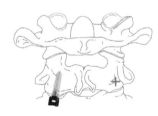	<ul><li>**Study pre-op MRI/MRA/CTA** to:<ol type="a"><li>determine course and anatomy of *vertebral artery* in foramen transversarium of C2.</li><li>Determine whether there is *enough bone* width between superomedial border of foramen transversarium and lateral border of spinal canal to accommodate safe passage of a long C2 screw.</li><li>Also note *location of carotid* in relation to anterior border of C2</li></ol></li><li>**Entry point:** superomedial portion of lateral mass of C2:<ul><li>3 mm above C2/C3 joint</li><li>3 mm medial from lateral border</li></ul></li><li>**Trajectory:**<ol><li>*Palpate* medial isthmus/lateral border of C2 spinal canal.</li><li>*Trajectory* should be as medial as possible but without violating lateral border of spinal canal:<ul><li>*Medial* 15°</li><li>*Superior* 25°</li></ul></li></ol></li><li>**Depth:** 25–30 mm</li><li>**Management of vertebral artery injury:** If brisk bleeding occurs, assume vertebral artery injury has occurred:<ol><li>Pack the drill hole with hemostatic agent and small amount of bone wax</li><li>Place screw and DO NOT instrument contralateral side</li><li>Abort procedure and proceed with angiography</li></ol></li></ul>

(Continued) ▶

Disease	Anatomy	Surgical technique

Odontoid screw

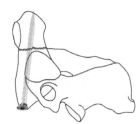

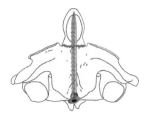

- **Contraindications:**
  a. Disrupted transverse ligament
  b. C2 body fracture
  c. Significant displacement of fragments
  d. Oblique fracture orientation of antero-cephalad to dorsocaudal
  e. Previous fracture nonunion, fracture older than 6 mo
  f. Inability to reduce fracture pre-op
  g. Poor pre-op fluoroscopic visualization. Use bite block and lateral displacement of endotracheal tube with oral gauze to improve visualization.
  h. Barrel chest
- **Entry point:**
  1. Use biplane fluoroscopy
  2. Prior to incision, reduce fracture via patient positioning with live fluoroscopy
  3. Skin incision at C5/C6
  4. *Screw entry point* at midpoint of anterior lip of inferior C2 endplate
- **Trajectory:**
  Aim for odontoid tip:
  – *Medial:* guided by fluoroscopy (0°)
  – *Superior:* guided by fluoroscopy
- **Depth:**
  – *Typical length: 35–40 mm*
  – *Use lag screw* to achieve reduction and compression of fracture line

Sublaminar wires with bone graft C1 - C2

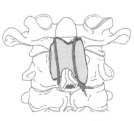

- Used primarily as a **salvage technique/ alternative** to screw-based fixation
- **Review CT** to confirm that there is no bifid lamina or laminar fractures.
- **Exposure:**
  1. Medial superior and inferior *C1 arch:*
     – Beware of location of sulcus arteriosus (vertebral artery).
     – Clear epidural space under C1
  2. Superior *C2 arch* and spinous processes
- **Wire passing:**
  1. Pass blunt needle with 0 silk under C1 arch
  2. Bend wire in half and tie the passed 0 suture to wire loop. Use suture to pull wire loop under C1 arch while constantly applying upward traction to keep wire opposed to inner bony surface of C1 lamina to avoid spinal cord compression
  3. Pass free ends of the wires through the wire loop and tighten on the C1 arch
  4. Thread free wire edges through predrilled holes in unicortical graft and secure free wire edges firmly around spinous process of C2
- **Bone graft:**
  1. *Unicortical graft.* Cortical surface placed dorsally.
  2. *Decorticate* inferior border of C1 lamina and superior border of C2 lamina/spinous process

Disease	Anatomy	Surgical technique
C1/C2 transarticular screw	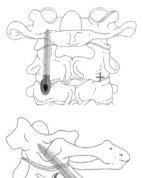	**Similar to C2 isthmus screw** but with a more cephalad trajectory • **Study pre-op MRI/MRA/CTA:** a. Determine course and anatomy of *vertebral artery* in foramen transversarium of C2. b. Determine whether there is *enough bone* width between superomedial border of foramen transversarium and lateral border of spinal canal to accommodate safe passage of long transarticular screw. c. Note location of *carotid* in relation to anterior border of C1 • **Entry point:** 1. Once bony landmarks are identified via midline incision, *separate stab incisions* may be required in order to achieve desired trajectories 2. *Starting point* is superior medial portion of lateral mass of C2: – 3 mm above C2/C3 joint – 3 mm medial from lateral border • **Trajectory:** 1. *Palpate* medial isthmus/lateral border of C2 spinal canal. 2. *Trajectory* should be as medial as possible but without violating the lateral border of spinal canal: – *Medial* 15° – *Superior:* superior border of anterior ring of C1 • **Depth:** 40 mm • **Management of vertebral artery injury:** If brisk bleeding occurs, assume vertebral artery injury has occurred: 1. Pack the drill hole with hemostatic agent and small amount of bone wax 2. Place screw and DO NOT instrument contralateral side 3. Abort procedure and proceed with angiography <div align="right">(*Continued*) ▶</div>

Disease	Anatomy	Surgical technique
C3–C7 lateral mass screw	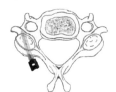 	• **Entry point:** From midpoint of lateral mass: – 1 mm medial – 1 mm inferior • **Trajectory:** May require removal of spinous processes to achieve lateral trajectory – *LATERAL* 30°: Good guide is that handle of drill/tap should be at least passed midline and on contralateral side – **Superior** 15–30°, parallel to facet joint. Palpate angle of facet joint with micro Penfield 4 • **Depth:** 10–15 mm • **CAUTION:** C6 and C7 lateral mass may be very small; place C6/C7 pedicle screws instead
C6/C7 pedicle screw	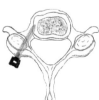	• **Review pre-op imaging:** a. Study *vascular anatomy:* Although foramen transversarium may be present at C6 or C7, it may not yet contain vertebral artery and may only contain veins b. Determine *size of pedicles.* • **Entry point:** From midpoint of lateral mass: – 2 mm lateral – 2 mm superior • **Trajectory:** 1. Consider *hemilaminectomy* for safety. 2. *Palpate* medial border of pedicle 3. *Trajectory:* – MEDIAL 30° – Superior 0° • **Depth:** 15 mm or longer (measure on CT) • **Management of vertebral artery injury:** If brisk bleeding occurs, and pre-op imaging confirms presence of vertebral artery at this level, assume vertebral artery injury has occurred: 1. Pack the drill hole with hemostatic agent and small amount of bone wax 2. Place screw, and DO NOT instrument contralateral side. 3. Abort procedure and proceed with angiography.

Pedicle screws	Anatomy	Surgical technique

Thoracic pedicle screws	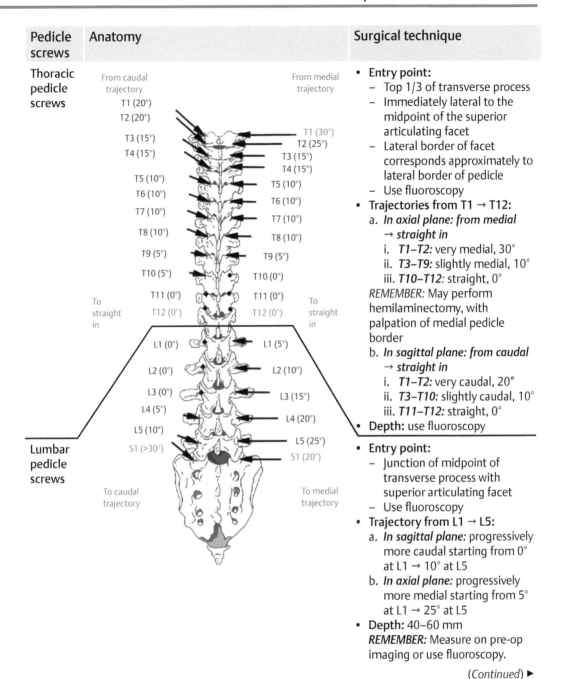 From caudal trajectory
	T1 (20°)
	T2 (20°)
	T3 (15°)
	T4 (15°)
	T5 (10°)
	T6 (10°)
	T7 (10°)
	T8 (10°)
	T9 (5°)
	T10 (5°)
	T11 (0°)
	T12 (0°)
	To straight in
	L1 (0°)
	L2 (0°)
	L3 (0°)
	L4 (5°)
	L5 (10°)
	S1 (>30°)
	To caudal trajectory
	
	From medial trajectory
	T1 (30°)
	T2 (25°)
	T3 (15°)
	T4 (15°)
	T5 (10°)
	T6 (10°)
	T7 (10°)
	T8 (10°)
	T9 (5°)
	T10 (0°)
	T11 (0°)
	T12 (0°)
	To straight in
	L1 (5°)
	L2 (10°)
	L3 (15°)
	L4 (20°)
	L5 (25°)
	S1 (20°)
	To medial trajectory
		• **Entry point:**
		  – Top 1/3 of transverse process
		  – Immediately lateral to the midpoint of the superior articulating facet
		  – Lateral border of facet corresponds approximately to lateral border of pedicle
		  – Use fluoroscopy
		• **Trajectories from T1 → T12:**
		  a. *In axial plane: from medial → straight in*
		    i. *T1–T2:* very medial, 30°
		    ii. *T3–T9:* slightly medial, 10°
		    iii. *T10–T12:* straight, 0°
		  REMEMBER: May perform hemilaminectomy, with palpation of medial pedicle border
		  b. *In sagittal plane: from caudal → straight in*
		    i. *T1–T2:* very caudal, 20°
		    ii. *T3–T10:* slightly caudal, 10°
		    iii. *T11–T12:* straight, 0°
		• **Depth:** use fluoroscopy

Lumbar pedicle screws		• **Entry point:**
		  – Junction of midpoint of transverse process with superior articulating facet
		  – Use fluoroscopy
		• **Trajectory from L1 → L5:**
		  a. *In sagittal plane:* progressively more caudal starting from 0° at L1 → 10° at L5
		  b. *In axial plane:* progressively more medial starting from 5° at L1 → 25° at L5
		• **Depth:** 40–60 mm
		  REMEMBER: Measure on pre-op imaging or use fluoroscopy.

(*Continued*) ▶

Pedicle screws	Anatomy	Surgical technique

S1 pedicle screws		• **Entry point:** Just inferior and lateral to S1 facet joint
		• **Trajectory:**
		  – *Medial:* 20°
		  – *Caudal:* point toward S1 promontorium
		• **Depth:** 35–40 mm
		REMEMBER: Measure on pre-op imaging or use fluoroscopy.

S2 alar screws		• **Entry point:** just medial to the midpoint of a line connecting the S1 and S2 foramina
		• **Trajectory:**
		  – *LATERAL* 40°
		  – *Caudally* parallel to superior endplate of S1
		• **Depth:** 50–60 mm
		• **Beware of anterior breach:** may lead to injury of pelvic vessels, viscera, lumbosacral plexus, or sympathetic chain

2.7.1 Ten Spinal Instrumentation Rescue and Salvage Techniques (Table 2.11 🔊) G

1. **Change trajectory**
   E.g.: T-spine pedicle screw: instead of transpedicular route use IN-OUT-IN technique through rib
2. Perform **laminectomy** to palpate internal landmarks
3. Add **fluoroscopy**; consider use of **intraoperative CT/navigation** if available
4. **Change fixation method:**
   E.g.: instead of pedicle screw, use wiring techniques, hook, or other techniques:
   • Occipital wires
   • Sublaminar wires
   • Spinous process wires
   • Supralaminar hooks
   • Infralaminar hooks
   • Pedicle hooks
   • Transverse process hooks
   • Iliac screws
   • Iliosacral screws
5. **Skip level:**
   E.g.: typical in scoliosis cases
6. **Add a level:** go one level above or below
7. Consider **unilateral instrumentation** only
8. Add **supplementary fusion in a different spinal column**
   E.g.: adding ACDF to a posterior cervical fusion
9. **Augment instrumentation:**
   a. use screw of greater diameter or rescue screw
   b. inject methyl methacrylate into osteoporotic bone prior to pedicle screw placement
10. If all else fails, **onlay fusion with external orthosis** (Halo, TLSO, etc.)

2.8 Pediatric Spine and Spinal Cord Injury Guidelines (Table 2.12) G

Potential AOD		a. **CT imaging** to determine condyle–C1 interval b. **MRI** for fluid within joint
Cervical spine evaluation	> 3 y of age	**DO NOT USE** cervical spine imaging after trauma IF: • Alert • No neurological deficit • No midline cervical tenderness • No painful distracting injury • No unexplained hypotension • Not intoxicated
	< 3 y of age	**DO NOT USE** cervical spine imaging after trauma IF: • Glasgow Coma Scale (GCS) > 13 • No neurological deficit • No midline cervical tenderness • No painful distracting injury • Not intoxicated • No unexplained hypotension • No motor vehicle accident • No fall from greater than 10 feet • No known or suspected non-accidental trauma

	If these criteria are **NOT** met	**USE** cervical spine imaging:
		a. Use **high-resolution CT** or cervical spine **radiographs**
		b. **For atlantoaxial rotatory fixation (AARF)** use three-position CT with C1–C2 motion analysis
		c. **Rule out ligamentous injury** via:
		  i. flexion/extension X-rays/fluoroscopy or
		  ii. MRI with STIR performed within 72 h of injury

Treatment of AARF		1. **Use reduction with manipulation** for AARF that has persisted for < 4 wk and that <u>does not reduce</u> spontaneously. Then place patient in **orthosis** 2. **Use halter, tong or halo traction** for patients with AARF that has persisted for > 4 wk. Then place patient in **orthosis** 3. **Internal fixation and fusion** for irreducible AARF or reduction that is not maintained once orthosis is removed

Synchondrosis		• Synchondrosis may be mistaken for fracture. But be careful: fracture may hide inside synchondrosis
		• **Management** of synchondrosis fractures is identical to bony fracture:
		  a. Reduction and external immobilization
		  b. Surgery only for persistent instability

Pseudosubluxation		• Common lateral cervical X-ray finding in children younger than 7 y. **Not pathologic** • When head is in flexed position, C2 moves anterior to C3 by 2–3 mm (> 3 mm may indicate pathologic subluxation) • **Swischuk's line:** anterior border of posterior arch of C2 should lie within 2 mm or less of a line drawn between the anterior borders of the posterior arches of C1 and C3. *More than 2-mm distance* is indicative of true subluxation rather than pseudosubluxation

SCIWORA
(spinal cord injury
without radiographic
abnormality)

- Patient presents with symptoms of spinal cord injury and normal imaging studies
- Treatment includes:
  - *Spinal immobilization* for up to12 wk
  - *Discontinue immobilization* if:
    a. Patient is asymptomatic
    b. Spinal stability confirmed on flexion extension X-rays
  - Patient should avoid high-risk activities for 6 mo

2/3 of cervical spine injury at age < 10 y occurs at the occiput–C2 level.

2.9 Scoliosis (Table 2.13) G

Type	Diagnosis	Other	Treatment

Degenerative scoliosis	**Exclude other causes of pain:**
	• peripheral vascular disease
	• knee or hip joint problems
	• neuropathy
	• kidney infection
	• pancreatitis
	• psychiatric disease
		Beware of pre-existing adolescent idiopathic scoliosis with super-imposed degenerative changes	1. **Nonoperative treatment:**
			• NSAIDs
			• Physical conditioning
			• Epidural steroid injections
			• Facet joint medial branch blocks
			 2. **Surgery:**
			• *Indications:*
			  a. Nonsurgical therapy fails
			  b. Cobb's angle > 30° with progression
			  c. Sagittal–vertical axis (SVA) > 5 cm
			  d. Lateral listhesis ≥ 6 mm
			  e. Rotation ≥ grade 2
			  f. Intercrest line below L4/L5 disk space
			• *If decompensated curve:*
			  – Consider restoration of sagittal balance (± osteotomy).
			  – *Goal of surgery* is:
			    a. to reduce the SVA
			    b. to achieve a pelvic incidence (PI) that is equal to the lumbar lordosis (LL) plus 11°

Congenital scoliosis:
1. **Failure of formation:** hemivertebra
2. **Failure of segmentation:** osseous bar connecting vertebrae
3. Greatest risk of progression when **both are present**
	1. **At diagnosis,** order:
	  a. MRI spine
	  b. Cardiac echo
	  c. Renal ultrasound
	2. **As long as no neurologic deficit,** follow patient with serial scoliosis films
	3. **If neurological deficit develops,** order:
	  a. MRI brain
	  b. MRI spinal cord
		"Growth is the enemy of congenital scoliosis"	1. **Nonoperative treatment** is ineffective
			2. **Surgical options:**
			  a. *Growth-preserving procedures:*
			    • growing rod
			    • hemiepiphysiodesis/ arthrodesis
			  b. *Trunk shortening procedures:* excision of hemivertebra and short segment fusion
			  c. *Long posterior fusion*

Type	Diagnosis	Other	Treatment

Infantile scoliosis: idiopathic in children younger than 3 y	1. **As long as no neurologic deficit,** follow patient with serial scoliosis films
	2. **If neurological deficit,** order:
	  a. MRI brain and spinal cord.
	  b. If MRIs are negative, proceed with EMG and metabolic bone workup
		If rib–vertebral angle difference > 20°, progression is likely	1. **Close follow-up** for progression in sagittal and coronal plane
			2. **Deformity > 30°:** serial body cast immobilization
			3. **If progression continues →** Surgery (growing rods)

Juvenile idiopathic scoliosis: 3–10 y	1. Full-length standing AP and lateral scoliosis **X-rays** ("3-ft-standing films") 2. **MRI entire spine**		1. **Curve < 20°** → Observation 2. **Progressive curve 20–40°** → Spinal orthosis 3. **Curve > 50°** → Surgery If child is younger than 8 y, consider instrumentation without fusion (growing rods)

Adolescent idiopathic scoliosis: > 10 y	1. Scoliosis **X-rays**
	2. ± MRI
		Definition:
		a. Patient 10–18 y
		b. Cobb's angle ≥ 10°
		  Female: male > 3:1
			1. **Cobb's angle < 20°** → Observation
			2. **Cobb's angle 20–40°:**
			  • *Bracing:* > 16 h daily
			  • *Until growth is complete* (no growth within 6 mo or 2 y after menarche); Risser's stages 4 to 5
			  • *Goal:* 50% curve correction in brace
			3. **Cobb's angle > 50°** → Surgery

Neuromuscular scoliosis	Full-length scoliosis standing AP and lateral X-rays or sitting if not ambulatory	**Underlying neural or muscular etiology for scoliosis** (i.e., cerebral palsy [CP] or Duchenne's muscular dystrophy)	• Consider **surgery** with progressive curve beyond 50° • **Medical morbidity** is significant in these patients, leading to higher surgical risk • **Preoperative evaluation** includes medical optimization (pulmonary, cardiac, etc.) • **Goals:** level pelvis, level shoulders

2.10 Tumors of Spine and Spinal Cord (Table 2.14) G

I. Extradural (50% of spine tumors)

Tumor	Presentation/ Demographics	Imaging/Other diagnostics	Other	Treatment
Metastasis	• Most common extradural spine tumor • **Most common histology:** a. Breast b. Lung c. Prostate	1. **MRI** 2. **PET scan** 3. **Biopsy of primary tumor**, if diagnosis is not established 4. **Oncologic workup**	a. Usually osteoclastic b. **OsteoBPlastic:** • Breast: women • Prostate: men	Treatment is ALWAYS PALLIATIVE A. **Limited to bone; no epidural component:** 1. Treat primary (*chemo*) 2. *Radiation therapy* (XRT) to spine lesion 3. Consider *vertebroplasty or surgical fusion* if instability present B. **With epidural component:** a. In patients *with poor prognosis* (usually < 6 mo) → consider XRT alone b. In patient *with good prognosis* (> 6 mo) →consider surgical resection (± stabilization - fusion as needed) + XRT IN REGARD TO SURGERY, REMEMBER: • **Surgery + XRT** is better than XRT alone • Prefer anterior or anterolateral approaches for anterior disease and laminectomy for disease limited EXCLUSIVELY to dorsal epidural space • **Surgery usually NOT indicated if:** a. Highly radiosensitive tumors (lymphoma, etc.) b. Complete paralysis > 8 h c. Inability to walk > 24 h • **Other indications for surgery:** a. Instability b. Neurologic deficit due to deformity or retropulsed bone c. Radioresistant tumor d. Tumor progression despite maximal XRT and chemotherapy

Tumor	Presentation/ Demographics	Imaging/Other diagnostics	Other	Treatment
Vertebral hemangioma AKA cavernous hemangioma 	• Most common primary spine tumor • **Incidence:** > 10% in general population	1. **MRI:** hyperintense on T1 and T2 2. **Bone scan:** cold 3. **Sagittal CT or X-ray:** lytic lesions with honeycomb vertical striations 4. **Axial CT:** lucent lesions with polka dot sign	• No malignant transformation • Only 1% symptomatic • **Histology:** – mature thin blood vessels replacing bone marrow – hypertrophic bone trabeculae	A. **Asymptomatic:** no treatment, no routine follow-up B. **Symptomatic with pain:** 1. Radiation therapy (< 40 Gy) 2. Embolization 3. Vertebroplasty 4. *Surgery:* for progressive neurological deficit from mass effect or lesions failing to respond to other treatment (strongly consider preoperative embolization) • **Suspicious for metastasis:** CT-guided biopsy (beware of bleeding!)
Chondrosarcoma	**Age > 50 y**	• Usually in thoracic vertebral body • Punctate calcification	May arise from osteochondroma	1. If suspected, perform **initial needle biopsy** with a marked track to excise during definitive surgery 2. **En bloc surgical resection** is best treatment option 3. May add **high-dose radiation therapy**
a. Osteosarcoma (old) b. Ewing's sarcoma (young)	• **Age < 10 y:** Ewing's sarcoma • **20s** likely Ewing's sarcoma • **Age 40+:** osteosarcoma	• Usually in lumbosacral vertebral body • Lytic and sclerotic regions coexist within same lesion	**Risk factors for osteosarcoma:** • Previous radiation • Paget's disease	• **Treatment:** 1. neoadjuvant chemotherapy THEN 2. en bloc resection • **Prognosis** depends on degree of histologic necrosis after chemo. The more the necrosis, the better.

(Continued) ▶

Tumor	Presentation/ Demographics	Imaging/ Other diagnostics	Other	Treatment
a. **Multiple myeloma** (disseminated) b. **Plasmacytoma** (focal lesion)	• **Age:** > 40 • Spine is the most common location	1. **MRI:** • **T1:** hypointense to marrow and hyperintense to muscle • **T2:** hyperintense 2. **Urine:** Bence–Jones proteins 3. Serum and urine **protein electrophoresis** (SPEP/UPEP)		1. **Palliative radical excision.** May be curative in cases of plasmacytoma 2. **Chemotherapy** 3. **XRT** 4. **Bone marrow transplant**
Aneurysmal bone cyst	• **Age** < 20 y • **Osteolytic lesion** with highly vascularized cavities with connective tissue/trabeculae inside surrounded by cortical bone	• Mostly cephalad spine • **Expansile** osteolytic mass • Thin **sclerotic margins** • **MRI:** − no enhancement − characteristic **fluid-fluid levels**	• Occurs with **open growth plate** • **Risk factors:** − Previous fracture − Previous bone tumor	• **Treatment options:** 1. Embolization 2. Curettage + bone grafting 3. En bloc resection after injection with fibrosing agents • **Recurrence rate:** 20%
Giant cell tumor/ osteoblastoma	• **Age:** 30–40 y • Female > male • **Malignant transformation** (5–10%): male >> female • **Benign metastasis** to lung etc. is possible	• Thoracic > cervical > lumbar • Nonsclerotic margins • **MRI:** partial enhancement with *soap bubble appearance*	• Occurs only with **closed growth plate** • It's similar to aneurysmal bone cyst, but slightly more aggressive behavior	• **Treatment options:** 1. Embolization 2. Curettage + bone grafting 3. En bloc resection • **Recurrence rate:** 50%

(Continued) ▲

Tumor	Presentation / Demographics	Imaging / Other diagnostics	Other	Treatment
a. **Osteoid osteoma** b. **Benign osteoblastoma**	• **Age:** 20–30 y • Presenting as pain for months **alleviated by aspirin** **Osteoid osteoma** 1. < 1 cm 2. Rarely in spine 3. Confined in bone 4. Lumbar > cervical 5. No malignant transformation 6. *Common location:* lamina, facet 7. *X-ray:* well demarcated 8. *Macroscopic appearance:* hardened bone	• Sharply demarcated with sclerosis • **Bone scan:** increased uptake	Both are histologically **benign identical lesions** with different behaviors **Benign osteoblastoma** 1. > 1 cm 2. Often in spine 3. More extensive, into spinal canal 4. Lumbar and thoracic > cervical 5. Very rare transformation to sarcoma 6. *Common location:* pedicle 7. *X-ray:* expansive, invasive 8. *Macroscopic appearance:* hemorrhagic soft purple mass	• **Treatment options:** 1. Observation 2. Complete surgical resection • High cure rate
Langerhans cell histiocytosis A disease spectrum including: 1. *Eosinophilic granuloma:* single lesion 2. *Hand–Schüeller–Christian disease:* • Chronic form • Typically < 5 y old 3. *Abt–Letterer–Siwe disease:* • Rare • Fatal • < 3 y old 4. *Hashimoto–Pritzker disease* • Rare • Self-limiting variant seen at birth	Painful osteolytic lesion in young person or child	• Lytic lesion without sclerosis • Punched out lesion with central density • **Single collapsed vertebral bone** (vertebra plana) in young person		a. Observation or b. **Intralesional injection of corticosteroids**

Tumor	Presentation/ Demographics	Imaging/ Other diagnostics	Other	Treatment
Osteochondroma	• **Age > 30 y** • 10% of primary bone tumors • 5% located in spine	• Exclusively posterior spine (typically cervical spinous process) • Often pedunculated appearance	**Arises from epiphyseal growth cartilage**	1. Observation 2. **Surgical resection**
Chordoma	Middle-aged patients	1. **CT:** lytic, destructive lesion with intratumoral calcifications 2. **MRI:** • Heterogeneous enhancement • Honeycomb appearance	**Arises in midline of spinal column from clivus to coccyx:** a. **Early middle age:** usually clivus b. **Older middle age:** usually sacrum	1. **Surgical resection** is primary treatment 2. **XRT/radiosurgery along with surgery for recurrences** • Very poor prognosis
II. Intradural extramedullary (40% of spine tumors)				
Meningioma	• **Age:** > 40 y • **Female: male = 9:1** • Commonly associated with neurofibromatosis type 2 (NF2)	• Most common: thoracic spine (80%) • **MRI:** − Extramedullary/intradural − Moderate homogeneous **enhancement with dural attachment tail**		**Complete surgical resection** including dura if possible **Prognosis:** very good; < 10% recurrence
Neurofibroma	Usually arises from **motor nerves** a. **Single localized neurofibroma:** usually sporadic b. **Plexiform neurofibroma:** usually NF1	1. **CT and X-ray:** • Bone erosion • Enlarged neural foramen 2. **MRI:** dense enhancement	1. Fusiform 2. Nonencapsulated 3. Diffuse 4. Cannot be dissected from parent nerve	**Surgical resection:** parent nerve usually embedded within tumor
Schwannoma	Usually arises from **sensory nerves**		1. Lobulated 2. Encapsulated 3. Well-circumscribed 4. Eccentric from parent nerve	**Surgical resection:** parent nerve fibers usually splayed around periphery of tumor

Tumor	Presentation/ Demographics	Imaging/ Other diagnostics	Other	Treatment
Dermoid	• Uncommon • Usually presents in patients younger than 1 y of age	**MRI:** usually resembles fat and CSF	**May be related to** previous myelomeningocele repair	**Surgery** for symptomatic lesion including those: a. with compressive symptoms or b. those causing aseptic meningitis
Epidermoid	• Uncommon • Usually presents in childhood • Female > male • Conus > rest of the cord	**MRI:** iso- or hyperintense compared to CSF on all sequences	a. **Congenital:** associated with spinal dysraphism b. **Acquired:** may be a late complication of lumbar puncture (1–20 y after)	**Surgery** for symptomatic lesion including those: a. with compressive symptoms or b. causing aseptic meningitis
Hemangioblastoma	• Uncommon • **Age 20–40 y** • **Presenting** usually with sensory changes or impaired proprioception • 1/3 associated with **von Hippel–Lindau disease**	**MRI:** • Diffuse cord expansion • Enhancing *nodule with extensive cyst* • Usually well demarcated • Very vascular		1. Perform **spinal angiography:** densely enhancing with draining vein 2. Consider **pre-op embolization.** 3. **Microsurgical resection** similar to arteriovenous malformation. **Prognosis:** excellent

Lymphoma	• Uncommon
	• **Age > 50 y**
	• **Associated with** immune compromised state:
	  – HIV
	  – Transplant, etc.
		MRI:
		• *T1:* hypointense
		• *T2:* hyperintense
		• Homogeneous enhancement
			Most common secondary to non-Hodgkin's lymphoma	**Radiotherapy plus steroids**
				
				Prognosis: poor

(Continued) ▲

Intramedullary (10% of spine tumors)

- **Common symptoms:**
  1. Weakness
  2. Loss of sensory faculties
  3. Possible bowel or bladder dysfunction
  4. Lhermitte's sign
- **Treatment guidelines:**
  1. **Asymptomatic lesions:** observation with close follow-up and repeat MRIs.
  2. **Symptomatic lesions + age > 65 y:** steroids ± XRT ± chemotherapy (biopsy if necessary)
  3. **Symptomatic lesions + age < 65 y:** surgery.
     Always start with biopsy and intra-op frozen section. Tailor further treatment based on frozen biopsy:
     a. *Circumscribed tumors such as ependymoma, hemangioblastoma, etc.:* attempt complete resection (followed by XRT if necessary)
     b. *Diffuse tumors such as astrocytoma:* stop at biopsy → then ± XRT ± chemotherapy

Tumor	Presentation/ Demographics	Imaging/ Other diagnostics	Other	Treatment

Astrocytoma	• Male > female
	• Children and young adults
		MRI
		• Cord expansion
		• Patchy enhancement
		• Usually eccentric in spinal cord
			• Most common intramedullary tumor in children and outside filum in adults
			• Thoracic > cervical cord
				A. Asymptomatic: observation
				B. Symptomatic:
				  1. Biopsy and duraplasty
				  2. XRT + chemotherapy
				
				Prognosis: poor

Ependymoma	• Male > female
	• Most common intramedullary tumor in adults
		MRI
		• Intense enhancement
		• Usually centrally located in spinal cord
		• Can be associated with cysts and hemorrhage
			• Most common intramedullary tumor at lower cord, conus, filum (typically myxopapillary type)
			• Cervical > thoracic Cord
			• Majority are:
			  – Low grade
			  – Slow growing
			  – Usually not highly vascularized
				1. **Surgically curable** disease with good plane between tumor and neural tissue (especially myxopapillary)
				2. **If subtotal resection:** XRT + chemotherapy
				
				Prognosis: good

2.11 Cases

2.11.1 Cervical Spine Fracture with Perched Facet

Chief complaint/History of present illness
- A 22 y/o woman presents to the ER following a rollover motor vehicle accident (MVA) with severe neck pain and weakness in her left upper extremity.

Physical examination
- Severe weakness in arm abduction at the shoulder (3/5).
- Hypesthesia of her shoulder region.

1. **Describe the C-spine computed tomography (CT) scans of the patient.**
   (See Table 2.2a: Cervical subluxation, locked or jumped facet joints).

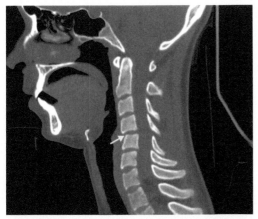

CT C-spine (midsagittal section) shows anterolisthesis of C4 over C5 (*arrow*).

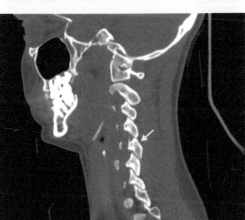

CT C-spine (sagittal section through facets) shows C4 facet dislocation over C5 (bowtie sign, *arrow*). See also the 3D reconstruction on next page.

Initial imaging

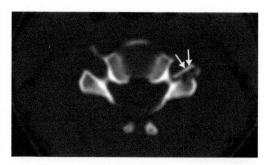

CT C-spine (axial section) shows "naked facet" sign bilaterally and fracture of the left transverse process (*arrows*).

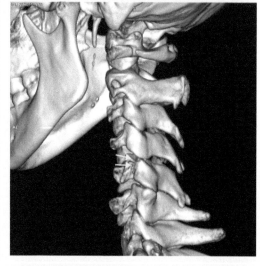

3D reconstruction of C-spine CT shows left C4 facet dislocation over C5 (*arrow*).

2. Would you like to obtain any further imaging studies?

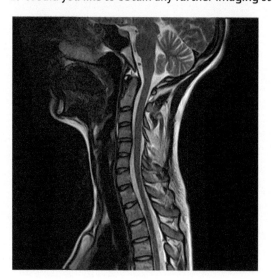

An MRI C-spine should be performed to rule out disc herniation. MRI C-spine showed no disc herniation and no spinal cord injury. (See Table 2.2a: Cervical subluxation, locked or jumped facet joints).

8. Postoperatively, the patient's arm abduction at the shoulder is found to be worse than preoperative and is now 2/5 strength. What is your plan?

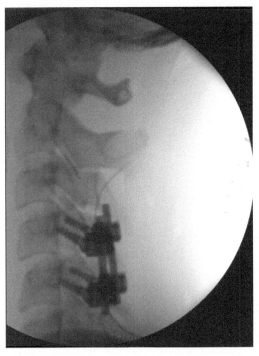

A postoperative X-ray of the cervical spine should be obtained to rule out misplacement of screws. The X-ray shows no screw misplacement (see the image on the left). A steroid taper should be considered, since deterioration is most likely secondary to C5 root irritation.a

9. Over the next few days the patient's deltoid weakness improves to 5–/5 strength and she is discharged. Two weeks later (3 weeks after surgery) the patient returns to your office with 3 days of sudden-onset severe pain in the contralateral shoulder and upper chest wall region radiating to her neck and scapula. The pain is relieved by adduction of the arm and flexing of the forearm. The patient also complains of progressive weakness of the upper extremity that presented 1 day after the onset of acute pain.

Physical examination	• Deltoid, supraspinatus, and infraspinatus strength 3+/5 biceps strength of 4/5. • Reflexes are diminished in left upper extremity.
Imaging studies	• Imaging studies of the cervical spine show excellent reduction of the previous anterolisthesis with no evidence of nerve root compression. • MRI of the shoulder: Within normal limits.

What's your plan?
The progression of symptoms (acute pain followed by weakness of proximal muscles of upper extremity without sensory deficit) and the clinical findings should raise the suspicion of Parsonage-Turner syndrome (PTS). Imaging of C-spine should be performed to rule out disc herniation or misplacement of screws. MRI of shoulder should also be obtained to rule out shoulder pathology. Finally, EMG/NCV studies of upper extremities will help solidify diagnosis. PTS is a self-limited disease treated with pain medications in the early stage (pain) followed by physiotherapy to improve muscle weakness. (See Table 1.4i).

3. **What is your diagnosis and treatment plan?**

The C-spine CT shows anterior C4 facet dislocation over C5 (perched facet). Since patient has neurological deficit (deltoid weakness) and MRI showed no disc herniation/injury a closed reduction with traction should be attempted followed by surgical stabilization. In this case the patient underwent posterior instrumented fusion. (See Table 2.2a: Cervical subluxation, locked or jumped facet joints, and Table 2.2c).

4. **What are the surgical approaches depending on presence of neurological deficits?**

   - Patient with neurological deficit: Closed reduction with traction + surgical stabilization (anterior/posterior/both).
   - Patient without neurological deficit: Open reduction (facet removal) + posterior instrumented fusion. (See Table 2.2a: Cervical subluxation, locked or jumped facet joints, and Table 2.2c).

5. **Describe the technique for C3-C7 lateral mass screw placement (entry point, trajectory, depth).** (See Table 2.10: C3-C7 lateral mass screw).

6. **How would your surgical plan be different, if the patient had an occluded vertebral artery?**

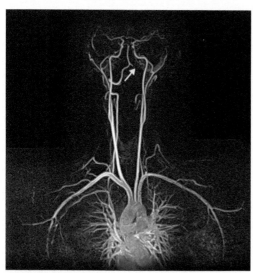

In a patient with an occluded vertebral artery, we should avoid putting in danger the contralateral patent vertebral artery. Thus, posterior decompression and reduction (by removal of the superior articulating facet of the inferior vertebra) should be followed by:

   - Anterior cervical discectomy and fusion (ACDF) or
   - Unilateral lateral mass screw placement ipsilaterally to the occluded vertebral artery plus subliminal or interspinous wires.

Some days after surgery patient should be treated with antiplatelet therapy for the occluded vertebral artery for around 3 months and then a repeat computed tomography angiogram (CTA) should be performed. (See Table 5.21b).

Magnetic resonance angiogram (MRA) of neck and head reveals occlusion of the left vertebral artery (*arrow*)

7. **Following the removal of the superior articulating facet of C5 and open reduction of the unilateral perched facet you have placed the C4 lateral mass screw successfully and are drilling the ipsilateral lateral mass of C5 to place screw at that level. You encounter severe hemorrhage of bright red blood. What is your diagnosis and treatment plan?**
   Vertebral artery injury. (See Table 11.2b).

2.11.2 Lumbar Disc Herniation with Cauda Equina Syndrome

1. Describe the lumbar spine MRI of the patient.

Chief complaint/History of present illness
- A 36 y/o construction worker is brought to the ER by his family because of severe low back and leg pain.

Physical examination
- Diffuse lower extremity weakness with 4/5 strength.
- Saddle hypesthesia.
- Normal anal sphincter tone.

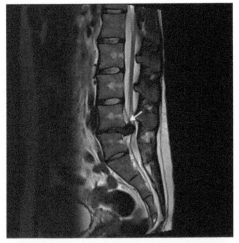

MRI L-spine (T2-weighted image, sagittal) shows very large disc herniation compressing the cauda equina (*arrow*).

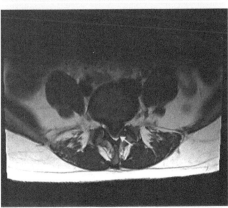

MRI L-spine (T2-weighted image, axial) shows very large disc herniation totally occluding the spinal canal compressing the cauda equina (*arrow*).

2. What are your concerns and how would you evaluate the patient's urinary function?

Patient may have developed cauda equina syndrome. His urinary function should be evaluated by measuring his postvoid residual urine volume. The patient is asked to empty his/her bladder completely. Then the residual urine volume can be measured either by ultrasound of the urinary bladder or by placing a Foley catheter to drain the remaining urine and measure the volume. (See Table 2.9: Cauda equina syndrome).

3. What is your plan?

Patient should undergo surgical decompression as soon as possible. (See Table 2.9: Cauda equina syndrome).

4. The patient is very concerned that he cannot feel his genital area. He wants to know if this will improve. Describe prognostic factors related to cauda equina syndrome.

Good prognostic factors for improvement are

- Surgery within 48 hours of symptom onset.
- Initial presentation without urinary retention (only motor, sensory, and saddle hypesthesia). (See Table 2.9: Cauda equina syndrome).

5. During surgery, you cannot find the large disc fragment. What is your plan?

- Confirm the correct level with X-ray (use pedicle as anatomic point for localization of disk fragment on imaging and for intra-op identification).
- Look for disc fragment in the axilla between the nerve root and the dural sac.
- Consider intradural fragment.

6. While you are performing your discectomy, the anesthesiologist reports that the patient has suddenly become hypotensive and tachycardic. What is your plan?

Retroperitoneal vessel injury should be ruled out. (See Table 11.2a).

7. The patient returns to your office 2 weeks after surgery for suture removal. There is a large palpable fluid-filled subcutaneous pocket with no drainage from the wound. Sterile aspiration with a 25-gauge needle reveals clear fluid. What is your plan?

Cerebrospinal fluid (CSF) leak is suspected. Since CSF is not leaking through the skin and if patient has no other complaints apply pressure corset for 3 months. (See Table 11.2f).

2.11.3 Cervical Spondylotic Myelopathy—Central Cord Syndrome

Chief complaint/History of present illness	• A 57 y/o woman presents with a 1-year history of gait unsteadiness, which has worsened over the past 3 months. Furthermore, she reports tingling in both her hands and clumsiness and she admits dropping objects more often lately.
Physical examination	• Spastic ataxic gait. • Normal strength in arms and legs but decreased fine motor control. • Sensation impaired in both hands, normal sensation in legs. • Symmetrically increased reflexes 3+ in both arms and 4+ in both legs with clonus. • Hoffman's sign positive bilaterally. • Babinski's sign positive bilaterally.

1. Describe the MRI films below.

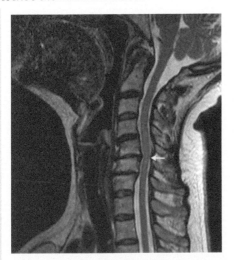

MRI cervical spine (T2, midsagittal section) shows C5-C6 stenosis with spinal cord compression with high cord signal at the level of stenosis (*arrow*). There is also a kyphotic deformity at the same level.

Imaging

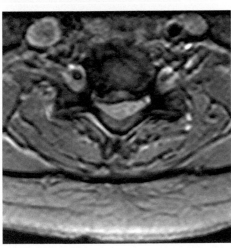

MRI cervical spine (T2, axial section at the level of C5-C6 disk space) shows disc or osteophyte especially to the right side with severe spinal cord compression.

2. What is the most likely diagnosis?
The most probable diagnosis is cervical spondylotic myelopathy based on the clinical presentation of the MRI of the cervical spine.

3. **What further studies should be performed and why?**
   - A CT scan of the cervical spine should be performed to look for ossified posterior longitudinal ligament, a calcified disc, and osteophytes (see image).
   - Plain X-rays of the cervical spine with flexion and extension films should be performed to rule out segmental instability. The X-rays did not reveal instability.

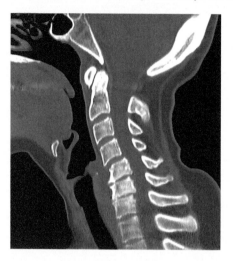 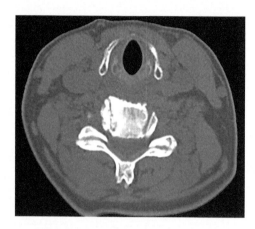

CT of the cervical spine (sagittal, axial) revealed no calcified ligaments or discs and no osteophytes.

4. **What is the treatment of cervical spondylotic myelopathy? What would you recommend to this patient and why?**

The treatment of cervical spondylotic myelopathy is surgery. The clinical presentation of the patient is consistent with cervical myelopathy attributable to spinal cord compression at the C5-C6 level. We should recommend the patient to undergo surgical decompression because the natural history of cervical myelopathy is progressive stepwise or gradual neurological deterioration. (See Table 2.6: Cervical myelopathy).

5. **What is the main objective of the surgical decompression? What are the predictors of poor prognosis?**

The main objective of surgical decompression is to arrest the progression of myelopathy. (See Table 2.6: Cervical myelopathy).

6. **What are the approaches for surgical decompression for cervical myelopathy?**
   - Anterior decompression (discectomy/corpectomy) and stabilization.
   - Posterior decompression (laminectomy) ± instrumented fusion.
     (See Table 2.6: Cervical myelopathy).

7. **Patient was scheduled for surgical decompression. Unluckily 1 week before the planned surgery she had a fall, which resulted in landing on her forehead and hyperextending her neck. After the fall the patient presented to ER complaining mainly about weakness of her upper extremities. She mentioned that she also felt her legs weak, but not as much as the arms. She denied bladder/bowel issues. Emergent CT and MRI of the cervical spine revealed no changes compared to the previous ones (see Section 2.3.3: Cervical Spondylotic Myelopathy—Central Cord Syndrome). Flexion/extension X-ray films of the cervical spine revealed no instability. The upper extremity weakness remained stable. What is this typical clinical presentation called?**

Central cord syndrome (motor deficit of extremities, upper extremities more affected). It's usually seen in patients with preexisting canal stenosis after a hyperextension cervical spine injury. (See Table 2.6: Central cord syndrome).

8. Would you offer surgical decompression to this patient and when? What are the general recommendations for timing of surgical decompression in central cord syndrome?
There is no instability as confirmed by the flexion/extension films. Patient is not deteriorating. We should recommend an elective surgery. (See Table 2.6: Central cord syndrome).

9. What approach for surgical decompression would you suggest and why?
There is only one level stenosis with anterior compression due to disc herniation. Furthermore, there is kyphotic deformity. Calcified disk and calcified posterior longitudinal ligament have been ruled out. Thus, an ACDF is the best option.

10. Describe the key procedural steps of an ACDF.
   (See Table10.11b).

11. During surgery you are informed about changes in neuromonitoring. What is your treatment plan?
   (See Table 11.2g).

12. Four days after surgery the patient complains about swallowing difficulty, which is getting worse. What urgent condition should you rule out and what further studies should be performed?

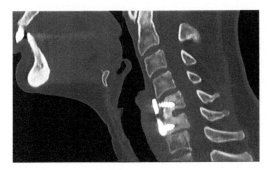

Hematoma should be ruled out. CT scan of the neck should be obtained. Urgent CT of cervical spine (see the image on the left) showed no hematoma. Furthermore, the alignment and the placement of the graft and instrumentation are good.
Typically, dysphagia is transient. (See Table 10.11d and Table 11.2e). In the presence of fever, esophageal injury should also be ruled out.

2.11.4 Spinal Epidural Abscess

Chief complaint/History of present illness	• A 75 y/o woman presents with 1-week history of back pain and progressive lower extremity weakness. She also reports several falls lately. She has not been able to walk for the past 24 hours. • Previous medical history is unremarkable.
Physical examination	• Temperature is 100.04 Fo (37.8 oC). • Patient not able to walk. • Lower extremity muscle strength: psoas, 3/5 bilaterally; rest of muscles, 2/5. • No bowel and bladder problems. • None of the lower extremity reflexes can be elicited. • Lower extremity hypesthesia below knees.

1. Describe the MRI of the patient.

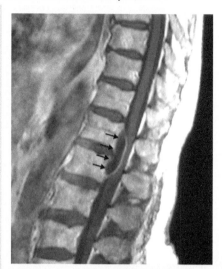

MRI thoracic—lumbar spine (enhanced T1-weighted image, sagittal) shows an extradural hypointense mass lesion (*arrows*) in the anterior epidural space extending from T12 to L1 vertebra with peripheral rim enhancement. There is marked compression of the spinal cord. Disk space and adjacent vertebrae look normal.

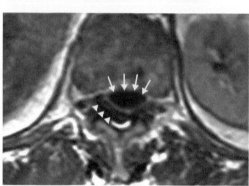

MRI thoracic—lumbar spine (enhanced T1-weighted image, axial) shows an extradural hypointense mass lesion (*arrows*) in the anterior epidural space with peripheral rim enhancement. There is marked compression of the spinal cord (*arrowheads*).

2. What is the differential diagnosis based on the MRI? What is the most likely diagnosis?
   - Differential diagnosis: Abscess, hematoma, metastasis/tumor, disc fragment.
   - Most likely diagnosis is epidural abscess.

3. What are the risk factors for spinal epidural abscesses? What are the most common causative pathogens?
   (See Table 2.8: Spinal epidural abscess).

4. What is the diagnostic workup for a spinal epidural abscess?
   - Laboratory tests (C-reactive protein [CRP], erythrocyte sedimentation rate [ESR], complete blood count [CBC] with differential).
   - Cultures (blood, urine).
   - MRI and CT of spine.
   - CT abdomen, pelvis

Imaging

5. What are the indications of nonsurgical treatment?

Indications of nonsurgical treatment are small abscess, no neurological symptoms, known causative pathogen, significant medical comorbidities. (See Table 2.8: Spinal epidural abscess).

6. How would you manage this patient and why? What are the goals of the surgery?

Patient should undergo abscess drainage and decompression of spinal cord due to significant size of abscess with marked spinal cord compression, causing rapid neurologic deterioration of 24 hours duration.

The main objective of the surgery is to decompress the spinal cord. Secondary goals are isolation of causative pathogen and stabilization (if required).

7. What are the treatment steps after abscess drainage? What is the duration of antibiotic therapy for spinal epidural abscess?

Intravenous (IV) antibiotics for 6 weeks followed by 6 weeks of oral (p.o.) antibiotics.

8. What is the management of a postoperative spinal infection?

(See Table 11.3c: Treatment of spinal infection).

Suggested Readings

Anderson DG, Vaccaro A. Decision-Making in Spinal Care. 2nd ed. New York, NY: Thieme; 2013

Bartanusz V, Harris J, Moldavsky M, Cai Y, Bucklen B. Short segment spinal instrumentation with index vertebra pedicle screw placement for pathologies involving the anterior and middle vertebral column is as effective as long segment stabilization with cage reconstruction: a biomechanical study. Spine 2015;40(22):1729–1736

Fehlings MG, Arvin B. Surgical management of cervical degenerative disease: the evidence relate to indications, impact, and outcome. J Neurosurg Spine 2009;11(2):97–100

Fehlings MG, Tetreault LA, Wilson JR, et al. A clinical practice guideline for the management of patients with acute spinal cord injury and central cord syndrome: recommendations on the timing (≤ 24 hours versus > 24 hours) of decompressive surgery. Global Spine J 2017;7(3, Suppl): 195S–202S

Gibbons KJ, Soloniuk DS, Razack N. Neurological injury and patterns of sacral fractures. J Neurosurg 1990;72(6):889–893

Hadley MN, Walters BC. Introduction to the guidelines for the management of acute cervical spine and spinal cord injuries. Neurosurgery 2013;72(Suppl 2):5–16

Kivioja J, Jensen I, Lindgren U. Neither the WAD-classification nor the Quebec Task Force follow-up regimen seems to be important for the outcome after a whiplash injury. A prospective study on 186 consecutive patients. Eur Spine J 2008;17(7):930–935

Lee JY, Vaccaro AR, Lim MR, et al. Thoracolumbar injury classification and severity score: a new paradigm for the treatment of thoracolumbar spine trauma. J Orthop Sci 2005;10(6):671–675

Lewkonia P, Paolucci EO, Thomas K. Reliability of the thoracolumbar injury classification and severity score and comparison with the denis classification for injury to the thoracic and lumbar spine. Spine 2012;37(26):2161–2167

Pekmezci M, Herfat S, Theologis AA, et al. Integrity of damage control posterior spinal fusion constructs for patients with polytrauma: a biomechanical investigation. Spine 2015;40(23): E1219–E1225

Pope MH, Panjabi M. Biomechanical definitions of spinal instability. Spine 1985;10(3):255–256

Radanov BP, Sturzenegger M, Di Stefano G. Long-term outcome after whiplash injury. A 2-year follow-up considering features of injury mechanism and somatic, radiologic, and psychosocial findings. Medicine (Baltimore) 1995;74(5):281–297

Samartzis D, Gillis CC, Shih P, O'Toole JE, Fessler RG. Intramedullary spinal cord tumors: part I—epidemiology, pathophysiology, and diagnosis. Global Spine J 2015a;5(5):425–435

Samartzis D, Gillis CC, Shih P, O'Toole JE, Fessler RG. Intramedullary spinal cord tumors: part i-epidemiology, pathophysiology, and diagnosis. Global Spine J 2015b;5(5):425–435

Savage JW, Moore TA, Arnold PM, et al. The reliability and validity of the thoracolumbar injury classification system in pediatric spine trauma. Spine 2015;40(18):E1014–E1018

Spitzer WO, Skovron ML, Salmi LR, et al. Scientific monograph of the Quebec Task Force on Whiplash-Associated Disorders: redefining "whiplash" and its management. Spine 1995; 20(8, Suppl):1S–73S

Vaccaro AR, Hulbert RJ, Patel AA, et al. Spine Trauma Study Group. The subaxial cervical spine injury classification system: a novel approach to recognize the importance of morphology, neurology, and integrity of the disco-ligamentous complex. Spine 2007;32(21):2365–2374

Vaccaro AR. Spine Surgery: Tricks of the Trade. 3rd ed. New York, NY: Thieme; 2016

3 Vascular Neurosurgery

3.1 Aneurysms

3.1.1 Nonruptured Aneurysms (Table 3.1a)   G

Risk factors for aneurysm formation	
History	• Previous subarachnoid hemorrhage (SAH) • Family history[a]
Habits	• Smoking[b, 1] • Ethanol • Cocaine
Associated pathology	• Hypertension • Endocarditis • Polycystic kidney[2] • Ehlers–Danlos • Marfan's • Moyamoya • Pseudoxanthoma elasticum • Aortic coarctation • Arterial venous malformation (AVM) • Fibromuscular dysplasia • Dissection with pseudoaneurysm • Vasculitis • Neurofibromatosis 1 (NF1) • Glucocorticoid remediable aldosteronism

[a]Two first- to third-degree relatives with intracranial aneurysms →8% risk of having unruptured aneurysm.
[b]Smoking is the most important modifiable risk factor.
Note: 5% of the population harbors an intracranial aneurysm

ISUIA (International Study of Unruptured Intracranial Aneurysms)[3]

ISUIA 1 (Retrospective) (Table 3.1b ◄)))   G

Yearly rupture risk for patients with unruptured intracranial aneurysms		
Aneurysms size (mm)	Risk of rupture / y	
	No previous bleed	Previous bleed
0–10	0.05%	0.5%
10–24	< 1%	< 1%
> 24	6%	

ISUIA 2 (Prospective)[4] (Table 3.1c) G

Five-year rupture risk for patients with unruptured intracranial aneurysms				
	Aneurysm size (mm)			
Location	<7	7–12	13–24	> 24
Cavernous ICA	0%	0%	3%	6.4%
Anterior circulation	0% (1.5% if previous bleed)	2.6%	14.5%	40%
Posterior circulation	2.5% (3.5% if previous bleed)	14.5%	18.4%	50%

90% develop in the anterior circulation	• Anterior communicating artery (ACom): 30% • Posterior communicating artery (PCom): 25% • Middle cerebral artery (MCA) bifurcation: 20% • Internal carotid artery (ICA) bifurcation: 8% • Other locations: 17%
Predictors for outcome	• **Age:** strong predictor of surgical outcome • **Size and location:** predict both surgical and endovascular outcomes

3.1.2 Ruptured Aneurysms: Spontaneous Subarachnoid Hemorrhage (Table 3.1d) G

Aneurysm size estimation on angiogram[5]

ICA diameter = 6 mm   MCA diameter = 4 mm

Note: Fifteen to 20% of SAH patients have negative angiograms → repeat angiogram reveals an abnormality in 1–2%. Eighty to 90% of spontaneous SAH is caused by rupture of cerebral aneurysm.

Imaging sensitivity	CTA	MRA
>5 mm aneurysm	95–100%	85–100%
<5 mm aneurysm	64–83%	56%

Note: SAH is visible on CT in 90% of patients within 24 hours and 60% of patients after 5 days, while xanthochromia may be present for up to 2 weeks BUT may not be present within first 2 hours.

Location of SAH depending on aneurysm[6] (Table 3.1e) G

Frequent aneurysms	Cistern
MCA	Sylvian
Ophthalmic	Carotid
PCom	Carotid
ACom	Lamina terminalis
Pericallosal	Callosal
Basilar apex	Interpeduncular
Posteroinferior cerebellar artery (PICA)	Lateral cerebellomedullary

SAH grades (Table 3.1f)   G

Grade	Hunt and Hess[7]		Mortality		World Federation of Neurological Surgeons (WFNS)[8]		
					Glasgow Coma Scale (GCS)	Major focal deficit (aphasia, hemiparesis)	Grade
1	Asymptomatic or mild headache	Slight nuchal rigidity	1%	5%	15	–	1
2	Severe headache	Cranial nerve (CN) deficit	5%	9%	13–14	–	2
3	Lethargy or	Mild focal deficit	19%	20%		+	3
4	Stupor	Dense deficit (hemiparesis)	40%	33%	7–12	±	4
5	Deep coma, moribund	Decerebrate rigidity	77%	77%	3–6	±	5

Note: Grade 0 in both classifications refers to intact aneurysm.
Hunt and Hess classification: Add 1 grade for serious systemic disease (e.g., hypertension, diabetes mellitus, chronic obstructive pulmonary disease) or severe vasospasm on arteriography.

Glasgow outcome scale[9] (Table 3.1g)   G

Score	Definition
5	Good recovery
4	Moderate disability (disabled but independent)
3	Severe disability (conscious but disabled/dependent)
2	Persistent vegetative state
1	Death

SAH Grades versus Glasgow outcome scale (Table 3.1h)   G

Hunt and Hess/WFNS	Glasgow outcome scale

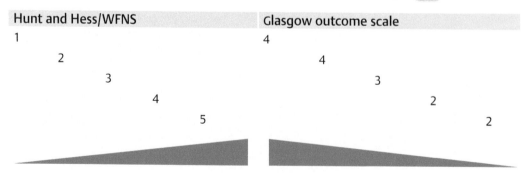

Rebleed rates (if not treated)[10] (Table 3.1i) G

0–24 h	4%
0–2 wk	20%
0–6 mo	50%
> 6 mo	3%

Note: Rebleed mortality is higher than 50%.

Basics for SAH[11] (Table 3.1j) G

ABCs	Airway—Breathing—Circulation
Lines	• Intubation • Central line • Arterial line • Ventriculostomy
Medication	• Phenytoin • Systolic blood pressure (SBP) control (nitroprusside sodium/not long acting) • Nimodipine (60 mg/4 h) • Gastrointestinal prophylaxis • Steroids for meningismus

Note: Xanthochromia 2 hours to 2 weeks after SAH.

3.1.3 Vascular Spasm

Vascular spasm prognosis (Fisher's grade)[12] (Table 3.1k) G

Grade	Blood on CT	Vasospasm risk (%)
1	No blood detected	21%
2	Diffuse or vertical layers < 1 mm thick	25%
3	Localized clot and/or vertical layer > 1 mm	37%
4	Intracerebral or intraventricular clot	31%

Note: Risk factors for clinical vasospasm also include smoking, low cardiac output, volume depletion, early spasm on angiogram, poor clinical grade, fever, hypertension, and sentinel bleed.
CT sensitivity for SAH ↓ at 24 hours.

Vascular spasm prognosis (Modified Fisher's grading)[13] (Table 3.1l) G

Grade	Blood on CT	Vasospasm risk (%)
1	Focal or diffuse *thin* SAH	24
2	Grade 1 + intraventricular hemorrhage (IVH)	33
3	Focal or diffuse *thick* SAH	33
4	Grade 3 + IVH	40

Vascular spasm estimation (TCD: Transcranial Doppler)[14] (Table 3.1m) G

Spasm	No	Mild/Moderate	Severe
Lindegaard's ratio (= velocity MCA:ICA)	<3	3–6	>6
Mean MCA velocity (cm/s)	<120	120–200	>200

Note: Lindegaard's ratio corrects the mean flow velocity for hyperemia (due to decreased blood viscosity from anemia, pressor use, increased cardiac output). TCD detectable changes in spasm may precede clinical symptoms by up to 24 to 48 hours.

Triple-H therapy (Table 3.1n) G

Consider ICP Monitoring + Baseline CT

Triple-H therapy	Targets	Medication
Hypervolemia	CVP: 10 cm H_2O P_{wedge}: 18 mm Hg	Crystalloids
Hemodilution	Hct:30%	
Hypertension	SBP: up to 220 mm Hg	Dobutamine (5µg/kg/min)

If no improvement after 60 min

add phenylephrine (2 µg/kg/min)

Note:
- Normal central venous pressure (CVP): 5 – 10 cm H_2O
- Normal pulmonary capillary wedge pressure (P_{wedge}): 6 – 12 mm Hg

3.1.4 Clipping versus Coiling $\boxed{G}$

ISAT (International Subarachnoid Aneurysm Trial)[15] (Table 3.1o)

Primary outcome	Modified Rankin scale 3–6 at 1 year (= death or dependence)

Dependent/Dead at 1 y	
Coiling	24%
Clipping	31%

Risk reduction with coiling		
Absolute	Total	7%
	Depending on age groups	<50 y: 3%
		>50 y: 10%
Relative	22%	

Treatment proposal	
Old patient + posterior circulation	Young patient + anterior circulation
↓	↓
coil	clip

Note: Coiling: lower risk of epilepsy versus higher risk of late rebleeding. Few basilar tip and middle cerebral aneurysms in study.

3.1.5 Aneurysm Surgery: General Recommendations

Aneurysm operative details/pearls[6,16,17] (Table 3.1p) $\boxed{G}$

Pre-op SAH grading: imaging/tests	• *If spasm on presentation:* coil or wait. • *Study angiogram:* for specifics and orientation of the aneurysm morphology. • *For very large aneurysms:* take into consideration mass effect, intramural calcification (perform CT to evaluate), intraluminal thrombosis, possibly trial balloon occlusion test (assess collateral flow).
Prerequisites for surgery	• Have emergency *suctions*. • Have *blood* available. • Have *etomidate* available. • Give *dexamethasone* (10 mg) and *mannitol* (1 g/kg).

(Continued) ▶

Operative technique	• Every artery has a safer surface to dissect.
	• Avoid retraction.
	• Ensure early *proximal control*.
	• *Clip first* (in case of multiple clipping) the deep, most inaccessible part of neck.
	• *When removing temporary clips*: remove distal clips first so as not to congest blood in aneurysm—open in situ first to see if it bleeds.
	• *At the end* always indocyanine green or Doppler.

Surgical options for fusiform aneurysms (Table 3.1q) G

1. Wrapping.

2. Clip reconstruction.

3. Trapping (± distal revascularization).

Attention to perforators!

Temporary clipping[18] (Table 3.1r ◀))) G

	Duration of temporary clipping	Further actions
Cooling to 35°C PLUS	<5 min	Nothing
	5–10 min	Etomidate: • Load (0.5 mg/kg) • Rebolus (0.1 mg/Kg)
	>10 min	• Etomidate protocol • Remove clip and reperfuse for 10 min • Consider circulatory arrest + deep hypothermia

Intraoperative rupture (Table 3.1s) G

• Large rescue suctions.

• Always have temporary clip preselected.

• Tell anesthesia.

• Tamponade (cottonoid—suction).

• Proximal control.

• Burst suppression (etomidate).

• Adenosine-induced circulatory arrest.[19]

Five to 10% of aneurysm cases.

Intraoperative papaverine for vessel in spasm (Table 3.1t) G

1. 30-mg papaverine in 9 mL of saline.
2. Dip cottonoid
3. Place cottonoid on spasm artery for 2 min.

Paine's point[20] (Table 3.1u) G

- From sphenoid ridge: 2.5 cm up + 2.5 cm anterior.
- 4.5-cm deep

3.1.6 Aneurysm Surgery: Details per Location

Proximal ICA (Paraclinoid[a]) aneurysms (Table 3.1v) G

Head position/craniotomy	Pterional craniotomy + aggressive drilling of sphenoid wing and orbital roof + possible drilling of anterior clinoid
Proximal control	a. Carotid in neck with pentothal-induced burst suppression: • Also permits retrograde suction–decompression of aneurysm + intra-opangiography • Expose cervical ICA in large and ruptured aneurysms <div align="center">OR</div>b. Balloon microcatheter endovascularly in cervical ICA: • Risk of thromboembolism and dissection
Distal control	ICA proximal to PCom
General surgical pearls	• *Retractor blade* on posterior aspect orbital cortex • *First cistern* to open is the carotid • *Clinoid*: semilunar flap → turned to protect ICA and aneurysm • *Dissect CN II* prior to clipping (march around)

Aneurysm-specific surgical pearls	• *Ophthalmic* (usually dome projects superiorly):
	   – Unroofing optic canal (early decompression of optic nerve)—medial clinoid—optic strut (last 5–7mm) → then open falciform ligament
	   – Protect the ophthalmic artery
	• **Superior hypophyseal** (usually dome projects inferomedially): more clinoid but no unroofing optic canal
	• **Lateral pointing:** aggressive removal clinoid

Notes:
- Attention to pneumatized clinoid or strut: possible delayed CSF fistula, infection.
- Intra-op digital subtraction angiography (DSA) is most useful.

[a]Paraclinoid: aneurysms at the origin of the ophthalmic artery, the origin of superior hypophyseal artery, the posterior carotid wall proximal to PCom (decreasing order of frequency).

PCom/anterior choroidal (Ach; supraclinoid) aneurysms (Table 3.1w) G

Head position/craniotomy	3. **Rotation:**
	  – 30 degrees (avoid having to pull temporal lobe)
	  – 45 degrees (if more exposure of posterior carotid cistern needed, such as in very large aneurysms)
	4. Neck hyperextension (maximizes frontal lobe displacement)
	5. Pterional craniotomy

Proximal control	• VERY PROXIMAL: falciform/carotid area (do it early in the subarachnoid exposure opening the proximal sylvian fissure) • Open the arachnoid binding the lateral aspect of optic nerve to the carotid artery • The removal of anterior clinoid is almost never necessary
Distal control	• PCom • Anterior cerebral artery (ACA) • MCA
General surgical pearls	• First step is to *identify the optic nerve* → then place frontal lobe retractor on the orbital cortex and progressively advance medially until over posterior aspect of gyrus rectus. • Do not pull temporal lobe • Most PCom aneurysms are treated by *clips applied* along the lateral aspect of carotid artery • *Find PCom* lateral and medial (Doppler it) → occlusion can lead to PCA infarct and anterior thalamoperforating lesion) • *Find and preserve ACh* (can be multiple or duplicated) → occlusion can lead to contralateral hemiparesis, hemisensory loss, hemianopsia • *Beware of CN III* when clipping (parasympathetic on surface)

Note: In patients presenting with CNIII palsies, there is no need to dissect the aneurysm sac from the nerve after clipping (the nerve will recover after evacuation of fundus).

ICA bifurcation aneurysms (Table 3.1x) G

Head position/craniotomy	Pterional craniotomy
Proximal control	• ICA (where depends on morphology → distal to ACh if possible)
Distal control	• A1 • MCA • PCom (depends on position of proximal control clip on ICA)

General surgical pearls	• *Begin* with superficial exposure of MCA bifurcation → continue with opening of horizontal segment lateral to medial following the inferior margin of M1
	• *Beware of perforators:* be careful of small perforating arteries on the posterior aspect of aneurysm
	• *Beware of where ACh* is (may hide under dome):
	  – Do not clip by mistake
	  – Always identify the ACh after the placement of clip
	• *Know what each A1 feeds and if Acom is patent* to know if you can sacrifice ipsilateral A1 with clip during rupture
	• Know the *proximity of lenticulostriate arteries to M1 origin*
	• *Clip* along axis M1

ACom aneurysms (Table 3.1y) G

Head position/craniotomy	• **Rotation**: 50 degrees (so you can see contralateral A1)
	• **Side:**
	  – For symmetric A1 → right-sided approach
	  – For asymmetric A1 → side of dominant A1
	• **Pterional craniotomy** (obtain good frontal exposure)
	• Consider **orbitozygomatic approach** for aneurysms pointing superiorly and posteriorly
	
	Regarding side, consider: hematoma, aneurysm from lateral aspect A1–A2 junction, multiple aneurysms, previous craniotomy

Proximal control	• Ipsilateral A1 + contralateral A1 • Place Gelfoam on contralateral A1 for easy identification during rupture
Distal control	• Ipsilateral A2 + contralateral A2 • *When removing clip:* REMOVE A2 BEFORE A1

(*Continued*) ▶

General surgical pearls	• *Find Heubner*: consider it the most medial of medial lenticulostri-ates—within 4 mm of ACom in 95% of patients
	• *Find A2* in interhemispheric fissure (have in mind orbitofrontal and frontopolar arteries)
	• *Know if A2 fills from both A1s* in case you must trap. Also evaluate preoperatively if there is a "third" A2.
	• Follow back side of A1 to A2 to avoid marching on dome.
	• *Gyrus rectus resection:* liberal (improves exposure of ipsilateral A2 and proximal neck—be careful to preserve the orbitofrontal and Heubner arteries)

Notes:
• The orientation of ACom varies from coronal to truly sagittal.
• Approaches: interhemispheric (difficulty in proximal control), subfrontal (careful with frontal sinus), transsylvian approach.
• Consider potential impact of the clip to the optic apparatus and contralateral A1.

MCA aneurysms (Table 3.1z ◀ᴺ)) G

Head position/craniotomy	• **Rotation:** 30 degrees (so that temporal lobe falls off)
	• Pterional craniotomy
Proximal control	M1
	• *Unruptur*ed aneurysms: distal to proximal opening of the sylvian fissure (follow initially the outer surface of superior trunk)
	• Ruptured *or proximal M1 aneurysms:* proximal to distal, beginning from ICA in carotid cistern (early proximal control requires retraction of frontal lobe)
Distal control	M2
General surgical pearls	• During pre-op planning, evaluate the potential need for revascularization preserving the parietal branch of *superficial temporal artery*
	• *MCA bifurcation* is in the most lateral aspect of the sphenoidal segment of sylvian fissure, 2 cm posterior to the anterior extent of the superior temporal gyrus
	• *For distal to proximal approach:* begin the dissection of the cortical fissure 3–4 cm posterior to the anterior limit of superior temporal gyrus
	• *For proximal to distal approach:* begin dissection of sphenoidal fissure, 2 cm medial to lateral edge of sphenoid ridge
	• Preserve all *perforating vessels of M1* (risk of capsular infarct). Also, be careful of *anterotemporal artery* (inferior surface M1)

Notes:
• The most common location is MCA bifurcation → the two M2s exit the bifurcation at 90 degrees from M1 and 180 degrees from each other.
• The arteries do not cross the sylvian fissure, so they can always be mobilized toward the frontal or temporal lobe versus sylvian veins, which are generally mobilized toward the temporal side.

Pericallosal aneurysms (Table 3.1aa)   G

Head position/craniotomy	• **Study Sagittal MRI:** define the relationship of aneurysm to corpus callosum • Unilateral interhemispheric approach anterior to coronal suture
Proximal control	• Can get there under aneurysm • Identify contralateral artery
Distal control	
General surgical pearls	• Make sure the *craniotomy* exposes at least part of the sagittal sinus • Avoid sacrificing veins draining into the sagittal sinus • *Do not pull on cingulate gyrus.* Avoid trauma to both cingulate gyri • *Lateral retraction* < 2.5 cm • May take some genu of the corpus callosum to get proximal

Notes:
• Pericallosal and callosomarginal send branches only to one hemisphere.
• The falx is thin anteriorly and widens posteriorly.

Basilar tip aneurysm (Table 3.1bb)

Head position/craniotomy	• **Rotation:** ~50 degrees rotation
	• **Neck:** Extend (maxillary eminence above orbital rim; balance between overlapping temporal lobe and overlapping ICA)
	• **Craniotomy:**
	  – Frontotemporal approach (usually right for right-handed parents) is a popular choice + performing additionally orbitozygomatic craniotomy is a possibility
	  – Subtemporal approach can also be used

Proximal control	Basilar below superior cerebellar artery (SCA)
Distal control	• PCom • P1 • SCAs
General surgical pearls	• Choose *left side* in case of ipsilateral oculomotor palsy, contralateral hemiparesis, coexistence of other aneurysms • Posterior clinoidectomy may be necessary • *Payne's point* → remove cerebrospinal fluid (CSF) • Use the *carotid–oculomotor triangle* • Resect *uncus* • *Temporary clip* lateral to oculomotor nerve • *May sacrifice PCom* (at P1–P2 junction). Use clips, not coagulation. Never sacrifice a fetal Pcom • Must see *perforators*

Notes: The most common in the posterior circulation. Ninety percent lie within 1 cm of dorsum sellae.

PICA aneurysms (Table 3.1cc)

Head position/craniotomy	• **Position:** three-fourths prone
	• **Rotation:**
	  – Neck flexed and rotated (45 degrees)
	  – Vertex inclined toward the floor (30 degrees)
	• **Skin incision:** "hockey sick"
	• **Craniotomy:**
	  – Suboccipital, far lateral approach
	  – Adequate exposure of craniocervical junction prior to dural opening (first suboccipital craniectomy → then C1 hemilaminectomy → finally resection of occipital condyle)

Proximal control	Vertebral proximal
Distal control	Vertebral distal (LOOK FOR IT MEDIALLY NOT CEPHALAD). Often difficult
General surgical pearls	POST-OP: assume lower CN issues: • Lateral: CN XI • Medial: CN XII • Superior: CN IX and X

Notes:
• Cervical PICA origins are not uncommon.
• Bypass options in case of vessel sacrifice include occipital–PICA or PICA–PICA bypass.
• Be careful of exposed mastoid air cells.

Vertebrobasilar (VB) junction aneurysms (Table 3.1dd)

Head position/craniotomy	• As in PICA • Lesion at the junction of proximal and middle thirds of clivus
Proximal control	Both vertebrals proximally
Distal control	**Basilar** • Expose between CNs VII/VIII and IX/X/XI • Complete or incomplete fenestration may be present
General surgical pearls	• Know *PCom circulation* so you can trap both vertebrals if necessary • Approach from side of lesion • There is no need to perform C1 hemilaminectomy

Note: The most technically demanding.

Anteroinferior cerebellar artery (AICA) aneurysms (Table 3.1ee)

Head position/craniotomy	• Far lateral suboccipital approach (with C1 hemilaminectomy) • Lesion at the junction of middle and inferior third of clivus
Proximal control	Basilar
Distal control	Basilar
General surgical pearls	• *AICA takeoff:* medial and superior to CN VI • *Place the instruments* between CNs IX to XI/VII and VIII/V

Notes:
• They are rare and usually treated endovascularly.
• The most common site for aneurysms of distal AICA is at the origin of the auditory artery.

3.1.7 Miscellaneous

Management of mycotic aneurysms[21] (Table 3.1ff) G

	Treatment
In general	1. **Antibiotics:** IV for 6 wk followed by p.o. for 6 wk 2. **Surgery or endovascular Tx:** consider if no response to medical treatment
Presentation with SAH	1. **Surgery:** if possible to sacrifice vessel or bypass 2. **Endovascular treatment[22,23]:** • Patient with high surgical risk • Candidate for cardiac surgery • Inaccessible/multiple intracranial aneurysms

Note: Follow-up for 1 year (may regrow!).

Treatment for IVH[24] (Table 3.1gg) G

• 1 mg (repeated every 8 hours) to 4 mg (repeated every 12 hours) intraventricular recombinant tissue plasminogen activator (rtPA)→ close ventriculostomy for 1 hour.

• Lower dose (3 mg/d) seems to have equal efficiency to higher dose.

Note: rtPA accelerates resolution of IVH with dose-dependent greatest effect in midline ventricles and least in postero-lateral ventricles[25]. Goal is to avoid communicating hydrocephalus.

3.2 Intracranial Hemorrhage

3.2.1 Spontaneous Intracerebral Hemorrhage (American Heart Association/American Stroke Association Guidelines 2015)[26] (Table 3.2a) G

Nonsurgical management	

Hemostasis	a. **Severe coagulation factor deficiency:** patients should receive appropriate factor replacement therapy
	b. **Severe thrombocytopenia:** patients should receive platelets
	c. ↑ **International normalized ratio (INR) due to Vitamin K antagonist:**
	  • Stop Vitamin K antagonist
	  • Replace Vitamin K–dependent factors → correct INR
	  • IV Vitamin K

Deep vein thrombosis (DVT) prophylaxis	Intermittent pneumatic compression from day of hospital admission
Blood pressure	For patients with SBP between 150 and 220 mm Hg without contraindication to acute ↓ blood pressure → ↓blood pressure to 140 mm Hg (can be effective for functional outcome improvement)
Seizure control	**Treat with antiseizure drugs:** • Patients with clinical seizures • Patients with mental state change + seizure findings on electroencephalogram (EEG)

Surgical management	

Supratentorial hemorrhage	• **Usefulness of surgery not well established:**
	
	  a. *STICH I:* no benefit of surgery over nonsurgical management regarding mortality or functional outcome (see Table 3.2b)[27]
	  d. *STICH II:* early surgery (hematoma evacuation and/or decompressive craniectomy) might provide small but clinically relevant survival advantage in conscious patients with lobar hemorrhages ≤1 cm from surface (see Table 3.2c)[28]
	  c. Consider hematoma evacuation as a **life-saving measure** in deteriorating patients

Infratentorial hemorrhage	• **Hematoma evacuation ASAP** for:
	  – Neurologically deteriorating patients
	  – Brainstem compression
	  – Hydrocephalus from ventricular obstruction
	  – ICH size ≥3–4 cm
	• Initial treatment of these patients with external ventricular drain (EVD) is not recommended

3.2.2 STICH trial (The International Surgical Trial in Intracerebral Hemorrhage)[27] (Table 3.2b)   G

Prospective study

Inclusion criteria	Spontaneous supratentorial ICH: • Arisen within 72 h • At least 2 cm on CT scan • GCS ≥ 5/15 • No obvious underlying cause

Conclusion: Treatment options depending on ICH depth from cortical surface	≤1 cm	Consider early surgery for patients with GCS ≥ 9/15 (noncomatose; median time from ICH onset to surgery in STICH: 30 h)
	>1 cm	Conservative medical treatment (may need surgery later)

Note: The STICH trial investigated the eventual benefit (death and disability after 6 months) from early surgical treatment. There was uniformly poor outcome in patients presenting in coma.

3.2.3 STICH II[28] (Table 3.2c)   G

Inclusion criteria	**Spontaneous superficial lobar hemorrhage:** • ICH within 1 cm from cortical surface • ICH volume 10–100 mL • Best GCS motor score ≥5–6 and eye score ≥2 → conscious • No IVH • No obvious underlying cause • Presentation within 48 h from ictus
Objective	To clarify if there is benefit from early (within 12 h) surgical treatment
Conclusion	*Possible* survival advantage (especially for those with GCS: 9–12/15)

3.3 Carotid Disease

3.3.1 Studies

Medical versus surgical treatment in symptomatic carotid stenosis (NASCET: North American SYMPTOMATIC Carotid Endarterectomy Trial)[29] (Table 3.3a) G

Carotid stenosis	Risk	
	At 2 y	At 5 y
>70%	• **Absolute risk reduction of ipsilateral stroke:** by 17%,[30] i.e., 26% stroke risk in medical patients versus only 9% stroke risk in surgical patients (26–9 = 17%) • **Relative risk reduction of ipsilateral stroke:** by 60%	Study interrupted because of evidence of treatment efficacy
50–69%		• **Absolute risk reduction of ipsilateral stroke:** by 6.5%, i.e., 22.2% stroke risk in medical patients versus 15.7% stroke risk in surgical patients (22.2–15.7 = 6.5%) • **Relative risk reduction of ipsilateral stroke:** by 30%
<50%	No benefit	No benefit

Notes:
* Study recommendation: do surgery before risk is 1%/waiting month.
* Study assumptions: estimated risk of disabling stroke or death associated with endarterectomy = 2%

Medical versus surgical treatment in asymptomatic carotid stenosis (ACAS/ACST: Asymptomatic Carotid Atherosclerosis Study/Asymptomatic Carotid Surgery Trial) (Table 3.3b) G

Carotid stenosis	Risk at 5 y
>60%	• **Absolute risk reduction of stroke or death:** by 6%, i.e., 11% stroke risk in medical patients versus 5% stroke risk in surgical patients[31] • Age < 75 y also benefits more from surgery[32]
<60%	No surgery

Note: Risk reduction applies if perioperative morbidity and mortality are less than 2%

CREST (Carotid Revascularization Endarterectomy versus Stenting Trial)[33] (Table 3.3c) [G]

Outcome at 30 d	Treatment		
	Stenting	Endarterectomy	
Stroke	4%	2%	overall equivalent risk rates
Myocardial equivalent	1%	2%	

Note: Individualized patient treatment based on pre-existing stroke and cardiac comorbidities, such as aortic arch/carotid artery tortuosity, vessel calcification, coronary artery disease, etc.

3.3.2 Treatment Options

Stenting (Table 3.3d) [G]

Indications for stenting

- Contralateral ICA occlusion
- "Hostile" neck:
    - For example, contralateral laryngeal nerve palsy.
    - Radiation therapy.
    - Previous carotid endarterectomy with recurrent stenosis.
- Tandem lesions
- Above C2.
- Medical comorbidity:
    - For example, congestive heart failure and/or severe left ventricular dysfunction.
    - Unstable angina.
    - Recent myocardial infarction.
    - Severe pulmonary disease.

Endarterectomy (Table 3.3e ◀)) [G]

Timing of carotid endarterectomy

Wake up post-op in PACU[a] with deficit	Immediate to OR
New deficit <2 h + loss of bruit	immediate to OR
New deficit <2 h + known stenosis >95%	immediate to OR
Crescendo symptoms	immediate to OR
Post-op deficit within hours/days	Immediate CT + CTA
Stroke >2 h	Wait 4 wk

[a]Postanesthesia care unit.

Key points for carotid endarterectomy: monitor/shunt/patch (Table 3.3f) G

1. Jugular is lateral and anterior to ICA	• **Planning the incision** beware of the following nerves coursing superiorly:
	  – Greatauricular nerve (possible paresthesia of ear)
	  – Marginal mandibular branch of facial nerve (possible drooping at corner of mouth and drooling)
	• **Incising the carotid sheath** beware of the vagus nerve located in most, but not all, patients in the posterior part (possible recurrent laryngeal nerve palsy with ipsilateral vocal cord paralysis)

2. Double ligate facial vein at level of bifurcation	
3. Work over omohyoid	**Section digastric** between mastoid and hyoid bone (posterior belly)
4. Find hypoglossal nerve and ansa	**Mobilize hypoglossal** after mobilizing ansa
5. Get distal and proximal to plaque	At time of **bifurcation exposure** → lidocaine to block sinus bradycardia
6. Shunt: • Sized to ICA • Heparinized saline • ICA first, then CCA	**Absolute indication** in case of pathologic EEG or other monitoring during the occlusion of carotid arteries (but first rule out anesthesia and increase SBP)
7. Before any clipping	5,000–10,000 IU IV heparin
8. Clamping • *Clamp on routine ICA:* ICA – CCA – ST – ECA • **Clamp on clot ICA:** NO ICA – CCA – ST – ECA • *Unclamp:* ECA – ST – CCA – ICA • *If after clamp still bleeding:* check ascending pharyngeal between ICA and ECA	
9. Track down intimal flaps	
10. Use patch graft to increase size of lumen	

Abbreviations: CCA, common carotid artery; ECA, external carotid artery; ICA, internal carotid artery; ST, superior thyroid.
Note: Also remember
• Possible glossopharyngeal nerve injury in high dissections of ICA (parallels the course of hypoglossal superiorly).
• Possible spinal accessory nerve injury by excessive lateral retraction.
Acetyl salicylic acid for 5 days pre-op. Hold for 24 hours post-op.

3.4 Stroke

3.4.1 Stroke Rate (Table 3.4a) G

First event	Elapsed time from first event		
	48 h	3 mo	2 y
After transient ischemic attack	5%	10%	40%
After amaurosis			20%

3.4.2 Stroke Syndromes (Table 3.4b) G

Artery	Territory	Symptoms
Anterior choroidal artery	• Visual apparatus + lateral geniculate nucleus	• Homonymous • Hemianopsia ⎤ ⎥ 3H's • Hemianesthesia ⎥ • Hemiparesis ⎦
	• Genu + posterior limb of internal capsule	
Heubner	• Caudate nucleus + putamen • Anterior limb of internal capsule	• Aphasia • Mild hemiparesis of face and arm

PICA
Five segments (first three must be preserved)
	• Wallenberg's syndrome (lateral part of medulla)	• Hiccups
		• Vomiting, vertigo, nystagmus (vestibular nuclei)
		  a. Ipsilateral:
		   – Horner's (descending sympathetic fibers)
		   – Dysphagia/hoarseness (nucleus ambiguous: CNs XI, X)
		   – Cerebellar signs (inferior cerebellar peduncle)
		   – Face Pain–temperature: (spinal trigeminal nucleus and tract)
		  b. Contralateral:
		   – Limbs and torso pain — temperature sensation (lateral spinothalamic tract)

BA bifurcation OR PCA (paramedian branches)	• Weber's syndrome (midbrain infarction)	• Ipsilateral CN III palsy • Contralateral hemiparesis

Abbreviations: BA, basilar artery; PCA, posterior cerebral artery.

3.4.3 Vertebral Insufficiency (5Ds) (Table 3.4c) $\boxed{\text{G}}$

1. Dizziness

2. Decreased vision

3. Diplopia

4. Dysarthria

5. Drop attack

3.4.4 Ischemic Stroke (American Heart Association/American Stroke Association Guidelines 2013 and Revision 2015, Adapted)[34,35] (Table 3.4d) $\boxed{\text{G}}$

Evaluation	a. NIH stroke scale (NIHSS; see Table 3.4i) b. Preferred modified NIH stroke scale (mNIHSS; see Table 3.4i)
Transport	Patients suspected to suffer from stroke should be transferred DIRECTLY to STROKE CENTER bypassing OTHER FACILITIES to minimize delay in treatment
Monitoring and ICU management	• Cardiac monitoring for ≥ 24 h • Supplemental O_2 for $SatO_2$ > 94% (NO supplemental O_2, unless patient is hypoxic) • Airway and ventilation support if needed • Treat hypovolemia with NaCl 0.9% • Treat cardiac arrhythmias • Antipyretic medication for temperature >38°C • Achieve normoglycemia (glucose 140–180 mg/dL)

iv rtPA (assure plasminogen activator) protocol (Table 3.4e)

Blood pressure (BP)	Eligibility for IV rtPA	• BP should be < 180/110 mm Hg, otherwise lower to and maintain < 180/110 mm Hg • Do not administer IV rtPA, if BP > 180/110 mm Hg
	BP after IV rtPA	• Maintain BP ≤ 180/105 mm Hg (close monitoring) • Treat if SBP > 180–230 mm Hg OR diastolic BP (DBP) > 105–120 mm Hg

iv rtPA protocol		1. **rtPA dose:** 0.9 mg/kg; administer 10% bolus over 1 min → 90% infusion over 60 min
		2. Admit to stroke unit
		3. **BP and neurological check:**
		  – Every 15 min during and after rtPA infusion for 2 h
		  – Every 30 min for 6 h
		  – Every hour until 24 h after rtPA
		• STAT noncontrast head CT and stop rtPA infusion IF:
		  – Patient develops severe headache
		  – Nausea or vomiting
		  – Worsening neurological examination
		• Delay placement of nasogastric (NG) tube, arterial line, or urinary catheter
		• CT or MRI at 24 h after rtPA before starting anticoagulants or antiplatelet therapy

Contraindications		• Improving symptoms • Heparin within previous 48 h • Gastrointestinal (GI)/genitourinary (GU) hemorrhage within past 21 d • Major surgery within past 14 d • ICH on CT/history of ICH • Stroke or serious head injury in the previous 3 mo • Arterial puncture at noncompressible site in the previous 7 d • Thrombin inhibitors or factor Xa inhibitors in the previous 2 d • Sustained SBP > 185 mm Hg • Sustained DPB > 110 mm Hg • Serum glucose < 50 mg/dL or > 400 mg/dL
Inclusion criteria for rtPA		• Age > 18 y • mNIHSS score ≥ 4 (measurable deficit)

Recommended treatment option depending on elapsed time from stroke (Table 3.4f) G

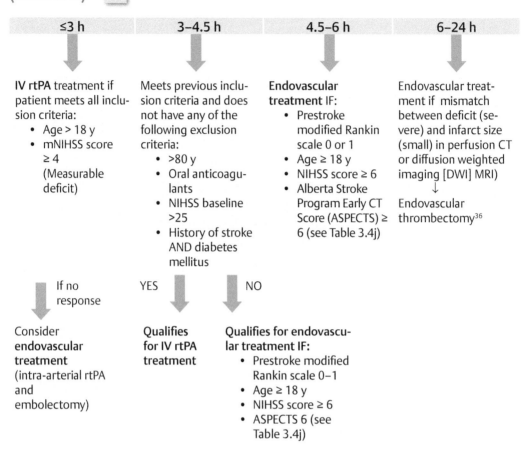

≤3 h	3–4.5 h	4.5–6 h	6–24 h

IV rtPA treatment if patient meets all inclusion criteria:
- Age > 18 y
- mNIHSS score ≥ 4 (Measurable deficit)

Meets previous inclusion criteria and does not have any of the following exclusion criteria:
- >80 y
- Oral anticoagulants
- NIHSS baseline >25
- History of stroke AND diabetes mellitus

Endovascular treatment IF:
- Prestroke modified Rankin scale 0 or 1
- Age ≥ 18 y
- NIHSS score ≥ 6
- Alberta Stroke Program Early CT Score (ASPECTS) ≥ 6 (see Table 3.4j)

Endovascular treatment if mismatch between deficit (severe) and infarct size (small) in perfusion CT or diffusion weighted imaging [DWI] MRI)
↓
Endovascular thrombectomy[36]

If no response

YES

NO

Consider **endovascular treatment** (intra-arterial rtPA and embolectomy)

Qualifies for IV rtPA treatment

Qualifies for endovascular treatment IF:
- Prestroke modified Rankin scale 0–1
- Age ≥ 18 y
- NIHSS score ≥ 6
- ASPECTS 6 (see Table 3.4j)

Other Treatments for Stroke (Table 3.4g)

Endovascular therapies (caution: intra-arterial rtPA is NOT Food and Drug Administration [FDA] approved)	Indications	• Symptom onset <6 h • MCA stroke • No contraindications to IV rtPA • Patients with large-artery occlusions who have failed to respond to iv rtPA
	Recommendations / guidelines	• Patients eligible for IV rtPA should receive iv rtPA even if intra-arterial treatments are considered • Stent retrievers are preferred over coil retrievers • Emergent extracranial carotid or vertebral angioplasty or stenting may be considered in dissection or cervical atherosclerosis
Anticoagulation and antithrombotic treatment	Not recommended for acute ischemic stroke	• Urgent anticoagulation for ischemic stroke including patients with ICA stenosis ipsilateral to ischemic stroke • Anticoagulation or aspirin <24 h after rtPA • Argatroban or other thrombin inhibitors • Clopidogrel • Tirofiban and eptifibatide
	Recommended	Aspirin 325 mg within 24–48 h after stroke onset
Volume expansion, induced hypertension	Not recommended	• Drug-induced hypertension • Albumin • Hemodilution by volume expansion • Vasodilatory agents (pentoxifylline)
	Use only in exceptional cases	Vasopressors only in exceptional cases for treatment of systemic hypotension producing neurological sequelae with close cardiac and neurological monitoring
Neuroprotective agents	Not recommended	• Induced hypothermia • Near-infrared laser therapy • Hyperbaric oxygen therapy EXCEPT for acute ischemic stroke from air embolism • Neuroprotective pharmacological agents
	Recommended	Continue statin therapy for patients already on statins

Surgical Therapies for Stroke (Table 3.4h)

Not recommended	Urgent or emergent carotid endarterectomy
Recommended	• Decompressive surgery for space-occupying cerebellar infarction • Decompressive surgery for malignant edema of cerebral hemisphere • EVD placement in patients with acute hydrocephalus secondary to ischemic stroke

Additional Care and Management (Table 3.4i)

Not recommended	• Nutritional supplements • Routine or prophylactic antibiotics • Routine placement of indwelling catheters
Recommended	• Comprehensive stroke care center including rehabilitation • Standardized stroke care order sets • Swallowing assessment before eating, drinking, or taking oral medications • Placement of nasal feeding tube or percutaneous endoscopic gastrostomy (PEG) for patients who cannot take solids or liquids • Early mobilization • Early intervention to prevent recurrent stroke • Aspirin for DVT prophylaxis if patient cannot receive anticoagulation • Antibiotics for suspected pneumonia or urinary tract infection

Patients Requiring ICU Care after Ischemic Stroke (Table 3.4j)

Indications	• Post-thrombolysis • Postinterventional treatment • Intracranial hematoma • Systemic hemorrhage • Craniotomy • Progressive neurological deterioration • Arterial dissections • Hypotension or need for iatrogenic hypertension • Cardiac complications

NIH Stroke Scale (NIHSS) and Modified NIH Stroke Scale (mNIHSS)[37] (Table 3.4i) G

Item		Score					
		0	1	2	3	4	unspecified
1a	level of consciousness (LOC)	alert	drowsy	obtunded	coma / unresponsive		
1b	LOC questions (month, age)	answers both	answers one correctly	answers neither			
1c	LOC commands (squeeze hands, blink eyes)	performs both tasks correctly	performs one task correctly	performs neither task			
2	gaze (extra-ocular movement)	normal	partial gaze palsy	total gaze palsy			
3	visual fields	no visual loss	partial hemianopia	complete hemianopia	bilateral hemianopia		
4	facial movement	normal	minor facial weakness	partial facial weakness	complete unilateral palsy		
5a	left arm motor 10 sec	no drift	drift before 10 seconds	falls before 10 seconds	no effort against gravity	no movement	amputation or joint fusion
5b	right arm motor 10 sec	no drift	drift before 10 seconds	falls before 10 seconds	no effort against gravity	no movement	amputation or joint fusion
6a	left leg motor 10 sec	no drift	drift before 5 seconds	falls before 5 seconds	no effort against gravity	no movement	amputation or joint fusion
6b	right leg motor 10 sec	no drift	drift before 5 seconds	falls before 5 seconds	no effort against gravity	no movement	amputation or joint fusion
7	limb ataxia (finger-nose, heel-shin)	absent	present in one limb	present in two limbs			amputation or joint fusion
8	sensory	normal	abnormal				
9	language (naming, reading or describing)	normal	mild aphasia	severe aphasia	mute or global aphasia		
10	dysarthria (eg. mama, tipp-top, thanks)	normal speech	mild to moderate, can be understood	severe, cannot be understood			intubated, other physical barrier
11	neglect	normal	mild	severe			

Notes: NIHSS max. score = 42, mNIHSS max. score = 31. The higher the score the more severe the stroke is.
In the mNIHSS 4 items of the original NIHSS were excluded (deleted with blue diagonal lines in the chart), thus increasing its inter-rater reliability.

ASPECT score[38] (Table 3.4j) G

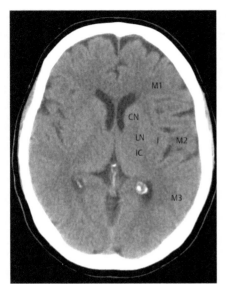

Location	Any evidence of early ischemic changes
Caudate (C)	−1
Insular ribbon (I)	−1
Internal capsule (IC)	−1
Lentiform nucleus (L)	−1
Anterior MCA cortex (M1)	−1

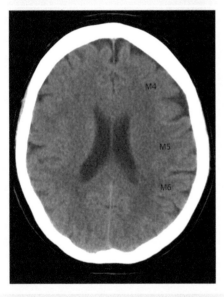

Location	Any evidence of early ischemic changes
MCA cortex lateral to the insular ribbon (M2)	−1
Posterior MCA cortex (M3)	−1
M4	−1
M5	−1
M6	−1

Notes:
- Middle cerebral artery (MCA) territory is divided into 10 regions of interest.
- The total initial score is 10 (= normal).
- The CT score identifies stroke patients unlikely to make an independent recovery despite thrombolytic therapy.

3.5 Moyamoya Disease

3.5.1 Moyamoya Disease (Table 3.5a)   G

Demographics	• More frequent among Japanese • Children and young adults
Presentation	• Pediatric patients present with ischemic stroke or TIA (80%) • Young adults present with hemorrhage (60%) • Headache • Seizures • Neurologic deficit and cognitive decline • Involvement of heart and kidneys is possible
Secondary moyamoya (moyamoyasyndrome)	• Thyrotoxicosis • Cerebral inflammation • Atherosclerosis • Down's syndrome, NF-1, Marfan's syndrome, Apert's syndrome
Imaging/other diagnostics	1. **DSA (or MRI–MRA with contrast)** — • Progressive (bilateral) stenosis of the distal carotids and stenosis of proximal ACA, MCA • Development of extensive compensatory collateral capillary network (looks like "puff of smoke") • Thickening of intima • No inflammation
	2. **MRI** — T1-weighted imaging (T1WI): multiple dot flow voids in basal ganglia (which enhance with contrast)
	3. **CT + contrast** — Multiple punctate dots in basal ganglia

3.5.2 Moyamoya Disease: Suzuki Stages in DSA (Table 3.5b)   G

Stage	DSA Findings
I	(Bilateral) stenosis of suprasellar ICA (bifurcation)
II	• Dilation of ACA, MCA, PCA • Collateral (moyamoya) vessels at brain base
III	Progression of ICA stenosis and moyamoya vessels
IV	• Progressive occlusion of circle of Willis and PCA • Reduction of moyamoya vessels • Presence of extracranial collaterals
V	Worsening of stage IV
VI	• No major cerebral arteries or moyamoya vessels • Extensive collaterals from ECA (external carotid artery)

3.5.3 Management of Moyamoya Disease (Table 3.5c) ⬚G

Medical (dubious effect)		• Antiplatelets • Vasodilators
	Indications	• Presence of mass effect (craniotomy to remove clot) • Suzuki stages II–IV • Patients with recurrent or progressive cerebral ischemic events and associated reduced cerebral perfusion reserve[39] in good neurological condition
	Revascularization	• Use external carotid circulation as donor supply to hypoperfused brain to prevent further ischemic injury[39] • DSA evaluates possible donor vessels and coexisting aneurysms
Surgical	Options	• **STA-MCA bypass (direct revascularization):** treatment of choice • **EDAMS (encephalo-duro-arterio-myosynagiosis):** anastomosis of temporalis muscle with blood supply to dura • **EMS (encephalo-myosynangiosis):** temporalis muscle with blood supply on brain • **EDAS (encephalo-duro-arterio-synangiosis):** STA and galeal cuff are sutured to a dural defect • Start aspirin on post-op day 1
	Timing for surgery	> 2 mo after the most recent symptomatic event
	Outcomes	• Surgery is more effective versus medical treatment[40,41] • There is effect on ischemia but not on the risk of hemorrhage • Relative risk reduction for cerebral infarction after direct revascularization: 70%[42]

3.6 Brain Arteriovenous Malformations

3.6.1 Spetzler–Martin Scale[43] (Table 3.6a) ⬚G

		Points
Size	>3 cm	1
	3–6 cm	2
	>6 cm	3
Location	Noneloquent	0
	Eloquent	1
Venous drainage pattern	Superficial	0
	Deep	1

3.6.2 AVM Rupture Rates (Table 3.6b)

Rapture rate per year	3–4%
Rapture Risk for first year posthemorrhage	Nonpregnant: 6% Pregnant: 26%
Mortality/y	1%
Mortality/bleed	10%
Morbidity/bleed	30%
Lifetime rupture risk (assuming 3%/y)	(105 – age)%

3.6.3 Multiple AVMs (Table 3.6c) G

1. **Wyburn - Mason syndrome** (AKA Bonnet – Dechaume – Blanc AKA retinoencephalofacial angiomatosis)
2. **Osler – Weber – Rendu syndrome** (AKA hereditary hemorrhagic telangiectasia): Epistaxis + vascular malformations (AVM/telangiectasia)

3.6.4 ARUBA Trial (A Randomized Trial of Unruptured Brain Arteriovenous Malformations)[44] (Table 3.6d) G

Objective	Investigated the risk of death and symptomatic stroke from unruptured brain arteriovenous malformation comparing two treatment modalities	
Groups	Interventional therapy group	**Medical management + prophylactic interventional therapy:** • Neurosurgery • Embolization • Stereotactic radiotherapy one of them OR combination
	Medical management group	Medical management alone
Included AVM characteristics	• Spetzler–Martin grade ≤ 4 • AVM diameter < 60 mm	
Findings	The randomization was interrupted (2013) due to superiority of the medical management group → outcome data for 223 patients (mean follow-up period: 33.3 mo)	
	Interventional therapy group	Medical management + prophylactic interventional therapy was associated with: • Higher number of strokes • Higher number of neurological deficits unrelated to stroke • Higher risk of death
	Medical management group	• Spontaneous rupture rate of 2.2%/y • Significantly lower risk of death or stroke

(Continued) ▶

Conclusion	Medical management alone is superior for prevention of death or stroke in patients with unruptured brain AVMs for a follow-up period of 33.3 mo
Criticism	For prophylactic interventional treatments, a mean follow-up period of 33.3 mo is:
	• Long enough for its complications to present
	• But not long enough for its eventual long-term benefits
	→ thus study continues its observational phase for at least 5 y

3.6.5 Treatment Based on Spetzler–Martin Scale (Table 3.6e) [G]

Scale	Treatment
1 + 2	Surgery
3	Either
4 + 5	Observation/γ knife

Note: Risk of rupture is increased, if (1) nidal aneurysm and (2) venous stenosis.

3.6.6 Timing for Other Treatment Modalities after AVM Embolization (Table 3.6f) [G]

a. **Surgery** → within days after embolization.

b. **Stereotactic radiosurgery** → wait 1 month after embolization

3.6.7 Surgery for AVMs

AVM principles (Table 3.6g) [G]

- In case of coexisting *aneurysm* → clip it first.
- Always obtain *post-op DSA* → take back to OR in case of residual.
- *Clip vein* prior to permanent sacrifice (to make sure no arteries, usually hidden under vein, remain).
- *Arterialized vein versus artery* → place temporary clip → observe distal color.
- *Pre-op propranolol*

Normal perfusion pressure breakthrough (Table 3.6h) [G]

- Treat like increased ICP including even barbiturates

3.7 Spinal Arteriovenous Malformations

3.7.1 Artery of Adamkiewicz (Arteria Radicularis Anterior Magna) (Table 3.7a) G

Level of origin	• T5–T8 (15%).
	• T9–L2 (85%) → T9–T12 (75%)
Side of origin	On the left (80%)

- "Hairpin turn" at its *anastomosis* with anterior spinal artery.
- Main *arterial supply* of spinal cord from T8 to conus.

3.7.2 Spinal AVMs (Table 3.7b) G

Type	Location	Treatment
Type I: dural AVM • IA: single arterial feeder • IB: ≥2 arterial feeders	Fistula at dura	1. Embolization OR 2. Surgery (proximal vein must be taken)
Type II: glomus	In spinal cord	1. Embolization (especially if single feeder) 2. Surgery (if ≥2 feeders)
Type III: juvenile	Everywhere (even invades vertebral body causing eventually scoliosis)	Natural history probably better than prognosis of any treatment
Type IV: pial (intradural perimedullary)	Fistula on pia	• Surgery (stop arteries) with exception of subtype III (embolization) • Feeders are too small for embolization

Note: Most common (80%) in adult is type I.

3.8 Dural Arteriovenous Fistula

3.8.1 Cranial Dural Arteriovenous Fistula (DAVF) (Table 3.8a) G

	Feeder	Treatment
Anterior	Ethmoidal	Open surgery
Transverse	• Tentorial • Occipital • Posterior auricular	Embolism ± surgery
Sagittal	Middle meningeal	Embolism ± surgery

Note: DAVF: external feeders versus AVM: internal feeders.

3.8.2 Borden's Classification[45] (Table 3.8b) G

Classification	Drainage
1	Into sinus only/or meningeal vein
2	Into sinus + leptomeningeal vein
3	Into only leptomeningeal vein

3.9 Carotid Cavernous Fistula

3.9.1 Carotid Cavernous Fistula (Table 3.9a) G

Usually involved venous structures	• Superior ophthalmic vein • Superior petrosal vein • Basilar plexus
Signs and symptoms	• Chemosis • Exophthalmos • Bruit • CN issues • Vision issues

3.9.2 Treatment of Carotid Cavernous Fistula (Table 3.9b) G

High flow (ICA straight to CS)	1. Transarterial balloon OR 2. Sacrifice ICA (if patient tolerates)

Low flow
  i. ICA branches
  ii. ECA branches
  iii. ICA + ECA branches
	1. Observe (50% spontaneously resolve) if:
	  • Normal CNs II, III, IV, VI +
	  • Eye pressure < 25 mm Hg
	    Otherwise
	2. Transvenous embolization

Abbreviations: CS, cavernous sinus; ECA, external carotid artery; ICA, internal carotid artery.

3.9.3 Workup for ICA Sacrifice (Table 3.9c) G

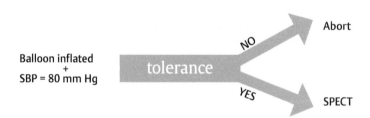

3.10 Sinus Thrombosis (Table 3.10a) ⓖ

Risk factors	• Pregnancy
	• Contraceptives
	• Dehydration
	• Hematologic disorders:
	   a. Proteins S, C deficiency
	   b. Antithrombin III deficiency
	   c. Factor V Leiden mutation

Treatment	1. Reverse underlying cause (hematologic workup) 2. Anticoagulation for 6 mo: heparin (not bolus) + coumadin 3. ± Transvenous thrombolysis

Note: Imaging findings: delta (CT noncontrast) versus empty delta (IV contrast CT).

3.11 Cerebral Arterial Dissection

3.11.1 Cerebral Arterial Dissection (Table 3.11a) ⓖ

Arteries	SAH	Ischemia due to:	Locations (where arteries are mobile)	Symptoms
Carotid artery	Possible	Occlusion + embolism	Pharyngeal portion of ICA	• Possible TIA, stroke • SAH • Ipsilateral (usually) headache • Carotidynia • Incomplete Horner (ptosis, miosis but no anhidrosis) • Bruits may be heard
Vertebral artery	If intradural	Occlusion + embolism (involvement of PICA will cause Wallenberg)	• C1–C2 junction • C6 (where it enters foramen transversarium) • Intracranial and dominant vertebral (when spontaneous)	• Possible TIA, stroke • SAH • Headache • Intradural: SAH • Extradural: 5Ds (see Table 3.4c)

Notes:
• Causes: (1) traumatic (much more common); (2) spontaneous (consider fibromuscular dysplasia, autoimmune diseases, Marfan's syndrome); and (3) iatrogenic.
• Angiogram: double lumen (pathognomonic)/string sign.
• MRI: crescent sign (bright signal in vessel wall on axial T2WI due to hematoma).

3.11.2 Treatment of Cerebral Arterial Dissection (Table 3.11b) $\boxed{G}$

Artery	Anticoagulation (for 3–6 mo)	Endovascular	Surgery
Carotid artery	a. **No bleeding risk** → heparin + coumadin b. **Bleeding risk** → acetylsalicylic acid/clopidogrel	Stent	Limited role
Vertebral artery	a. **No SAH** → as in carotid: anticoagulants b. **SAH** → stent OR sacrifice (remember PICA; no anticoagulants)		

Note:
- Indications for endovascular: (1) ineffective or contraindicated medical therapy and (2) symptomatic flow limiting stenosis.
- Acute ICA occlusion or acute dissection + cerebral vascular accident → give tPA because likely distal embolus is present (get CTA first).

3.12 Surgical Tips

3.12.1 Non Critical Sinuses (Table 3.12a) $\boxed{G}$

- Anterior one-third of superior sagittal sinus.
- Inferior sagittal sinus.
- Nondominant transverse and sigmoid sinus.

3.12.2 Eloquent Brain (Table 3.12b) $\boxed{G}$

- Speech, visual, sensory, motor.
- Deep structures: thalami, internal capsule.
- Brainstem.
- Cerebellar nuclei, peduncles.

3.13 Cases

3.13.1 Subarachnoid Hemorrhage with Aneurysm

Chief complaint/History of present illness	• A 43 y/o female presents to the ER with sudden onset of severe headache.
Physical examination	• Her neurological examination is significant for lethargy, nuchal rigidity with severe headache, and confusion.

Imaging

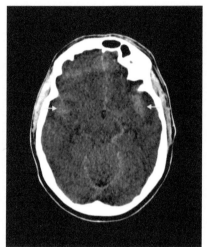

CT brain shows subarachnoid hemorrhage (SAH) in the interhemispheric fissure, in the Sylvian fissure bilat`erally (*arrows*), and in the basal cisterns.

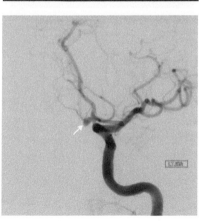

Digital subtractive angiography of brain shows an anterior communicating artery (ACom) aneurysm (*arrow*).

1. **What is your diagnosis?**
   Subarachnoid hemorrhage due to aneurysm rupture.

2. **What are the patient's Hunt and Hess and Fisher grades?**
   Patient presents with headache, nuchal rigidity, lethargy, and confusion without cranial nerve (CN) deficit, thus the Hunt and Hess grade is 3. The CT brain shows localized clot in bilateral Sylvian fissures, thus the Fisher grade is 3. (See Table 3.1f, Table 3.1k, and Table 3.1l).

3. **What is your initial management?**
   Patient should be assessed in ER in ABC (airways, breathing, and circulation) order and stabilized. The appropriate IV and arterial lines should be placed. Then the patient should undergo CT brain and CTA brain, which will allow diagnosis. The patient should then be admitted to intensive care unit (ICU). Planning of definitive treatment to secure the aneurysm should be made (either via craniotomy or via endovascular approach). Appropriate medications should be administered. (See Table 3.1j).

4. **Describe the operative treatment of an ACom aneurysm via craniotomy.**
   (See Table 3.1x, Table 10.1b, and Table 10.2b).

5. **As you are performing the final dissection around the aneurysm, an intraoperative rupture of the aneurysm dome occurs. What is your plan?**
   (See Table 3.1r).

6. **The patient has an uncomplicated postoperative course until day 8 when she starts to develop an acute hemiparesis and change in mental status. A CT brain is unremarkable with the exception of postoperative changes. What is your diagnostic and treatment plan?**
   Patient's neurological deficits are attributed to vascular spasm. Patient should undergo transcranial doppler which will reveal increased middle cerebral arterial (MCA) velocities with increased Lindegaard ratio indicative of vascular spasm. (See Table 3.1m). Triple H therapy should be considered (hypervolemia, hemodilution, hypertension). (See Table 3.1n).

7. **Following your treatment the patient has resolution of hemiparesis and returns to her baseline mental status. She again becomes more stuporous 3 days later. Her CT scan of the brain and TCDs are normal but her serum Na+ level is 124 mEq/mL. What is your diagnosis and treatment plan?**
   Patient's neurological deterioration is attributed to hyponatremia most commonly due to cerebral salt wasting. Hyponatremia should be corrected in ICU, but not too rapidly due to the risk of pontine myelinolysis. Normal saline should be administered. In severe cases hypertonic saline solutions may be required and the flow should be titrated based on serum sodium. Patient should be monitored closely in ICU. Avoid fluid restriction in SAH patients because it is related to vasospasm and brain ischemia. (See Table 5.28a).

3.13.2 Spontaneous Intracerebral Hemorrhage

Chief complaint/History of present illness	• A 40 y/o female patient presents with sudden onset of hemiparesis and hemihypesthesia on the left side that started 2 hours before being brought to the ER. • Relevant past medication history: Birth control pills.
Physical examination	• Her condition is stable except for hypertension with a blood pressure of 190/120. • Right-sided hemiparesis and hemihypesthesia.

Imaging

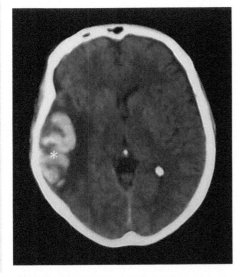

CT brain (axial section) shows intracerebral hemorrhage (*asterisk*) in the right temporoparietal area compressing the ipsilateral lateral ventricles without midline shift.

1. **What is your diagnosis and initial treatment plan?**

   Patient should be assessed in ER in ABC order and stabilized. The appropriate IV and arterial lines should be placed. CT revealed an intracranial hemorrhage in the right temporoparietal area. Patient should be admitted to the ICU and the systolic blood pressure should be lowered to 140 mm Hg preferably using continuous IV agents. Treat with anticonvulsants only if patient presents with clinical seizures or with mental status change and seizure findings on electroencephalogram (EEG). Check prothrombin time/international normalized ratio (PT/INR), activated partial thromboplastin time (aPTT), and platelets and treat when needed. If patient takes any antiplatelet or anticoagulant, their action should be reversed. (See Table 5.29).

   Due to young age of the patient, she should undergo further investigation with MRI and CTA/MRA to rule out underlying pathology, which might have caused the hemorrhage. Measures for intracranial pressure (ICP) control should also be taken. (See Table 3.2a).

2. **What are some causes of intracerebral hemorrhage?**
   - Vascular lesions (aneurysm, arteriovenous malformation [AVM], cavernoma).
   - Venous thrombosis.
   - Tumors (primary, secondary).
   - Mycotic aneurysms.
   - Hypertension.
   - Amyloid angiopathy.

3. **Following your initial treatment the patient's level of consciousness deteriorates. What is your treatment plan?**

   If the level of consciousness deteriorates, we should consider measures for ICP control first and if the patient does not respond, only then should we proceed with hematoma evacuation. Studies have not shown a benefit of surgery for supratentorial intracranial hematomas compared to medical treatment for life-threatening hematomas. If the brain is not swollen after the hematoma is removed, the bone flap can be replaced. (See also Table 3.2a: Surgical management).

4. **Post procedure the patient mental status is improved. On the second day after the procedure the patient starts to become obtunded again. CT brain shows no hemorrhage, no hydroceph-alus but significant swelling of the ipsilateral hemisphere with 1 cm midline shift. What is your initial management plan?**
Head of bed should be elevated at 30°. Mannitol should be administered. If mannitol is contrain-dicated consider saline 3%. (See Table 5.8b).

5. **Despite your management efforts the patient continues to deteriorate and is now obtunded requiring immediate intubation. Repeat CT does not show hydrocephalus or hemorrhage but increased midline shift to 1.5 cm. What is your treatment plan?**
Patient should undergo a decompressive craniectomy with large >12 cm decompression. (See Table 10.9b).

3.13.3 Ischemic Stroke

Chief complaint/History of present illness	• A 58 y/o man presents with right-sided hemiparesis and aphasia. According to his family the patient was last normal 3.5 hours ago. • No history of oral anticoagulants, diabetes mellitus, or previous stroke.
Physical examination	• Motor strength is normal in the left upper and lower extremities. • Motor strength is 3/5 in the right upper extremity and 2/5 in the right lower extremity. • Left gaze preference. • Slight right facial palsy. • Global aphasia. • NIHSS score: 20.

1. **What are the first management measures of an acute ischemic stroke?**
First the patient should be stabilized (ABC). Then he can be assessed for neurological deficits. (See Table 3.4d).

2. **What diagnostic study are you going to order first? What other imaging studies could solidify the diagnosis of ischemic stroke?**
   • A noncontrast head CT should be done as soon as the patient is stabilized to rule out intracra-nial hemorrhage, which is a contraindication for IV recombinant tissue plasminogen activator (rtPA). Furthermore, head CT can rule out other causes of neurological deficit (e.g., tumor). (See Table 3.4e).
   • Other imaging studies that could be done to confirm diagnosis of ischemic stroke are: CTA/MRA (can reveal the occluded vessel), CT perfusion/MRI diffusion perfusion. Imaging should not delay the onset of IV rtPA therapy, thus CTA and CT perfusion are generally preferred.

3. **Which vessel is most likely occluded based on the clinical symptoms? Describe the clinical symptoms when occlusion is located in (a) anterior choroidal artery, (b) recurrent artery of Heubner, (c) posterior inferior cerebral artery (PICA), and (d) basilar artery bifurcation/posterior cerebral artery.**
Based on the clinical symptoms the left proximal MCA artery is most likely occluded. (See Table 3.4b, Table 12.11, and Table 12.12).

4. **What is the time period after ischemic stroke onset within which IV rtPA protocol can be applied? What are the inclusion criteria and what the exclusion criteria for IV rtPA protocol treatment?**
   Intravenous rtPA protocol is recommended for treatment of acute ischemic stroke within a time frame of up to 3 hours after onset of neurological symptoms. This time window can be extended up to 4.5 hours with the addition of some exclusion criteria. (See Table 3.4f).

5. **Describe the IV rtPA protocol (dosage). What are the contraindications?**
   (See Table 3.4e).

6. **What is your plan for this patient?**
   After stabilizing the patient, a noncontrast-enhanced head CT scan should be performed as soon as possible. If intracerebral hemorrhage is ruled out, patient should receive IV rtPA protocol, since the time window recommended for IV rtPA treatment can be extended up to 4.5 hours from symptoms onset. Furthermore, the patient meets none of the exclusion criteria. (See Table 3.4e and Table 3.4f).

7. **During IV infusion of rtPA the patient vomits and his neurological status worsens. What is your plan?**
   Intravenous infusion should be discontinued immediately and a noncontrast-enhanced head CT should be performed as soon as possible to rule out intracranial hemorrhage. No hemorrhage has been revealed on head CT. (See Table 3.4e).

8. **What can be used to reverse the effects of rtPA?**
   - Cryoprecipitate.
   - Tranexamic acid or e-aminocaproic acid (if cryoprecipitate is contraindicated). (See Table 5.29).

9. **What are the criteria for endovascular treatment?**
   Pre-stroke modified Rankin Scale ≤1, NIHSS score ≥6, ASPECTS ≥6, ≥18 years old, no response after IV rtPA within 4.5 hours from stroke onset, ICA or proximal MCA occlusion. (See Table 3.4f and Table 3.4g).

10. **Patient does not respond to IV rtPA treatment. What is your plan?**
    Endovascular thrombectomy could be considered. A CTA should be performed to reveal the occluded vessel. Endovascular thrombectomy is indicated for ICA or proximal MCA occlusion. Furthermore, the patient should meet the rest of the above-mentioned criteria. Keep in mind that if acute ischemic stroke patients are eligible for IV rtPA, then they should receive IV rtPA first even if endovascular treatments are considered. (See Table 3.4f and Table 3.4g).

11. **How is the NIHSS score calculated? What are the minimum and maximum scores possible? Which items of the original NIHSS were excluded in the modified NIHSS?**
    The maximum possible NIHSS score is 42 and the minimum is 0 (normal examination). The higher the score the more severe the stroke is. NIHSS score is associated with clinical outcome. (See Table 3.4i).

12. Patient did not respond to the mechanical thrombectomy. Two days after stroke onset the patient deteriorates and he is intubated. Right pupil is 3 mm and reacts normally to light whereas his left pupil is 4 mm and reacts sluggishly to light. Emergent noncontrast-enhanced head CT is performed which shows malignant left MCA infarction with significant midline shift (see image). What is your plan?

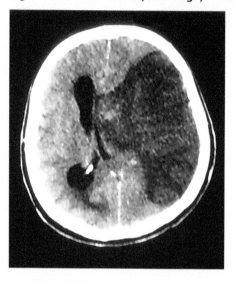

Large decompressive craniectomy with dural expansion should be considered. Decompressive craniectomy is recommended in patients younger than 60 years with unilateral MCA infarcts (> 50% of MCA territory) with neurological deterioration (not alert) within 48 hours of stroke onset despite medical treatment.

13. Describe the key procedural steps of decompressive craniectomy. What are the indications of decompressive craniectomy?
    Conditions with medically refractory increased ICP (traumatic brain injury [TBI], ischemic stroke). (See Table 10.9b).

References

[1] Juvela S. Natural history of unruptured intracranial aneurysms: risks for neurysm formation, growth, and rupture Acta Neurochir Suppl 2002; 82:27–30

[2] Nurmonen HJ, Huttunen T, Huttunen J, et al. Polycystic kidney disease among 4,436 intracranial aneurysm patients from a defined population. Neurology. 2017; 89(18):1852–1859

[3] International Study of Unruptured Intracranial Aneurysms Investigators. Unruptured intracranial aneurysms: risk of rupture and risks of surgical intervention. N Engl J Med. 1998; 339(24):1725–1733

[4] Wiebers DO, Whisnant JP, Huston J, III, et al; International Study of Unruptured Intracranial Aneurysms Investigators. Unruptured intracranial aneurysms: natural history, clinical outcome, and risks of surgical and endovascular treatment. Lancet. 2003; 362(9378):103–110

[5] Rai AT, Hogg JP, Cline B, Hobbs G. Cerebrovascular geometry in the anterior circulation: an analysis of diameter, length and the vessel taper. J Neurointerv Surg. 2013; 5(4):371–375

[6] Lawton MT. Seven aneurysms: Tenets and Techniques for clipping. New York, NY: Thieme Medical Publishers; 2011

[7] Hunt WE, Hess RM. Surgical risk as related to time of intervention in the repair of intracranial aneurysms. J Neurosurg. 1968; 28(1):14–20

[8] Drake CG. Report of World Federation of Neurological Surgeons Committee on a Universal Subarachnoid Hemorrhage Grading Scale. J Neurosurg. 1988; 68(6):985–986

[9] Jennett B, Bond M. Assessment of outcome after severe brain damage. Lancet. 1975; 1(7905):480–484

[10] Jane JA, Winn HR, Richardson AE. The natural history of intracranial aneurysms: rebleeding rates during the acute and long term period and implication for surgical management. Clin Neurosurg. 1977; 24:176–184

[11] Connolly ES, Jr, Rabinstein AA, Carhuapoma JR, et al; American Heart Association Stroke Council. Council on Cardiovascular Radiology and Intervention. Council on Cardiovascular Nursing. Council on Cardiovascular Surgery and Anesthesia. Council on Clinical Cardiology. Guidelines for the management of aneurysmal subarachnoid hemorrhage: a guideline for healthcare professionals from the American Heart Association/american Stroke Association. Stroke. 2012; 43(6):1711–1737

[12] Fisher CM, Kistler JP, Davis JM. Relation of cerebral vasospasm to subarachnoid hemorrhage visualized by computerized tomographic scanning. Neurosurgery. 1980; 6(1):1–9

[13] Frontera JA, Claassen J, Schmidt JM, et al. Prediction of symptomatic vasospasm after subarachnoid hemorrhage: the modified fisher scale. Neurosurgery. 2006; 59(1):21–27, discussion 21–27

[14] Lindegaard KF, Nornes H, Bakke SJ, Sorteberg W, Nakstad P. Cerebral vasospasm diagnosis by means of angiography and blood velocity measurements. Acta Neurochir (Wien). 1989; 100(1–2):12–24

[15] Molyneux AJ, Kerr RS, Yu LM, et al; International Subarachnoid Aneurysm Trial (ISAT) Collaborative Group. International subarachnoid aneurysm trial (ISAT) of neurosurgical clipping versus endovascular coiling in 2143 patients with ruptured intracranial aneurysms: a randomised comparison of effects on survival, dependency, seizures, rebleeding, subgroups, and aneurysm occlusion. Lancet. 2005; 366(9488):809–817

[16] Samson DS, Batjer HH, White J, Trammell TJ, Eddleman CS. Intracranial Aneurysm Surgery: Basic Principles and Techniques. New York, NY: Thieme Medical Publishers; 2012

[17] Nussbaum ES. Video Atlas of Intracranial Aneurysm Surgery. New York, NY: Thieme Medical Publishers; 2013

[18] Samson D, Batjer HH, Bowman G, et al. A clinical study of the parameters and effects of temporary arterial occlusion in the management of intracranial aneurysms. Neurosurgery. 1994; 34(1):22–28, discussion 28–29

[19] Luostarinen T, Takala RS, Niemi TT, et al. Adenosine-induced cardiac arrest during intraoperative cerebral aneurysm rupture. World Neurosurg. 2010; 73(2):79–83, discussion e9

[20] Paine JT, Batjer HH, Samson D. Intraoperative ventricular puncture. Neurosurgery. 1988; 22(6, Pt 1):1107–1109

[21] Brust JC, Dickinson PC, Hughes JE, Holtzman RN. The diagnosis and treatment of cerebral mycotic aneurysms. Ann Neurol. 1990; 27(3):238–246

[22] Ducruet AF, Hickman ZL, Zacharia BE, et al. Intracranial infectious aneurysms: a comprehensive review. Neurosurg Rev. 2010; 33(1):37–46

[23] Chapot R, Houdart E, Saint-Maurice JP, et al. Endovascular treatment of cerebral mycotic aneurysms. Radiology. 2002; 222(2):389–396

[24] Findlay JM, Grace MG, Weir BK. Treatment of intraventricular hemorrhage with tissue plasminogen activator. Neurosurgery. 1993; 32(6):941–947, discussion 947

[25] Webb AJ, Ullman NL, Mann S, Muschelli J, Awad IA, Hanley DF. Resolution of intraventricular hemorrhage varies by ventricular region and dose of intraventricular thrombolytic: the Clot Lysis: Evaluating Accelerated Resolution of IVH (CLEAR IVH) program. Stroke. 2012; 43(6):1666–1668

[26] Hemphill JC, III, Greenberg SM, Anderson CS, et al; American Heart Association Stroke Council. Council on Cardiovascular and Stroke Nursing. Council on Clinical Cardiology. Guidelines for the management of spontaneous intracerebral hemorrhage: a guideline for healthcare professionals from the American Heart Association/American Stroke Association. Stroke. 2015; 46(7):2032–2060

[27] Mendelow AD, Gregson BA, Fernandes HM, et al; STICH investigators. Early surgery versus initial conservative treatment in patients with spontaneous supratentorial intracerebral haematomas in the International Surgical Trial in Intracerebral Haemorrhage (STICH): a randomised trial. Lancet. 2005; 365(9457):387–397

[28] Mendelow AD, Gregson BA, Rowan EN, Murray GD, Gholkar A, Mitchell PM; STICH II Investigators. Early surgery versus initial conservative treatment in patients with spontaneous supratentorial lobar intracerebral haematomas (STICH II): a randomised trial. Lancet. 2013; 382(9890):397–408

[29] Barnett HJM, Taylor DW, Haynes RB, et al; North American Symptomatic Carotid Endarterectomy Trial Collaborators. Beneficial effect of carotid endarterectomy in symptomatic patients with high-grade carotid stenosis. N Engl J Med. 1991; 325(7):445–453

[30] Barnett HJ, Taylor DW, Eliasziw M, et al. Benefit of carotid endarterectomy in patients with symptomatic moderate or severe stenosis. North American Symptomatic Carotid Endarterectomy Trial Collaborators. N Engl J Med. 1998; 339(20):1415–1425

[31] Endarterectomy for asymptomatic carotid artery stenosis. Executive Committee for the Asymptomatic Carotid Atherosclerosis Study. JAMA. 1995; 273(18):1421–1428

[32] Halliday A, Harrison M, Hayter E, et al. 10-year stroke prevention aher successful Carotid endarterectomy for asymptomatic stenosis (ACST-1): a multicentre randomised trial. Lancet. 2010; 376(9746):1074–1084

[33] Brott TG, Hobson RW, II, Howard G, et al; CREST Investigators. Stenting versus endarterectomy for treatment of carotid-artery stenosis. N Engl J Med. 2010; 363(1):11–23

[34] Jauch EC, Saver JL, Adams HP, Jr, et al; American Heart Association Stroke Council. Council on Cardiovascular Nursing. Council on Peripheral Vascular Disease. Council on Clinical Cardiology. Guidelines for the early management of patients with acute ischemic stroke: a guideline for healthcare professionals from the American Heart Association/American Stroke Association. Stroke. 2013; 44(3):870–947

[35] Powers WJ, Derdeyn CP, Biller J, et al; American Heart Association Stroke Council. 2015 American Heart Association/American Stroke Association Focused Update of the 2013 Guidelines for the Early Management of Patients With Acute Ischemic Stroke Regarding Endovascular Treatment: A Guideline for Healthcare Professionals From the American Heart Association/American Stroke Association. Stroke. 2015; 46(10):3020–3035

[36] Nogueira RG, Jadhav AP, Haussen DC, et al; DAWN Trial Investigators. Thrombectomy 6 to 24 hours after stroke with a mismatch between deficit and infarct. N Engl J Med. 2018; 378(1):11–21

[37] Meyer BC, Lyden PD. The modified National Institutes of Health Stroke Scale: its time has come. Int J Stroke. 2009; 4(4):267–273

[38] Barber PA, Demchuk AM, Zhang J, Buchan AM. Validity and reliability of a quantitative computed tomography score in predicting outcome of hyperacute stroke before thrombolytic therapy. ASPECTS Study Group. Alberta Stroke Programme Early CT Score. Lancet. 2000; 355(9216):1670–1674

[39] Smith ER, Scott RM. Surgical management of moyamoya syndrome. Skull Base. 2005; 15(1):15–26

[40] Fukui M. Current state of study on moyamoya disease in Japan. Surg Neurol. 1997; 47(2):138–143

[41] Vilela MD, Newell DW. Superficial temporal artery to middle cerebral artery bypass: past, present, and future. Neurosurg Focus. 2008; 24(2):E2

[42] Kim T, Oh CW, Kwon OK, et al. Stroke prevention by direct revascularization for patients with adult-onset moyamoya disease presenting with ischemia. J Neurosurg. 2016; 124(6):1788–1793

[43] Spetzler RF, Martin NA. A proposed grading system for arteriovenous malformations. J Neurosurg. 1986; 65(4):476–483

[44] Mohr JP, Parides MK, Stapf C, et al; international ARUBA investigators. Medical management with or without interventional therapy for unruptured brain arteriovenous malformations (ARUBA): a multicentre, non-blinded, randomised trial. Lancet. 2014; 383(9917):614–621

[45] Borden JA, Wu JK, Shucart WA. A proposed classification for spinal and cranial dural arteriovenous fistulous malformations and implications for treatment. J Neurosurg. 1995; 82(2):166–179

4 Oncology (Brain)

4.1 Astrocytomas (Table 4.1a) Ⓖ

Tumor	Presentation/ demographics	Imaging/other diagnostics	Other	Treatment
Astrocytomas with better prognosis: a. **Grade I:** • Pilocytic astrocytoma • Subependymal giant cell astrocytoma b. **Grade II:** • Pleomorphic xanthoastrocytoma	See following table "Other Astrocytic Tumors" (Table 4.1b)			
Diffuse astrocytoma: (Grade II)	1. Young adults presenting with seizures 2. Focal neurologic deficits are less common (compared to high grade lesions) 3. May be an incidental finding (investigating trauma, headache etc.) 4. They represent 20% of astrocytomas	1. **Imaging:** a. **MRI:** ↑ intensity in T2 weighted images. Typically a frontal lobe lesion with no or minimal enhancement b. **CT:** ↓ density 2. **Histology:** nuclear atypia and pleomorphism	**Subtypes of diffuse astrocytomas:** 1. **Fibrillary** (most common) 2. **Gemistocytic** (> 20 gemistocytic cells per high power field associate with worse prognosis) 3. **Protoplasmic**	**Mainstay of treatment is:** 1. **Maximal Surgical resection** *that can be safely accomplished.* Consider awake craniotomy for lesions involving eloquent brain. Early resection is superior to biopsy and observation (5-y survival rate of 74 vs. 60%)[1] and should be preferred even for incidental findings[2]

Tumor	Presentation/ demographics	Imaging/other diagnostics	Other	Treatment
				2. **Radiation therapy.** Dose: 50 Gy in 2-Gy fractions over 6 wk. There is data suggesting that postoperative (early) radiation prolongs progression-free survival but does not prolong overall survival.[3] May choose not to give adjuvant radiation post-op in patients who fulfill several of the following criteria:

- Age < 40 y
- Lesion not crossing midline
- Initial tumor size < 5 cm
- No pre-op neuro deficit
- Gross total resection with isocitrate dehydrogenase (IDH) mutation

If adjuvant radiation is not given, then perform very close follow-up.

Prognosis:

a. More favorable for:
  - Gross total resection
  - Young age (< 40 y)
  - Karnofsky's performance score > 80
  - Location in noneloquent brain
  - Maximal tumor diameter < 4 cm
  - Mutations in IDH1 and IDH2

  If above criteria are met, then a 5-y survival rate of 97% may be expected.[4]

b. **Five-year survival rate:**
  - Gross total resection: 70%
  - Subtotal resection: 40%

c. **Overall median survival is 8 y**

(Continued) ▲

Tumor	Presentation/ demographics	Imaging/other diagnostics	Other	Treatment
				d. **Recurrent tumor** may be of the same or higher grade (III or IV) compared with initial tumor. ***Treat with:*** • *Surgical re-resection* if possible, particularly in the presence of mass effect • *Radiation therapy* if it had not been administered initially or significant time has passed since administration • *Chemotherapy* may be a good option for those who have not received it before. Investigative clinical treatment protocols may be preferable for patients having previously received chemotherapy.
Anaplastic astrocytoma: (Grade III)	1. Mean patient age at presentation: ~50 y 2. 30% of astrocytomas	1. There is usually enhancement and edema on imaging 2. **Histology:** nuclear atypia and mitoses	From a "low-grade" astrocytoma or de novo	**Treatment options for anaplastic astrocytomas (grade III) and glioblastomas (grade IV) are the same** Current treatment for patients < 70 y is surgery **PLUS** radiation **PLUS** chemotherapy 1. **Open surgery** *is preferred when gross total resection is possible.* Partial resection carries risk of postoperative hemorrhage and edema and there is no survival benefit.[5] Gross total resection is associated with improved survival.[6] 2. **Stereotactic biopsy** should be preferred when: • Gross total resection cannot be safely achieved • Elderly patients, usually those older than 70 y (young age is the most important positive prognostic factor) • Karnofsky's performance scale < 70 • Multiple lesions Target the most suspicious region for high-grade lesion based on MRI.

Tumor	Presentation/ demographics	Imaging/other diagnostics	Other	Treatment

				3. **Radiation therapy** of tumor and the margin of Increased signal in T2 weighted image (T2WI) signal[7] within 6 wks from surgery or biopsy
				Total dose is 60 Gy administered as 2 Gy for 5 d/wk for 6 wsk (30 fractions)
				4. **Chemotherapy**: Temozolomide: (alkylating agent)
				  a. Within 6 wks from surgery or biopsy.
				  b. Dose[8]: 75 mg/m^2/d until the completion of radiation therapy
				  c. A month after the end of radiation therapy, initiate 5d of daily treatment every 4 wks for a total of 6 cycles with 150 to 200 mg/m^2/d
				Possible side effect: myelosuppression.
				Methylation of O^6-methylguanine-DNA methyltransferase (MGMT) gene is a good prognosticator for tumor response to temozolomide
				(Continued) ▶

Tumor	Presentation/demographics	Imaging/other diagnostics	Other	Treatment

Glioblastoma: (Grade IV)	1. The most common primary tumor of brain with mean patient age at presentation: ~55 y for de novo lesion and ~45 y for progression from lower grade
	2. 50% of astrocytomas
	3. Multifocal in 5%
	4. Rarely:
	  • CSF dissemination
	  • Metastases
	5. **"Butterfly glioma":** invasion of contralateral hemisphere through corpus callosum
		1. **MRI:** typically deep frontotemporal lesion with irregular enhancement
		2. **Histology:** microvascular proliferation, necrosis
			1. Subtypes:
			  • Giant cell GBM (better prognosis)
			  • Gliosarcoma: 2% of GBMs typically in temporal lobe with sarcoma component and metastases
			  • Epithelioid GBM
			2. **Genetic syndromes associated with GBM:**
			  a. Turcot's
			  b. Li-Fraumeni
			  c. Neurofibromatosis 1 (NF1)
				5. **Recurrence:**
				  a. Consider **surgical resection** if it can be safely performed and Karnofsky's performance scale is > 70
				  b. **Carmustine-impregnated wafers,** placed in tumor bed, marginally increase survival but have a high complication rate (wound healing, malignant edema, etc.). May be considered for recurrence if not already used in primary resection.[9]
				  c. Consider **stereotactic radiosurgery** for patients with no indication for surgery
				  d. Consider **chemotherapy** (temozolomide or other agents)
				6. **Prognosis:** For both grades III and IV, prognosis is more favorable for:
				  a. Gross total resection
				  b. age < 50 y
				  c. MGMT gene methylation (predicts response to alkylating chemotherapy)
				  d. IDH1 and IDH2 gene mutations
				
				Overall prognosis:
				• ***Anaplastic astrocytoma:*** median survival 2–3 y
				• **GBM:**
				  a. IDH wild-type GBM (typically de novo ~90% of cases): median survival (with complete treatment) 15 mo.[10]
				  b. IDH-mutant GBM (usually history of prior low grade glioma and younger age: 10% of cases): median survival (with complete treatment) 31 mo.[10]

4.1.1 Other Astrocytic Tumors (Table 4.1b) G

Tumor	Presentation/demographics	Imaging/other diagnostics	Other	Treatment

Pilocytic (juvenile) astrocytoma: (Grade I)	1. Pediatric patients and young adults, usually younger than 20 y
	2. Almost 30% of pediatric gliomas
		1. **MRI:** frequently enhancing mural nodule and cyst
		2. **Predilection for:**
		• cerebellar hemispheres
		• hypothalamus, optic nerves chiasm
		• brainstem
				1. **Surgical resection:** the nodule (and the enhancing components) should be resected
				2. **Biopsy** in optic chiasm lesion (for optic nerve involvement: surgical resection)
				3. **Recurrence:** repeat surgical resection
				4. **Radiation therapy in:**
				  a. Inoperable recurrence
				  b. Optic chiasm involvement
				Prognosis:
				• 10-y survival rate of 85%
				• 20-y survival rate of 70%

Subependymal giant cell astrocytoma (Grade I)	1. Age < 20 y 2. Associated with tuberous sclerosis 3. Hydrocephalus 4. Seizures	**MRI:** lesion arising in the ventricular wall near the foramen of Monro: • With heterogeneous signal on T1WI and T2WI • With significant contrast enhancement • may be cystic		**Consider surgical resection in:** a. Progressive growth b. mass effect symptoms-hydrocephalus
Pleomorphic xanthoastrocytoma: (Grade II) **Anaplastic pleomorphic xanthoastrocytoma:** (Grade III)	1. Pediatric patients and young adults with supratentorial, superficially located lesion (subpial astrocytes) 2. Seizures	**MRI:** • typically cystic lesion • with mural nodule • in temporal lobe	Increased number of mitoses or necrosis compared to typical grade II pleomorphic xanthoastrocytoma	**Surgical resection** **Prognosis:** 5-y survival rate of 80% 1. **Surgical resection** 2. **Radiation therapy**

4.1.2 Oligodendrogliomas and Oligoastrocytomas (Table 4.1c) ⑥

Overall better prognosis than astrocytic tumors

Tumor	Presentation/demographics	Imaging/other diagnostics	Treatment
Oligodendroglioma: (Grade II)	1. Adults of 40 y (there is also a second peak in pediatric patients 6–12 y of age) 2. See "For all the above tumors"	a. **MRI:** • Infiltrative lesion in cortex and subcortical white matter of frontal lobe (followed in frequency by temporal lobe) • Cystic component may be present • Lesion may enhance • **T2WI:** hyperintense • **Diffusion weighted imaging (DWI):** no diffusion restriction b. **CT:** hypodense lesion *with calcifications* (in 70–90%) **Histology:** • "Fried egg" cytoplasm (artifact of fixation with formalin) • "Chicken wire" (fine network of branching capillaries; vascular pattern	1. **Surgical resection** 2. **Chemotherapy:** a. **PCV:** procarbazine, carmustine and vincristine is the mainstay of treatment b. **Temozolomide.** Less toxicity and side effects (particularly nausea) but ongoing study for comparison with PCV in effectiveness. 3. **Radiotherapy:** typically not a first-line treatment in newly diagnosed patients. Initial studies showed that adding radiation to surgery and chemo increased progression-free survival, but did not increase overall survival. Employed primarily as a second-line therapy for recurrences. Nonetheless, there are new data suggesting that adding radiation to chemo on first diagnosis may increase survival in: a. Patients younger than 40 y with subtotal resection b. Patients older than 40 y.[11] **Prognosis:** • 1p/19q co-deletion (combined loss of heterozygosity) predicts response to chemotherapy and longer survival • Improved survival also for: – Young age – Frontal lobe lesion – No enhancement – Complete resection • **5-y survival rate:** 70%. **Overall median survival of 12 y**

Tumor	Presentation/ demographics	Imaging/other diagnostics	Treatment
Anaplastic Oligodendroglioma: (Grade III)	1. Age > 40 y 2. See "For all the above tumors"	1. Contrast enhancement does not reliably distinguish grade II oligodendroglioma from grade III lesions 2. **MRS** may help distinguish oligodendroglioma from anaplastic subtype: presence of lipid/lactate peak in the latter	1. **Surgical resection** 2. **Chemotherapy** 3. **Radiation therapy** **Prognosis:** • 1p/19q co-deletion predicts response to chemotherapy and longer survival • **5-y survival rate:** 40%. *Overall median survival of 4y*
Oligoastrocytoma: (Grade II)	1. Patients 30–50 y old 2. See "For all the above tumors"	Two types of cells (oligodendroglioma + diffuse astrocytoma)	Treatment similar to anaplastic oligodendrogliomas **Prognosis:** • 1p/19q co-deletion predicts response to chemotherapy and longer survival • Depends on the extent of astrocytic component • **5-y survival rate:** 60%. **Overall median survival of 6y**
Anaplastic oligoastrocytoma: (Grade III)	1. Patients is 30–50 y old 2. See "For all the above tumors"	1. As above 2. Nuclear atypia, pleomorphism, increased mitoses	Treatment is similar to oligoastrocytoma. Prognosis is worse than oligoastrocytoma
For all the above tumors	**For all the above tumors, symptoms include:** 1. Seizures (in almost 70% of cases) 2. Headache 3. Focal neurological deficit 4. Hemorrhage		**For all the above tumors:** 1. Mutations in IDH1 and IDH2 (detected by immunohistochemistry and MRS) are associated with improved prognosis.[12] 2. Presence of astrocytic component worsens prognosis 3. Antiepileptics. Routinely given, even prophylactically, for all patients with oligodendroglial tumors

4.2 Ependymomas (Table 4.2) G

Tumor	Presentation/demographics	Imaging/other diagnostics	Other	Treatment

Subependy-moma (Grade I)	1. Patient are 40–60 y of age
	2. Typically asymptomatic
	3. may present due to obstructive hydrocephalus
		1. Small, usually < 2 cm (vs. subependymal giant cell astrocytomas, which are typically large)
		2. **Location frequency:**
		  • 4th ventricle in 60%
		  • Lateral ventricles in 40%
		3. No enhancement or edema in MRI (isointense on T1WI and hyperintense on T2WI)
		4. **Histology:** epithelial membrane antigen (EMA) negative (vs. positive in ependymomas)
				1. **Close follow-up** in asymptomatic patients
				2. **Treat hydrocephalus** if present
				3. **Surgical resection** is uncommon and is reserved for symptomatic mass effect and growing lesions with atypical behavior
				
				Prognosis: excellent. A very slowly growing lesion that usually remain asymptomatic

Tumor	Presentation/demographics	Imaging/other diagnostics	Other	Treatment
Ependymoma (Grade II)	1. **Pediatric patients:** • Posterior fossa lesion (floor of the 4th ventricle) • Hydrocephalus with subsequent ↑ICP and cranial nerves palsies (CNVI, VII) 2. **Adults:** • **intramedullary spinal lesion:** The subtype presenting in the filum is typically of myxopapillary histology and is a much more benign variant (grade I). • It may also present, less commonly, as a supratentorial lesion frequently with cystic component 3. "**Drop metastasis**" (spine) may present along with the cranial lesion and should be ruled out 4. Associated with NF2	1. **MRI** of entire neuraxis to exclude seeding. 2. Lesion may be: • lobulated • cystic • with calcifications • with varying enhancement 3. Lesions rarely may also present outside the CNS (mediastinum, ovaries and other) 4. **Histology:** Glial fibrillary acidic protein (GFAP) positive (vs. choroid plexus papillomas and metastatic carcinomas that are negative)	1. **Grade II variants:** a. Cellular b. Papillary ("classic form") c. Clear cell d. Tanycytic 2. **Myxopapillary ependymoma** of the filum is a grade I lesion)	1. **Surgical resection** is the mainstay both for cranial and spinal lesions. Extent of resection affects survival.[13] Due to frequent invasion of obex, complete resection is often impossible in children. 2. **Radiation:** For patients with cranial lesions, who are older than 3 y include: a. Fractionated radiation at resection bed b. Spinal radiation in case of drop metastasis. Ependymomas are very radiosensitive. Spinal ependymomas (both intramedullary and myxopapillary of the filum) are typically cured via surgery and do not require radiation 3. **For cranial lesions, consider:** • postoperative (2 wks postop) lumbar puncture for CSF cytology or • MRI of neuraxis to exclude drop metastasis **Prognosis:** 5-y survival: a. Pediatric patients 30% b. Adults near 80% c. Myxopapillary > 95%
Anaplastic ependymoma (Grade III)	Commonly a posterior fossa lesion in pediatric patients	1. MRI: contrast enhancement 2. Histology: pleomorphism, mitoses, endothelial proliferation, necrosis		1. **Surgical resection** 2. Followed by **radiation therapy** to the primary site and spinal metastases.[13,14] **Worse prognosis for:** a. age < 3 y b. subtotal resection.[13] **Chemotherapy** could be considered as a treatment option for ependymomas in order to delay radiation therapy in very young children.[15]

Note: Ependymoblastoma is a pediatric grade IV malignant lesion classified in primitive neuroectodermal tumors (PNETs).

4.3 Brainstem Gliomas (Table 4.3a) G

Tumor	Presentation/ demographics	Imaging/ other diagnostics	Treatment

1. **Mesencephalic/ tectal:** a benign subtype of brainstem gliomas
2. **Pontine:**
Diffuse pontine glioma: the most common pediatric brainstem tumor
3. **Medullar**
	1. Pediatric patients
	2. Multiple cranial nerve palsies
	3. Long tract signs
	4. Vertical and rotatory nystagmus
	5. Decreased alertness
	6. Hydrocephalus
		MRI:
		1. Typical presentation of **diffuse lesion** is hypointense on T1WI, hyperintense on T2WI with no contrast enhancement. Enhancement and necrosis is related to higher grade lesions
		2. **Pilocytic (focal) lesion** presents with enhancement
			1. **Radiation therapy** is the primary treatment for brainstem gliomas (50 Gy for 6 wk, 5 d/wk)
			2. **No biopsy** for diffuse lesions. Perform brain MRS (differential diagnosis includes, encephalitis, acute disseminated encephalomyelitis [ADEM], demyelination)
			3. **Surgery only for:**
			a. Hydrocephalus
			b. Dorsal exophytic lesion (usually pilocytic astrocytoma).
			Remember:
			• Use monitoring
			• Beware of the fourth ventricle floor (identify facial and hypoglossal colliculus)
			4. **Dexamethasone**
			5. **Chemotherapy.** Recently, in addition to standard chemotherapy, chemoembolization has been employed.
			
			Prognosis for diffuse lesions:
			• Survival of 6–12 mo
			• *Better prognosis for:*
			a. Tectal gliomas:
			  – A benign subtype of brainstem gliomas
			  – Usually does not require any intervention except for shunting due to obstruction of aqueduct of Sylvius
			b. Cystic and focal exophytic lesions

Focal or diffuse			

Note: Higher-grade lesions are more frequent in lower brainstem, while lower-grade lesions are more frequent in upper brainstem

4.3.1 Optic Apparatus/Hypothalamic Gliomas (Table 4.3b) G

Tumor	Presentation/demographics	Imaging/other diagnostics	Other	Treatment

Typically a pilocytic astrocytoma	1. Children typically younger than 5 y of age
	2. Disturbance of vision (visual acuity or field defects)
	3. Endocrine dysfunction (hypopituitarism, precocious puberty)
	4. Hydrocephalus and/or psychobehavioral symptoms (large lesions involving the 3rd ventricle and/or limbic system)
		1. **MRI brain:** the lesion infiltrates the optic apparatus (typically no displacement). Hyperintense on T2WI with various enhancement
		2. Consider MRA for suprasellar lesions
		3. Evaluate vision and endocrine function
		4. **Classification:**
		  • **Stage 1:** optic nerves only
		  • **Stage 2:** chiasm involved
		  • **Stage 3:** hypothalamic involvement
			1. **Association with NF1** (*REMEMBER:* repeated ophthalmologic evaluation for NF1 patients).
			2. May be bilateral.
				1. Asymptomatic nonprogressing lesions may be **followed closely** (imaging, vision, and endocrine function).
				2. **Chemotherapy** (carboplatin and vincristine among other regimens) for symptomatic or progressive tumor
				3. **Radiation therapy** (stereotactic radiosurgery, external beam radiation) for:
				  a. Older children (age >3 y)
				  b. Progression during chemotherapy
				  c. Relapse after chemotherapy
				4. Consider **surgical resection** for:
				  a. Unilateral lesion anterior to chiasm with no useful vision.
				  b. Shunt placement for suprasellar expansion causing hydrocephalus
				
				Prognosis:
				a. **worse for:**
				  • Location posterior to chiasm
				  • Young age
				  • Pilomyxoid astrocytoma subtype
				b. **Better for:**
				  • NF1 patients.
				  • 10-y survival rate is approximately 85% with treatment[16]

4.4 Choroid Plexus Tumors (Table 4.4) G

Tumor	Presentation/ demographics	Imaging/other diagnostics	Other	Treatment

Choroid plexus papilloma (Grade I)	1. **Usually children < 2 y** with *supratentorial* lesion and signs of ↑ ICP (macrocrania, tense fontanelle etc.).
	 2. **Adults** usually present with *infratentorial* lesion
	 3. **Anatomic location:**
	   a. 50% in lateral ventricles (atrium, left >right)
	   b. 40% in 4th ventricle and cerebellopontine angle (CPA)
	   c. 5% in 3rd ventricle (roof)
	   d. 5% in multiple sites
	 4. **Presents typically with hydrocephalus**
		MRI:
		 • strongly enhancing lobulated intraventricular lesion usually associated with hydrocephalus
		 • Cauliflower shape
			Very frequent in first year of life	**Surgical resection**
				 Prognosis: 5-y survival: ~90%

Atypical choroid plexus papilloma (Grade II)	As above	1. **MRI:** similar to choroid plexus papilloma + possibly hemorrhage-necrosis 2. **Histology:** Two or more mitoses per 10 high-power fields (related to recurrence)		**Surgical resection** **Prognosis:** • *Higher recurrence rate* as compared to grade I lesions • *Intermediate 5-y survival rate* between grade I and III lesions

Tumor	Presentation/demographics	Imaging/other diagnostics	Other	Treatment

Choroid plexus carcinoma (Grade III)	As above	1. **MRI:** similar to atypical choroid plexus papilloma + frequently ependymal, brain invasion and edema
		2. **Histology:** More than 5 mitoses per 10 high-power fields
		3. **Immunohistochemistry:** if positive epithelial membrane antigen (EMA) or carcinoembryonic antigen (CEA), consider metastatic lesion rather than primary choroid plexus tumor
				1. **Surgical resection** (the most important prognostic factor)
				2. **After partial surgical resection** consider:
				  a. Chemotherapy
				  b. Radiation therapy (not in children < 3 y of age).[17,18,19]
				
				Prognosis:
				• **5-y survival rate:** ~50% after complete surgical resection
				• **Worse outcome:**
				  a. CSF seeding
				  b. Brain invasion
				  c. TP53 gene mutation

	For all the above tumors: 80% of choroid plexus tumors present in children < 2 y of age	**For all the above tumors:** 1. Imaging cannot reliably distinguish between different grades 2. **Perform preoperatively MRI of entire spine** (there is risk of CSF seeding, higher with grade III lesions)	**For all the above tumors:** Associated with: • Li–Fraumeni syndrome • Aicardi's syndrome	**For all the above tumors:** 1. Always consider **surgery** for residual tumor or recurrence 2. **Possible complication:** postoperative subdural collections (fistula between ventricles and subdural space) that may require shunting 3. **Hydrocephalus** may not resolve completely postoperatively.

4.5 Neuronal and Mixed Neuronal–Glial Tumors (Table 4.5) G

Tumor	Presentation/demographics	Imaging/other diagnostics	Other	Treatment
Dysembryoplastic neuroepithelial tumor (DNT or DNET) (Grade I)	1. Children and young adults (<20 y of age) with pharmacoresistant epilepsy 2. temporal (or frontal) lesion 3. Very slow growth	1. MRI: a. Wedge-shaped cystic supratentorial cortical lesion b. No edema with usually no enhancement (or punctate enhancement) c. Typically hyperintense on T2WI 2. Associated with cortical dysplasia		Surgical resection for pharmacoresistant epilepsy: a. Resect epileptogenic foci b. Duration of intractable seizures is inversely correlated to improvement after surgery
Ganglioglioma: (GRADE I)	Children and young adults with seizures and temporal lobe lesion	Frequently cystic lesion with enhancing mural nodule and calcifications	Neuronal (ganglion) + astrocytic (glial) cells: some correlate prognosis with the astrocytic component	Surgical resection Prognosis: 10-y survival rate of 85%
Anaplastic ganglioglioma: (Grade III)				1. Surgical resection 2. Radiation therapy Prognosis: not significantly worse
Central neurocytoma: (Grade II)	1. Young adults with large ventricles 2. Symptoms of ↑ICP	1. MRI and CT: a. "Bubbly" lesion originating in septum pellucidum, within the lateral and 3rd ventricles in the vicinity of foramen of Monro b. Contrast enhancement c. Usually calcifications 2. Histology: "Fried egg" cell appearance similar to oligodendroglioma, but no IDH mutations or 1p19q deletions		1. Surgical resection: The 2-year and 4-year recurrence rates in pts w/ MIB-1 labeling >4% are 50% and 75% respectively 2. Stereotactic radiosurgery if MIB-1 is elevated (> 2%) and no gross total resection has been achieved 3. Chemotherapy in recurrence and inoperable tumors Prognosis: complete surgical resection is a cure.

Tumor	Presentation/demographics	Imaging/other diagnostics	Other	Treatment

Paraganglioma	1. Middle-age patients and slow growth
	2. Possibly catecholamine release with severe hypertension/cardiac arrhythmias
	3. Cranial nerves palsy
	4. **Based on location:**
	  a. *Carotid body tumor* (carotid bifurcation):
	    • Painless mass in neck that may affect cranial nerves X and XII or cause narrowing of internal carotid artery (ICA) with accompanying cerebrovascular events
	    • *Angiogram:* splaying of bifurcation
	    • 5% are bilateral
	  b. *Glomus tympanicum* (auricular branch of vagus):
	    • Most common tumor of middle ear
	    • Very vascular
	    • Hearing loss-tinnitus
	    • Lower cranial nerves palsy and possibly cranial nerve VII
		1. **Laboratory workup:**
		  a. Plasma metanephrines
		  b. 24-h urine collection for metanephrines and catecholamines
		  c. Clonidine suppression test
		2. **Otoscopic examination** for glomus tympanicum (red mass that pulsates behind eardrum)
		3. **Angiogram** helps differentiate glomus from vestibular schwannoma and evaluates the possibility to sacrifice the jugular vein during surgery
			Paraganglion cells	1. **Surgical resection:**
				Consider preoperative embolization 24–48 h before surgery in selected cases. There is a risk of significant edema following embolization Following surgery, there is postoperative risk of lower cranial nerve dysfunction (tracheostomy or gastrostomy may be needed)
				2. **Radiation therapy** (40 Gy in 15 fractions): Controls growth but does not cause shrinkage. Consider in large tumors or patients who cannot tolerate surgery.
				
				REMEMBER: If the tumor secrets catecholamines prior to embolization or surgery pretreat:
				  a. 2 wks with alpha-blockers:
				    • phenoxybenzamine 10 mg orally twice daily to maximum 50 mg twice daily
				    • phentolamine IV in acute hypertensive crisis)
				  b. 24 h with beta-blockers : propranolol 5–10 mg four times daily
				Alpha blockers should precede beta blockers (to prevent hypertension and ischemic heart disease)
				
				Prognosis: 5-y survival rate of 90%
				
				(Continued) ▲

Tumor	Presentation/demographics	Imaging/other diagnostics	Other	Treatment
	c. *Glomus jugulare* (jugular foramen, superior vagal ganglion): • Very vascular • Hearing loss–tinnitus • Lower cranial nerves palsy + possibly cranial nerve VII palsy d. *Glomus intravagale* (inferior vagal ganglion): rare e. *Pheochromocytoma* (adrenal medulla and sympathetic chain): If age < 50 y perform genetic testing mainly to exclude: • von Hippel–Lindau • multiple endocrine neoplasia type 2A (MEN2A) and MEN2B • neurofibromatosis			

4.6 Embryonal Tumors (Table 4.6) G

Tumor	Presentation/demographics	Imaging/other diagnostics	Other	Treatment
Medulloblastomas: (Grade IV)	1. Typically pediatric pts (peak age: 7 y) and young adults with lesion arising from: • the roof of the 4th ventricle (vs. ependymoma arising from floor) • in cerebellar hemisphere (older children, adults) 2. **May present with:** a. Hydrocephalus b. ↑ICP signs c. Gait disturbance and Truncal ataxia d. Truncal ataxia 3. Frequently **drop metastases** (up to 1/3 of cases) 4. Rarely metastases (higher frequency with large cell subtype) 5. Preterm children are at increased risk	1. **MRI:** • **T2WI:** heterogeneous • **DWI:** restricted diffusion • significant contrast enhancement 2. **CT:** hyperdense lesion 3. **MRI of entire spine with contrast** to rule out drop metastases preoperatively or at least 2–3 wk postoperatively (not earlier because of blood) 4. **Histology:** "Small round blue cell neoplasm"	1. Most common malignant pediatric brain tumor 2. Based on molecular subgroup (*medulloblastomas genetically defined:* WHO classification 2016)[20]: • Medulloblastoma WNT • Medulloblastoma SHH • Medulloblastoma Group 3 • Medulloblastoma Group 4	1. **Surgical resection:** a. Lesion on the 4th ventricle floor and brainstem is not resected to prevent poor neurological outcome b. Consider external ventricular drain (EVD) preoperatively *REMEMBER:* a. *Gross total resection:* no residual tumor b. *Near-total resection:* < 1.5 cm² residual tumor c. *Subtotal resection:* > 1.5 cm² residual tumor 2. **Lumbar puncture** for cytology before craniotomy if no hydrocephalus 3. Consider treatment of **hydrocephalus** (shunt carries a risk of seeding) 4. **Craniospinal radiation therapy** for age > 3 y: • **Dose:** 10–15 Gy to tumor bed and 35–40 Gy to neuraxis over 6 wks • Consider lower dose to neuraxis after gross total resection

(Continued) ▲

Tumor	Presentation/ demographics	Imaging/other diagnostics	Other	Treatment
				5. **Chemotherapy** (lomustine, vincristine, cisplatin): • Children < 3 y • Residual tumor > 1.5 cm^2 • Metastases • Recurrence **Prognosis** a. *Prognosis worse for:* • Male patient • Residual tumor > 1.5 cm^2 • Age < 3 y • Metastases • Loss of 17q, amplification of c-myc and ERBB2 overexpression b. *Prognosis based on WHO classification:* • Medulloblastoma: WNT EXCELLENT (90% long-term survival LTS) • Medulloblastoma: SHH GOOD: (60–85% LTS as long as no TP53 mutation) • Medulloblastoma: Group 3 POOR: (< 50% LTS) • Medulloblastoma: Group 4 GOOD: (75% LTS) ERBB2-protein negative tumors have a better prognosis

Tumor	Presentation/demographics	Imaging/other diagnostics	Other	Treatment
Neuroblastoma: (tumor of the sympathetic nervous system)	1. Most common in children (may be congenital)	**CRANIAL workup:**	**Esthesioneuroblastoma** (olfactory neuroblastoma):	• Neuroblastomas are very radio- and chemosensitive.
a. *Peripheral:* the primary tumor is located in the adrenal glands, paraspinal or periaortic regions, where sympathetic nervous tissue is present	2. 65% of patients present with disseminated disease frequently spreading to bone (with pain)	6. *MRI brain:* supratentorial enhancing lesion with possibly hemorrhagic, necrotic, cystic component	• Malignant tumor usually in older adults (> 50 y)	• Treatment includes a **combination** of surgery, radiotherapy, and chemotherapy.
	3. Skull may be involved:	7. *CT brain/orbit* to evaluate skull invasion	• Originates from the olfactory neural crest cells	• **Prognosis** is age dependent:
	• "Raccoon eyes" (involvement of orbits)	8. Consider *bone scan and PET* for metastatic disease	• Possible extension inside the cranial vault	a. 5-y survival rate for children of age < 1y is 55%
b. *Cerebral:*	• Palpable calvarial mass		• Surgical resection, usually endoscopic	b. Significantly worse for older children
• Primary cerebral neuroblastoma (PNET)	4. Possibly palpable abdominal or paraspinal mass		• *Prognosis:* 7-y expected survival	
• metastases from peripheral neuroblastomas	5. There is association **with:**			
	• Opsoclonus myoclonus syndrome (paraneoplastic)[21]			
	• NF1			

4.7 Vestibular Schwannoma (Table 4.7) G

Presentation/demographics	Imaging/other diagnostics	Other	Treatment
Patients at the 4th–6th decade of life with: 1. Ipsilateral sensorineural loss of hearing (high-tone loss and difficulty in discriminating words) 2. High-pitched tinnitus 3. Disequilibrium 4. *Tumor > 2 cm may also present* with (compression of adjacent structures): • Facial numbness • Facial weakness (usually late symptom) • Otalgia • Brainstem symptoms • Dysgeusia • Lower cranial nerve symptoms • Hydrocephalus (tumor >4 cm) • Represents **80% of CPA tumors**. Second most common is meningioma.	1. **MRI brain:** • Lesion presents heterogeneous enhancement and may be cystic • *When large:* "ice cream on cone" shape • *When small:* "filling defect" within the increased signal CSF of internal acoustic canal (high-resolution T2WI) 2. **CT brain:** enlarged internal auditory meatus (normal diameter: 5–8 mm). Meningiomas cause hyperostosis and decrease of the diameter of the internal auditory canal 3. **Audiometric tests:** a. Pure-tone audiogram b. Speech discrimination c. When the lesion is small (<1.5 cm): • *ENG* (electronystagmography) for superior vestibular nerve • *VEMP* (vestibular evoked myogenic potential) for inferior vestibular nerve • *ABR* (auditory brain responses): prognosis for preservation of hearing	1. It is a grade I lesion presenting in the CPA and arising from Schwann cells of the superior division of the vestibular nerve (transition zone between central and peripheral myelination). 2. The 2nd most common intracranial schwannoma is from trigeminal nerve 3. Associated with loss of a tumor suppressor gene on the long arm of chromosome 22 4. Facial nerve is displaced anteriorly (75% of cases), followed (in frequency) by superiorly, inferiorly, posteriorly 5. **"50/50 rule"** to define serviceable hearing: • pure-tone audiogram threshold ≤ 50 dB • speech discrimination score ≥ 50%	1. **Tumors < 1.5 cm with perfect hearing:** consider close follow-up *REMEMBER:* a. No further growth is expected if no growth has been documented in the first 5 y from diagnosis b. 60% of vestibular schwannomas are slow growing (< 1 mm/y) 2. **Tumors < 1.5 cm with serviceable hearing:** a. Close follow-up b. Stereotactic radiosurgery 3. **Tumors > 1.5 cm:** a. *Stereotactic radiosurgery* for: • Lesions up to 3 cm with no mass effect • Residual post-op lesions (12–16 Gy, depending on weather hearing is serviceable) b. Consider *fractionated radiotherapy* for even larger lesions with no mass effect and significant patient comorbidity Approximately 18–24 mo are necessary for radiation therapy to present its full effect

Presentation/ demographics	Imaging/other diagnostics	Other	Treatment

• **NF2:**
1. Bilateral vestibular Schwannomas
2. An early diagnosis of vestibular schwannoma (<40 y of age) should initiate investigation on possible coexistence of NF2
	4. **Histology:**
	a. *Antoni A pattern* (cellular, fibrillary elongated appearing tissue)
	b. *Antoni B pattern* (less cellular microcystic tissue)
			Surgery vs. radiation therapy:
			a. *Radiation therapy* appears to be superior to surgery at preserving hearing (particularly when dose to 50% isodose is kept below 13 Gy)
			b. *Surgery* is superior at controlling vertigo/disequilibrium
			c. Their results appear ***comparable for:***
			  • Facial nerve preservation
			  • Trigeminal nerve function
			  • Tumor control (a temporary increase in dimension may be observed with radiation therapy)
			4. **Tumors > 3 cm or with symptoms of mass effect:**
			Surgery (always with intraoperative monitoring). Choice of approach depends on several factors including:
			  • Tumor size
			  • Tumor anatomy
			  • Hearing in ipsilateral ear
			  • Hearing in contralateral ear
			  • Surgeon preference
			Surgical approaches:
			a. *Retrosigmoid:*
			  • Good for hearing preservation
			  • Wide angle of view
			  • Beware of cerebellar retraction
			  • Not good for purely intracanalicular tumors
			b. *Translabyrinthine:*
			  • No preservation of hearing
			  • Superior facial nerve preservation
			  • Excellent for avoiding cerebellar retraction in large tumors
			c. *Subtemporal:*
			  • Improved hearing preservation
			  • Slight increase in facial nerve palsy. Facial nerve encountered first in this approach
			  • Excellent approach for purely intracanalicular tumors

(Continued) ▲

Presentation/demographics	Imaging/other diagnostics	Other	Treatment

			Post-op complications
			1. *Facial nerve palsy* (frequency increasing with size of tumor):
			   a. Natural tears when needed and at least every 2 h
			   b. Eye lubricant ointment before bedtime and tape the eye shut
			   c. If no immediate recovery is expected (or if also sensation is impaired because of CNV dysfunction), then perform tarsorrhaphy in the first days
			   d. If no return of function is expected or in case of no improvement in the 1st year, a hypoglossal-facial anastomosis can be considered
			2. *Vestibular nerve dysfunction* (frequency increasing with size of tumor): nausea, vomit, and disequilibrium (they are self-resolving)
			3. *Brainstem dysfunction:* persistent ataxia
			4. *Lower cranial nerves palsy:* risk of aspiration
			5. *CSF leak*
			6. *Headaches* due to:
			   • chemical meningitis from subdural bone drilling. Irrigate well after drilling to minimize risk
			   • attachment of muscle onto dura in craniectomy site. Perform craniotomy instead of craniectomy to decrease this risk.
			
			Remember:
			   a. Treat preoperatively coexistent **hydrocephalus.** May also present post-op (even years later)
			   b. Preserving the facial nerve/brainstem function is more important than the degree of resection (considering the possibility of post-op radiation therapy and that this is a histologically benign tumor)
			   c. *Chemotherapy:* avastin has been used for NF2 vestibular schwannomas
			   d. *Preoperatively* note the location and size of the jugular bulb and sigmoid sinus, as well as the degree

4.8 Meningiomas (Table 4.8) G

Tumor	Presentation/demographics	Imaging/other diagnostics	Other	Treatment

Meningioma: (Grade I)
 	
Subtypes:
• *Meningothelial (syncytial)*: the most common
• *Fibrous (fibroblastic)*
• *Transitional*
• *Psammomatous*
• *Angiomatous*: abundant blood vessels
• *Microcystic*: may present cysts having an atypical radiologic presentation)
• *Secretory*: significant perilesional edema that may complicate treatment
• *Lymphoplasmacyte-rich meningioma*: significant lympho-plasmacytic infiltrates in the tumor and clinical presentation that resembles an inflammatory process with peripheral blood abnormalities
• *Metaplastic*: mesenchymal differentiation of various extent (bone, cartilage, fat may be observed)
	1. Very common (15%) primary intracranial tumor presenting usually in female adults
	2. **Presentation**
	  a. Frequently asymptomatic
	  b. Neurological deficit depending on location
	  c. Seizures (supratentorial tumor)
	  d. Foster–Kennedy syndrome in olfactory groove meningiomas (anosmia + ipsilateral optic atrophy + contralateral papilledema)
	3. **Multiple meningiomas** are associated with NF2
		1. **MRI:**
		  • dural-based enhancing lesion with variable edema.
		  • *T1WI*: isointense
		  • *T2WI*: hyper or isointense
		  • *"Dural tail"* (which may also be observed in pleomorphic xanthoastrocytoma)
		REMEMBER: Check patency of dural sinuses (consider MRV-based on location of lesion)
		2. **CT:** hyperostosis of adjacent bone and calcification of lesion may be present
			1. They arise from arachnoid meningothelial "cap" cells
			2. **Genetics:**
			  a. Monosomy 22 (up to 70% of tumors)
			  b. 1p and 14q deletions (associated with more aggressive behavior)
			  c. Association with NF2
			3. Associated with radiation
				1. **Follow up for:**
				  a. Asymptomatic tumor
				  b. No progressive growth
				  c. Low life expectancy
				  • After first diagnosis, repeat MRI after 3–4 mo (to exclude rapid growth) and then follow annually for 3 y.
				  • Pregnancy and breast cancer may cause growth.
				2. **Surgical resection for:**
				  a. Symptomatic
				  b. lesions with progressive growth
				
				Surgical technique:
				  a. Consider preoperative embolization with particulate agents
				  b. Deprive early the tumor of its blood supply
				  c. Internal decompression maintaining the capsule ("if you can debulk, you should debulk")
				  d. Avoid healthy brain retraction
				  e. Drill (remove) any attached bone
				  f. *Maintain venous drainage:*
				    • Superior sagittal sinus can usually be safely occluded anterior to coronal suture but never posteriorly to the vein of Trolard
				    • The dominant transverse sinus should be preserved

Tumor	Presentation/ demographics	Imaging/other diagnostics	Other	Treatment

		3. **Digital subtraction angiography (DSA):**
		• May be needed based on anatomic location and/or for pre-op embolization
		• "Sunburst" or radial appearance. Enhancement presents in early arterial phase and persists ("come early, stay late")
		• External carotid artery feeders with the exception of:
		  a. Olfactory groove (fed by the ethmoidal branches of ophthalmic artery, which is a branch of ICA)
		  b. Supra and parasellar lesions
		4. **Frequent anatomic locations** (90% are supratentorial):
		• **Adults:**
		  a. *Parasagittal:* Grading for meningioma invasion of superior sagittal sinus[22]:
		    – *Type I:* attachment to lateral wall of sinus
				It is safer to:
				• Leave residual tumor in sinus than sacrifice sinus
				• Close follow-up of remnant
				• Stereotactic radiosurgery in case of growth
				3. **Consider focal radiation therapy/ radiosurgery:**
				  a. For tumors < 3 cm
				  b. For patients with contraindication to surgery
				  c. For surgically inaccessible lesion
				  d. For growing residual tumor
				  e. After recurrence
				  f. For atypical or anaplastic meningioma after surgical resection
				
				REMEMBER: Stereotactic radiosurgery has overall disease stabilization rate of 89% and complication rate of 7%[23]
				
				Prognosis:
				• Most important for preventing recurrence is extent of resection
				• Ki-67/MIB-1 inversely correlates with prognosis
				• *Worse prognosis for:*
				  a. 1p and 14q deletions
				  b. Lack of progesterone receptors are associated with more aggressive behavior

Tumor	Presentation/ demographics	Imaging/other diagnostics	Other	Treatment

		– *Type II*: lateral recess invasion
		– *Type III*: lateral wall invasion
		– *Type IV*: lateral wall and roof invasion
		– *Type V*: total occlusion of sinus with contralateral wall spared
		– *Type VI*: total occlusion with invasion of all walls
		b. **Convexity**
		c. **Tuberculum sellae** (chiasmal syndrome: optic atrophy + bitemporal hemianopsia)
		d. **Sphenoidal ridge**:
		  – Pterional or lateral third
		  – Alar or middle third
		  – Clinoidal or medial third
		Multiple meningiomas in 9% of pts (frequently associated with history of radiation or NF2).		

(Continued) ▲

Tumor	Presentation/ demographics	Imaging/other diagnostics	Other	Treatment

		• *Children:*
		  a. Intraventricular
		  b. Posterior fossa
		5. **Rare anatomic locations:**
		  a. Intraosseous (skull)
		  b. Subcutaneous
		6. **Metastases** (lung, liver, lymph nodes, heart): usually grade III meningiomas
		7. Consider **hemangiopericytoma** if the lesion is growing more rapidly than expected
		8. **Histology:** psammoma bodies (calcified whorls)
		9. **Immunohistochemical stains:**
		  a. EMA
		  b. Vimentin
				Recurrence rate:
				a. Based on *WHO grade:*
				  • 9% for grade I meningioma
				  • 29% for grade II atypical meningioma
				  • 70% for grade III anaplastic meningioma
				b. Based on *Simpson grade* (10 year recurrence rate depending on extent of resection)[24]:
				  • *Grade I:* complete (even sinus) → 10%
				  • *Grade II:* complete but only coagulation of dural attachment → 20%
				  • *Grade III:* complete but without coagulation → 30%
				  • *Grade IV:* partial (residual tumor) → 40–80%
				  • *Grade V:* simple decompression/biopsy → 100%
				Treatment of recurrence:
				a. Repeat surgical resection and/or
				b. Focal radiation therapy

Tumor	Presentation/demographics	Imaging/other diagnostics	Other	Treatment
Atypical meningioma (Grade II) *Other grade II meningiomas:* • Chordoid • *Clear cell:* young adults with lesion in spinal canal or posterior fossa	5% of meningiomas	• Brain invasion and mitotic count of 4 or more/10 high-power fields.[10] • Can also be diagnosed based on the presence of 3 out of 5 of the subsequent features: 1. Spontaneous necrosis 2. Sheeting (loss of whorling or fascicular architecture) 3. Prominent nucleoli 4. High cellularity 5. Small cells (clusters with high nuclear-to-cytoplasmic ratio)[10]		1. **Surgical resection** 2. **Radiation therapy** after both total and subtotal resection.[25] *Prognosis:* a. 5-y survival rate of 30% b. Metastases in 5% of cases
Anaplastic (malignant) meningioma (Grade III) *Other grade III meningiomas:* • Papillary • Rhabdoid	1–3% of meningiomas	1. **MRI:** • Necrosis • Tumor invades brain • significant edema 2. **CT:** osteolysis may be present	**Two subtypes exist:** • Arising de novo • Progressing from lower grade tumor	1. **Surgical resection** 2. **Radiation therapy** after both total and subtotal resection.[25] 3. **No effective chemotherapy** exists *Prognosis:* a. *Gross total resection* appears to confer an overall survival advantage (overall median survival of 3.2 y compared to 1.3 y for subtotal resection) b. Patients with *de novo tumor* have a better survival[26] c. *Metastases* in 30% of cases

4.9 Mesenchymal, Non-meningothelial Tumors (Table 4.9) [G]

Tumor	Presentation/ demographics	Imaging/other diagnostics	Other	Treatment
Hemangiopericytoma: • Grade I (solitary fibrous tumor, very rare) • Grade II • Grade III (anaplastic)	Adults aged 40–50 y with usually supratentorial lesion	**MRI:** • May be difficult to differentiate from meningioma (dural-based lesion frequently presenting "dural tail") • Contrast enhancement • Bone erosion • Flow voids • *No hyperostosis and no Ca^{++} (vs. meningioma)*	1. **Sarcoma** originating from pericytes surrounding blood vessels 2. Almost 30% **metastasize** (lung, bone, liver, lymph nodes)	1. **Surgical resection** followed by **radiation therapy** 2. **Chemotherapy** for metastases and recurrence **Prognosis:** • Frequent local recurrence after treatment • 10-year survival rate of ~40% • Mean survival after metastases: 2 y
Hemangioblastoma: (Grade I)	1. **Adult** (2nd – 4th decade) non metastatic lesion of the posterior fossa presenting with mass effect (it is the most common primary posterior fossa lesion in adults) 2. May also be found within brainstem or spinal cord (thoracic or cervical) 3. Except for CNS, may also present in *retina* (ask for ophthalmic examination) 4. Exclude coexisting **polycythemia** (the tumor secrets erythropoietin)	1. Perform **MRI of entire neuraxis** (exclude coexisting lesions): • Signal voids (vascular lesion) • Possibly hemosiderin surrounding lesion (indicating previous hemorrhage) • frequently cystic component (slightly hyperintense in T1WI in comparison with CSF) and with enhancing mural nodule • may also be solid with no cyst in 40% of cases 2. Consider **angiography:** • avascular cyst and highly vascular nodule • Usually performed if pre-op embolization is indicated	**Three types:** 1. Juvenile 2. Transitional 3. Clear cell	1. Surgical resection (possibly en block): when a nodule exists, it has to be identified and excised; otherwise, the cyst will recur (part of the content of the nodule's vessels leaks, forming the cyst). The cyst wall is typically non-neoplastic and may be left behind 2. Consider **preoperative embolization** (rarely needed). **Prognosis:** • Recurrence in 20% of cases • 10-y survival rate of 85%

Tumor	Presentation/ demographics	Imaging/other diagnostics	Other	Treatment
	5. Consider von Hippel–Lindau disease: • At least 25% of hemangioblastomas • Typically presents earlier in life			
Hemangioma	1. **Benign lesion of:** a. Skull (frontal, parietal) b. Spine (usually vertebral body in low thoracic or lumbar) 2. **Diagnosed because of:** a. Cosmetic reasons b. Bleeding after scalp injury c. Back pain in spinal lesions	**CT/MRI brain:** • "Honeycomb" or "sunburst" pattern (trabecular) • Outer table of skull > inner with nonbeveled and nonsclerotic margins • Extradural	Capillary and cavernous formations on histology	**Surgical resection** en block (excision of involved skin may also be necessary)
Osteoma	Benign lesion usually in females	**CT/MRI brain:** Homogeneous lesion of outer skull table	**Differential diagnosis:** fibrous dysplasia (benign lesion presenting with replacement of bone by connective tissue)	**Surgical resection if:** a. Mass effect b. Cosmetic reasons

4.10 Hematologic Tumors (Table 4.10) G

Tumor	Presentation/ demographics	Imaging/other diagnostics	Other	Treatment
Lymphoma	a. **Primary** (typically parenchymal), usually associated with: • Immunosuppression • HIV (responsible for the increase in lymphoma incidence) • Epstein–Barr virus • Autoimmune diseases (rheumatoid arthritis and lupus) b. **Secondary** (typically leptomeningeal), usually non-Hodgkin's 1. **Lymphomas present with:** a. B symptoms (fever, weight loss, night sweats) b. Carcinomatous meningitis (multiple cranial nerve palsies) c. Mass effect and often neuropsychiatric symptoms 2. Association with uveitis 3. B-cell much more frequently than T-cell 4. **Mean age** is 60 y in immunocompetent patients and 35 y for patients with immunodeficiency	1. **MRI brain:** a. *Primary:* • single or multiple periventricular subependymal, corpus callosum or basal ganglia lesions that enhance homogenously (may also present as dural mass). • AIDS-related lesion is typically multicentric b. *Secondary:* Leptomeningeal enhancement, enhancing dural mass possibly with bone involvement (parenchymal lesion may also be present) 2. **CT brain:** hyperdense (helpful for diagnosis) 3. **Lumbar puncture** (lymphomatous cells) 4. **Workup for systemic lymphoma** (when not already known): a. Check lymph nodes b. CT chest and abdomen c. MRI spine d. Testicular ultrasound e. Bone marrow biopsy f. Ophthalmologic evaluation	Immunodeficiency is a significant risk factor	1. **Steroids** (they may cause the lesion to disappear: "ghost tumor"). They may increase diagnostic difficulty when administered before biopsy (lysis of tumor cells) 2. **Surgery** only for: a. Stereotactic biopsy. (Lumbar puncture cannot define the subtype) b. Reservoir placement (for intrathecal chemotherapy) c. Life-threatening brain herniation 3. **Whole brain radiation therapy** (40–50 Gy). Very radiosensitive tumor 4. **Chemotherapy** (methotrexate): improves outcome when combined with radiation therapy. Consider intrathecal chemotherapy for concurrent brain and leptomeningeal disease REMEMBER: In HIV patients toxoplasmosis is the most common cause of enhancing brain mass. For these patients, administer antitoxoplasmosis treatment upon radiographic diagnosis for 2 wks. If no improvement after 2 wks, then a biopsy should be performed.

Tumor	Presentation/ demographics	Imaging/other diagnostics	Other	Treatment
				Prognosis: • Median survival of a few months without treatment and up to 4 y with treatment • Leptomeningeal involvement and AIDS are associated with worse prognosis
Multiple myeloma	1. Multiple bone lytic lesions in patient with pain. Skull involvement is less frequent than vertebrae. 2. Immunosuppression (risk of infection) 3. Reduced hematopoiesis 4. Osteoporosis with fractures and hypercalcemia 5. Hyperviscosity syndrome or renal failure 6. Compression in spinal canal	1. **MRI/CT:** enhancement and bone involvement (CT is superior in evaluating extent of lesion) 2. **Diagnostic tests:** a. *24-h urine* (kappa Bence Jones protein) b. *Serum and urine electrophoresis* (M-protein: monoclonal IgG or IgA) c. Blood count and coagulation	• Plasma cells (single clone) • **Plasmacytoma:** – Single lesion – Electrophoresis is negative for M-protein – Marrow biopsy is negative for myeloma – Up to 60% of these patients will present myeloma in 5 y.	1. **Radiation therapy** 2. **Surgery** for mass effect symptoms or spine instability or plasmacytoma 3. **Chemotherapy** (may also be given intrathecally) 4. **Autologous stem cell transplant** **Prognosis:** Average life expectancy is 3 y (heterogeneous, varying from 1–10 y).

4.11 Langerhans Cell Histiocytosis (Table 4.11) G

Presentation/ demographics	Imaging/other diagnostics	Other	Treatment
a. **Unifocal (eosinophilic granuloma):** tender lytic bone lesion (usually parietal) that involves both skull tables *REMEMBER:* Possible dura involvement b. **Multifocal (uni- or multisystem):** • Various organs may be involved (bone, skin, lymph nodes, liver spleen, lung) • Associated with repeated respiratory infections 1. Children and young adults 2. **REMEMBER:** Diabetes insipidus is the most frequent initial sign of Langerhans cell histiocytosis in the CNS[27]	1. **CT:** hypodensity within bone destruction 2. **MRI:** a. Possibly thick infundibulum that enhances b. Rarely other brain Involvement 3. Consider **bone scan and PET scan** to stage disease and evaluate response to therapy	**Letterer–Siwe disease:** a. Fulminant histiocytosis b. Multiple organ involvement c. First years of life d. Fatal	1. **Surgical resection** of isolated bone lesions (remember involvement of dura) 2. Consider **radiation therapy** and **chemotherapy** for systemic involvement including stalk **Prognosis:** excellent for localized disease[28]

4.12 Pineal Tumors (Table 4.12a) Ⓖ

Tumor	Presentation/ demographics	Imaging/other diagnostics	Other	Treatment

	For all tumors described below:
	1. Hydrocephalus (obstructive)
	2. Gaze palsy and Parinaud's syndrome
		For all tumors described below:
		1. **MRI spine** (exclude drop metastases)
		2. **Lumbar puncture** for CSF markers (differential diagnosis)
		3. Consider **angiography** when surgical resection is indicated
				For all tumors described below:
				1. See treatment in tables:
				  • "Germ cell tumors"
				  • "Pineal region lesion treatment algorithm"
				2. Treat hydrocephalus if present

Pineocytoma (Grade I)	Children and young adults	**MRI:** a. A cyst may be present b. Enhancement (may be peripheral) c. Peripheral calcification		Surgical resection **Prognosis:** 5-y survival rate of 90%

Pineal parenchymal tumor of intermediate differentiation
(Grade II or III)
	1. Middle aged adults
	2. Rarely CSF seeding
		1. **MRI:**
		  a. *T1WI:* Iso- or hypointense
		  b. *T2WI:* isointense with gray matter (with small cystic foci)
		  c. Enhancing
		  d. Commonly extension in adjacent structures
		2. **CT:** hyperdense mass
				1. Surgical resection
				2. Radiation therapy

(Continued) ▶

Tumor	Presentation/demographics	Imaging/other diagnostics	Other	Treatment

Pineoblastoma (Grade IV) (is considered a PNET)	1. Children
	2. CSF seeding in almost 50%
	3. May metastasize
		1. MRI:
		  a. Usually iso- or hypointense on T2WI
		  b. Heterogeneous enhancement, necrosis, hemorrhage
		2. CT:
		  a. Hyperdense
		  b. Calcification
			Associated with:
			  a. Familial bilateral retinoblastoma ("trilateral retinoblastoma")
			  b. Familial adenomatous polyposis
				1. **Surgical resection**
				2. **Radiation therapy** (craniospinal) if age >3 y
				3. **Chemotherapy**
				Prognosis: median survival of 2 y

Papillary tumor of the pineal region (Grade II or III)	1. Children and young adults 2. Rare	**MRI:** moderate enhancement (heterogeneous)		1. **Surgical resection** 2. **Radiation therapy** (focal) **Prognosis:** 5-year survival rate of 70%

Pineal cyst: A glial cyst that is frequently an incidental finding. May present with hydrocephalus. Follow with MRI every year if cyst < 2 cm. Surgical resection for symptomatic lesion.

Note: See Table 4.12b for tumors in pineal location. Germ cell tumors are the most frequent in this region.

4.12.1 Germt Cell Tumors (Table 4.12b) G

Tumor	Presentation/demographics	Imaging/other diagnostics	Other	Treatment
For all tumors described below: all are malignant with the exception of mature teratomas	For all tumors described below: 1. **Midline mass:** a. Suprasellar b. Pineal region c. Contemporarily: "Synchronous germ cell tumor" 2. Usually seen in children and young adults with: a. *Suprasellar lesion:* • Visual deficits • Hypopituitarism • Diabetes insipidus b. *Pineal lesion:* • Hydrocephalus • Gaze palsy • Parinaud's syndrome 3. May present with precocious puberty because of LH (luteinizing hormone) effect of beta-human chorionic gonadotropin (β-hCG)	For all tumors described below: 1. Markers are in blood and CSF (perform lumbar puncture) 2. **MRI spine** to rule out drop metastases 3. Consider **angiography** when surgical resection is indicated for a pineal lesion	For all tumors described below: There is association with Down syndrome and also syndromes with additional X chromosome	For all tumors described below: **STEP 1** *Treat hydrocephalus,* try to avoid seeding: a. Consider endoscopic third ventriculostomy (may also allow for biopsy and CSF sampling) b. Consider temporary EVD instead of third ventriculostomy if: • Open surgical resection is an option • Planning radiation therapy and chemotherapy for germinoma (regression of tumor is expected in days) **STEP 2** *Biopsy:* a. Endoscopic b. Stereotactic c. Open (preferred by many because of risk of hemorrhage) Biopsy is the treatment choice for all lesions except for those with significant increase of alpha-fetoprotein (AFP) or β-hCG, indicating nongerminomatous germ cell tumor → proceed directly to surgical resection (step 3) **STEP 3** *Surgical resection:* a. For lesion with characteristics of teratoma on MRI and no significant elevation of AFP or β-hCG b. For nongerminomatous germ cell tumor (significant increase of AFP or β-hCG)

(Continued) ▲

Tumor	Presentation/ demographics	Imaging/other diagnostics	Other	Treatment
				STEP 4 **Radiation therapy and chemotherapy:** a. As the only treatment for germinoma b. As adjuvant therapy for nongermino- matous germ cell tumor **REMEMBER:** Markers are mainly useful in assessing response to treatment and recurrence
Germinoma		1. **Markers:** • *β-hCG:* positive in 10–50% • *AFP:* negative • *PLAP* (placental alkaline phosphatase): positive (when an isolated finding it is suggestive of germinoma) 2. **MRI brain:** • *T1WI:* isointense • *T2WI:* hypointense with enhancement 3. **CT brain:** hyperdense	**The most common:** a. Germ cell tumor b. Pineal tumor	1. **Radiation therapy** to entire neuraxis (30 Gy) and 15 Gy to primary site[29] 2. **Chemotherapy** **Prognosis:** 5-y survival rate is 90%
Embryonal carcinoma		Markers: • *β-hCG:* negative • *AFP:* positive • *PLAP:* negative	Nongerminomatous germ cell tumor	1. Surgical resection followed by 2. Radiation (craniospinal) and 3. Chemotherapy (bleomycin, vinblastine, cisplatin, carboplatin, etoposide) **Prognosis:** 5-y survival rate is 40–70%
Yolk sac tumor (endodermal sinus tumor)		Markers: • *β-hCG:* negative • *AFP:* positive (significantly elevated) • *PLAP:* negative	Nongerminomatous germ cell tumor	1. Surgical resection followed by 2. Radiation (craniospinal) and 3. Chemotherapy (bleomycin, vinblastine, cisplatin, carboplatin, etoposide) **Prognosis:** 5-y survival rate is 40–70%

Tumor	Presentation/demographics	Imaging/other diagnostics	Other	Treatment
Choriocarcinoma	Primary or metastatic	**Markers:** • *β-hCG:* positive • *AFP:* negative • *PLAP:* negative	1. Nongerminomatous germ cell tumor 2. Highly hemorrhagic	1. **Surgical resection** followed by 2. **Radiation** (craniospinal) and 3. **Chemotherapy** (bleomycin, vinblastine, cisplatin, carboplatin, etoposide) **Prognosis:** 5-y survival rate is 40–70%
Teratoma: • Mature teratoma (all 3 germ cell layers are fully differentiated) • Immature teratoma • Teratoma with malignant transformation		1. **Markers:** • *β-hCG:* negative • *AFP:* negative for mature and positive for immature subtype • *PLAP:* negative • *CEA:* possibly elevated 2. **MRI brain may present:** • Cysts • calcification (↓ T2WI signal) • fat (↑ T1WI signal) • irregular enhancement	1. Nongerminomatous germ cell tumor 2. **Characteristic feature:** presence of all 3 embryonic germ cell layers (endoderm, mesoderm, ectoderm)	a. **Mature teratoma:** Surgical resection confers excellent prognosis. b. **Immature teratoma:** 1. **Surgical resection** followed by 2. **Radiation therapy** (craniospinal) and 3. **Chemotherapy** (bleomycin, vinblastine, cisplatin, carboplatin, etoposide)

4.12.3 Pineal Region Lesion Treatment Algorithm (Table 4.12c) G

Step 1	Step 2	Tumor	Treatment
1. Serum/CSF markers: • β-hCG • AFP **REMEMBER:** • MRI spine • Treat hydrocephalus when present avoiding seeding if possible (consider 3rd ventriculostomy and EVD)	Consider **biopsy/resection:** • If either tumor marker (β-hCG, AFP) is positive (nongerminomatous germ cell tumor) or • If meningioma/primary pineal tumor is suspected **Surgical approaches to pineal region:** 1. **Occipital transtentorial:** preferred when the vein of Galen is inferiorly displaced. Be careful with retraction of occipital lobe! 2. **Supracerebellar infratentorial approach:** preferred when vein of Galen is superiorly displaced. 3. **Transventricular** (through posterior superior temporal gyrus): used when there is dilation of the ventricles and an eccentric lesion. Be very careful of venous injury!	**Meningioma** (velum interpositum; tumor may be heavily calcified) **Pineoblastoma** (usually displaces pineal calcium to periphery) **Pineocytoma** (usually displaces pineal calcium to periphery) **Nongerminomatous germ cell tumor** (usually engulfs pineal calcium)	**Surgery** is primary treatment 1. **Radiation** therapy (craniospinal) if age > 3 y 2. **Chemotherapy** **Prognosis:** median survival of 2 y **Surgery** is primary treatment **Prognosis:** 5-y survival rate of 90% 1. **Radiation therapy** (craniospinal) 2. **Chemotherapy** (bleomycin, vinblastine, cisplatin, carboplatin, etoposide) **Prognosis:** 5-y survival rate is 40–70%
	One may consider directly **radiation therapy:** • If both tumor markers (β-hCG, AFP) are negative (may also consider checking for PLAP) and • If germinoma is suspected	**If complete resolution:** It was likely a germinoma **If not:** It was likely mixed histology	Consider **chemotherapy** **Prognosis:** 5-y survival rate is 90% **Biopsy** **Prognosis:** Worse prognosis is expected

4.13 Pituitary Adenomas (Table 4.13) G

Tumor	Presentation/ demographics	Imaging/other diagnostics	Other	Treatment
		For all the above adenomas		

Prolactinoma	1. The most frequent adenoma (usually females): prevalence 30%
	2. Infertility:
	  a. *Males*: impotence, decreased libido, rarelygal actorrhea and gynecomastia
	  b. *Females*: amenorrhea, galactorrhea (Forbes–Albright syndrome)
	3. Bone loss
		1. **Workup:** see "For all the above adeno-mas" at the end of the table
		2. **Prolactin (PRL) levels:**
		  • *< 25 ng/mL*: normal/
		  • *25–150 ng/mL*: pituitary stalk compression (compression of stalk causes increased levels of **PRL** by loss of inhibition)
		  • *> 150 ng/mL*: prolactinoma
		  REMEMBER: when there is strong clinical suspicion but no hyperpro-lactinemia, consider "hook effect" (the excess of PRL impairs adequate immune complex formation with falsely low results). Ask for dilutions of the sample and recheck
		3. **Differential diagnosis of hyperprolactinemia:**
		  a. Pregnancy and lactation
		  b. Medication (dopamine receptor antagonists as phenothiazines and metoclopramide, tricyclic antidepressants, H² antagonists, verapamil, etc.)
		  c. Renal failure
		  d. Cirrhosis
		  e. Primary hypothyroidism
		  f. Empty sella syndrome
		  g. Macroprolactinemia (polymerization of PRL molecules of no clinical im-portance in asymptomatic patient).
			Arises from lactotrophs (cells)	*The only adenoma that may be cured without surgery!!*
				1. **Dopamine agonists** is the treatment of choice (results are expected in 6–8 wks):
				  a. *Bromocriptine (dopamine agonist)*: initial dose of 1.25 mg/d and gra-dually increase
				  Side effects: headache, nausea, and vomiting (self-resolving) REMEM-BER: there is risk of rapid growth when treatment is disrupted
				  b. *Cabergoline*: initial dose 0.25 mg, twice/wk and gradually increase (typically to 0.5–1 mg twice/wk)
				
				REMEMBER: target of treatment is PRL < 20 ng/mL. There is ~30% probability of normal PRL levels after discontinuation of dopamine agonists. Consider discon-tinuation of treatment with dopamine agonist (progressively), if the lesion is no longer visible on MRI. Close follow-up especially in the 1st year

Tumor	Presentation/ demographics	Imaging/other diagnostics	Other	Treatment
		For all the above adenomas		2. **Surgical excision** for: 　a. significant neurologic deficit (due to mass effect that has not resolved adequately or rapidly enough with dopamineagonist treatment. Most tumors shrink in size within 3–6 mo) 　b. no response/ no tolerance/ contraindication (certain psychiatric conditions) to medical treatment 　c. CSF leak because of tumor shrinkage 　*REMEMBER:* persistent post-op slight hyperprolactinemia may be due to stalk injury. Close follow-up with no treatment 3. **Radiation therapy** may (rarely) be considered when all the above had no result or are contraindicated.

Tumor	Presentation/demographics	Imaging/other diagnostics	Other	Treatment
		For all the above adenomas		
Adrenocorticotropic hormone (ACTH) adenoma (*AKA Cushing's disease*)	1. Cushing's disease (usually females): prevalence 10% 2. **Hypercortisolism** due to increased secretion of ACTH from the pituitary adenoma with subsequent: a. increased weight (frequently typical centripetal deposition of fat with "buffalo hump" and "moon facies") b. hypertension c. hyperglycemia d. hypokalemic alkalosis e. atrophy of skin with purple striae (trunk) and hyperpigmentation (ACTH has melanocyte-stimulating hormone cross-reactivity) f. depression, g. emotional lability h. fatigue (muscle wasting) i. hirsutism j. acne	**Workup:** 1. **MRI:** Usually microadenomas (lesion <1 cm) 2. **Histology:** Basophilic 3. **Lab tests:** • 8 a.m. serum cortisol levels • 24-h urine free cortisol 4. Consider **low-dose dexamethasone suppression test:** administer 1 mg dexamethasone orally at 11 p.m. and check serum cortisol at 8 a.m. next morning → cortisol >10 µg/dL is abnormal *In case of pituitary adenomas cortisol is not suppressed with low dose dexamethasone.*	1. Arises from corticotrophs 2. Most common cause of *Cushing's syndrome:* exogenous steroids	*A surgical disease!!* 1. **Transsphenoidal surgical resection** is the treatment of choice: • remission in 85% of microadenomas and 65% of macroadenomas • recurrence or persistence of symptoms are also treated with surgery (cure in 50–60% of cases). • Consider: a. ***Hemihypophysectomy***, if localization of lesion is difficult b. ***total hypophysectomy*** in selected persistent cases 2. **Radiation therapy** (fractionated radiotherapy or stereotactic radiosurgery) in patients who cannot tolerate surgery or in selected recurrent cases. *REMEMBER:* response evolves slowly (usually 1–2 y)

(Continued) ▲

Tumor	Presentation/demographics	Imaging/other diagnostics	Other	Treatment

For all the above adenomas

Presentation/demographics

3. **Nelson's syndrome:**
   a. Pituitary enlargement after bilateral adrenalectomy
   b. Increased ACTH
   c. Hyperpigmentation

4. **REMEMBER:** *similar symptoms may be caused by:*
   a. **Ectopic ACTH secretion** (as in certain tumors: small cell lung carcinoma, thymoma, carcinoid, medullary thyroid carcinoma and pheochromocytoma)
   b. Cortisol secretion by **adrenal tumor**
   c. **Corticotropin-releasing hormone (CRH) secretion** (hypothalamic or ectopic).

Imaging/other diagnostics

5. If ectopic ACTH secretion is suspected then:
   a. CT abdomen
   b. **High-dose dexamethasone suppression test:**
      i. Define baseline cortisol level at 8 a.m.
      ii. Administer 8 mg orally at 11 p.m. and recheck cortisol level at 8 a.m. next morning.
      iii. If cortisol levels after the test are reduced to < 50% of baseline → Cushing's disease (pituitary origin) vs. with ectopic secretion of ACTH/adrenal tumors, there will be no significant variation
      After high dexamethasone dose cortisol is suppressed in case of pituitary tumors, but is not suppressed in case of ectopic ACTH secretion.
   c. **CRH stimulation test:**
      0.1 µg/kg IV CRH will increase ACTH and cortisol only in Cushing's disease.
      After CRH stimulation, ACTH and cortisol levels increase in case of pituitary tumors, but do not increase in case of tumors with ectopic ACTH secretion.

Treatment

3. **Bilateral adrenalectomy:**
   • in intractable or life-threatening Cushing's disease (nonsatisfactory results with surgical excision of pituitary adenoma).
   • With adrenalectomy, *lifelong replacement* is needed including mineralocorticoids.
   • There is a 30% risk of Nelson's syndrome, which is treated with total hypophysectomy or radiation of the pituitary

4. **Medical treatment** (adjuvant therapy):
   a. **Ketoconazole** (antifungal that inhibits steroid synthesis in adrenal glands): 200–600 mg twice/day (75% of patients subsequently have normal cortisol levels).
   Side effects: hepatotoxicity (usually resolves after drug withdrawal)
   b. **Mitotane**
   c. **Metyrapone**

Tumor	Presentation/ demographics	Imaging/other diagnostics	Other	Treatment
		For all the above adenomas		
		6. **Bilateral inferior petrosal sinus sampling (BIPSS):** • Cushing's disease: ACTH in sinus to peripheral ACTH ratio > 1.4:1 • Sensitivity is increased with CRH stimulation. • BIPSS *can also lateralize the lesion* in pituitary gland (important for successful resection), but the presence of the circular sinus allows aspiration of sinus blood from the contralateral side. Consequently, this test is not highly specific. 7. **Assessment of the function of hypo-thalamic-pituitary-adrenal axis:** a. *Insulin tolerance test* (in a normal patient, hypoglycemia induced by insulin causes cortisol increment; consequently, cortisol increment may be expected to be normal under stress conditions) → Peak cortisol < 16 μg/dL means inadequate response and supplementary steroid treatment is needed b. *Cosyntropin test:* after stimulation with cosyntropin, a peak cortisol level > 18 μg/dL is normally expected. Otherwise cortisol reserve is not satisfactory		**Indicative of cure:** a. Morning cortisol of < 5 μg/dL on the first 2 postoperative days b. Morning cortisol < 8 μg/dL after low-dose dexamethasone suppression test on the 3rd postoperative day **REMEMBER:** If no treatment, the median survival is less than 5 y

(*Continued*) ▲

Tumor	Presentation/ demographics	Imaging/other diagnostics	Other	Treatment
		For all the above adenomas		

Growth hormone (GH) adenoma	• 2nd most frequent functional adenoma after prolactinoma (prevalence 15%)
	
	1. **Adults (usually males)** → **acromegaly:**
	  a. Frontal bossing, prognathism, hands and feet increase in size
	  b. Hypertension and cardiac abnormalities
	  c. Glucose intolerance
	  d. Macroglossia (soft tissue swelling)
	  e. Sleep apnea
	  f. Peripheral nerve entrapment
	  g. Colon cancer (there is significantly higher risk)
	2. **Children (before closure of epiphyseal plates)** → **gigantism**
		Workup:
		1. **MRI:** Usually macroadenomas (lesion >1 cm)
		2. **Histology:** acidophilic
		3. **Lab tests:**
		  i. *GH serum levels:* normal is < 5 ng/mL and secretion is pulsatile. Not the most reliable indicator of acromegaly.
		    REMEMBER: GH > 40 ng/mL is difficult to cure
		  ii. *IGF-1 (insulin-like growth factor 1 AKA somatomedin C) serum levels:* more specific and useful than GH levels. Normal values change based on age.
		4. **Oral glucose suppression test** (OGST; 75 g of oral glucose load):
		  • Lowest level of GH in the first 2 h should normally be < 1 ng/mL (otherwise patient suffers from acromegaly).
		  • Used primarily to monitor response to treatment than for diagnosis.
		5. **Colonoscopy** at the time of diagnosis and appropriate follow-up intervals after the diagnosis
		6. Evaluation by **cardiologist**
			Arises from somatotrophs	*A surgical disease!*
				1. **Transsphenoidal surgical resection** is the treatment of choice. Normal post-op values:
				  • Normal IGF-1
				  • GH < 5 ng/mL (baseline)
				  • GH < 1 ng/mL after glucose suppression test
				2. **Medical treatment** is not curative (supportive treatment in persistent cases):
				  a. *Octreotide* (somatostatin analog that also helps as preoperative treatment): 100μg three times/day (wait 4 wks for results).
				    Side effects: cholelithiasis, nausea, abdominal pain, diarrhea
				  b. **Dopamine agonists**
				  c. **GH antagonists** (Pegvisomant): not an initial treatment
				3. **Radiation therapy:** consider if the above fail

Tumor	Presentation/ demographics	Imaging/other diagnostics	Other	Treatment
		For all the above adenomas		

Thyroid-stimulating hormone (TSH) adenoma	1. The least frequent (prevalence is 1%)
	 2. **Secondary hyperthyroidism:**
	 • Palpitations
	 • Hyperactivity
	 • Anxiety
	 • No tolerance of heat
	 • Sweating
	 • Tremor
	 • Loss of weight
		Lab tests: Elevated T3/T4 with elevated or normal TSH (not reduced as expected)	Aggressive tumor	1. **Transsphenoidal surgical resection is** the treatment of choice
				 2. **Radiation therapy** for poor results after surgical excision
				 3. If the above fail, consider:
				   a. Octreotide
				   b. Bromocriptine
				 REMEMBER: TSH adenomas have the worst treatment outcome.

• Follicle-stimulating hormone (FSH) adenoma • Luteinizing hormone (LH) adenoma	1. Mass effect symptoms 2. Affected sexual and reproductive function	Lab tests: • FSH • LH • Testosterone • Estradiol levels		Transsphenoidal surgical resection is the treatment of choice

Nonfunctional adenoma (null cell)	1. 25% of adenomas
	 2. Incidental finding
	 3. Mass effect symptoms
	 4. pituitary insufficiency
				1. **Close follow-up in:**
				   a. All asymptomatic microadenomas
				   b. Stable asymptomatic macroadenomas
				 2. **Transsphenoidal surgical resection** in all other cases

(Continued) ▲

Tumor	Presentation/demographics	Imaging/other diagnostics	Other	Treatment
		For all the above adenomas		

	1. Pituitary adenomas represent 10 – 15% of **intracranial tumors.**
	2. Adults at the 3rd – 4th decade of life with **following presentation:**
	  a. *Incidental findings*
	  b. *Mass effect on* (if lesion is large):
	    • *Optic chiasm above sella:* bitemporal hemianopia
	    • *Prefixed optic chiasm:* homonymous hemianopia (optic tract compression)
		1. **MRI brain and pituitary:**
		  • *Normal pituitary gland* enhances early (lack of blood brain barrier), while the adenoma enhances in a delayed manner.
		  • *Neurohypophysis:* high intensity on T1WI
		  • *Stalk deviation* may help identify a side of a microadenoma
		  • If MRI is contraindicated, ask for a CT with contrast and coronal cuts
		2. **Evaluation of anterior pituitary gland function:**
		  a. PRL (midmorning)
		  b. GH
		  c. IGF-1 (more reliable than GH)
		  d. *8 a.m. cortisol* (best for detecting hypocortisolism):
		    • >14 µg/dL is normal
		    • < 6 µg/dL indicates hypocortisolism
			1. They arise from adenohypophysis
			2. Microadenoma if lesion < 1 cm
			3. Preoperative diabetes insipidus should question on the diagnosis of adenoma
				1. **Replacement hormone** treatment when appropriate based on endocrinologic evaluation:
				  • Always correct cortisol levels first before administration of thyroid hormones (risk of adrenal crisis)
				  • *Need for cortisol replacement* may be clarified by:
				    – Cosyntropin stimulation
				    – Discontinuing steroids for 24–48 h and checking cortisol levels (6 a.m.): >10 µg/dL is considered normal
				  • *Normal cortisol replacement dose:* 20 mg hydrocortisone in the morning and 10 mg in the evening. Increase dose when patient is under stressful condition
				  • Consider **thyroid and testosterone replacement**

Tumor	Presentation/ demographics	Imaging/other diagnostics	Other	Treatment

For all the above adenomas

Presentation/demographics:

- *Postfixed optic chiasm:* loss of vision in ipsilateral eye (compression of optic nerve) and superior temporal quadrantanopia in contralateral eye (anterior Wil- brand's knee)
- Symptoms from *CN III, IV, V1, V2, VI compression*
- Proptosis or chemosis (invasion of cavernous sinus)
- Rarely obstructive hydrocephalus
- c. *Pituitary gland insufficiency* (affecting the pituitary hormones with following order: GH > FSH, LH > TSH > ACTH) REMEMBER: In single hormone deficiency, think of autoimmune hypophysitis (frequently ACTH or ADH deficiency and thickening of the stalk).
- d. *Symptoms from the over-secretion of the corresponding hormone* as described above (65% of adenomas are functional)
- e. *Headache*
- f. *CSF rhinorrhea*

Imaging/other diagnostics:

- e. 24 h urine free cortisol (the best for detecting hypercortisolism)
- f. ACTH
- g. TSH, T3, T 4 h. FSH,LH
- h. Testosterone (males)
- i. Estradiol (females)
- j. Blood glucose (fasting): will be reduced in hypoadrenalism
2. **Visual fields** (for macroadenomas compressing optic chiasm)
3. Consider **CT chest/abdomen** if an ectopic secretion is suspected
4. **Histology:**
   - a. *Basophilic:* ACTH, TSH, and FSH/LH adenomas
   - b. *Acidophilic:* GH, PRL adenomas
   - c. *Chromophobic:* Null cell, PRL adenomas

Treatment:

2. **Surgery:**
   - Indicated for all symptomatic lesions causing mass effect symptoms or endocrinologic dysfunction with the exception of prolactinomas)
   - *Surgical approaches:*
     - a. *Transsphenoidal:* microscopic or endoscopic (the latter offers improved visualization, minimal invasiveness, less complicati- on,and reduced hospital stay but has a steep learning curve)[31]
     - b. *Transcranial* (in significant suprasellar or middle fossa expansion or after failed trans- sphenoidal surgery):
       - – Subfrontal
       - – Subtemporal
       - – Pterional (right side unless coexistent pathology on left or worse left eye function or mainly left extension of tumor)
       - – Orbitozygomatic
       - – Anterior transcallosal
   - *Post-op complications include:*
     - a. *Pituitary insufficiency:* treat with replacement therapy

(Continued) ▶

Tumor	Presentation/ demographics	Imaging/other diagnostics	Other	Treatment
		For all the above adenomas		

g. **Pituitary apoplexy:** hemorr-hagic necrosis of a pituitary adenoma *presenting with:*
- sudden headache
- pituitary insufficiency
- neurologic deficit
- altered mental status
- symptoms similar to subarachnoid hemorrhage (SAH; when blood is in chiasmatic cistern)
- hydrocephalus
- hypothalamic symptoms.

Treatment:
- Steroids
- Early transsphenoidal decompression for patients with significant neuro-ophthalmological deficits

Prognosis: Frequently excellent recovery.[30]

b. *Diabetes insipidus:*
- Diagnosis: Urine output > 250 mL for 1–2 h and specific gravity < 1.005 frequently with accompa-nying elevation of serum sodium
- Treatment:
  i. Try fluid replacement.
  ii. When replacement with IV/oral fluids is not sufficient, adminis-ter desmopressin SQ/IV (2–4 µg) twice/day (or 10 times this dose intranasally, if nasal packs have been removed) or vasopressin.
- Patterns of diabetes insipidus:
  i. Transient (up to 36 h post-op)
  ii. Prolonged (rarely permanent but may take months to normalize)
  iii. *"Triphasic response":*
     • Diabetes insipidus of short duration (injury to neurohy-pophysis)
     • Normalization or SIADH (ADH deposits are released from hypothalamus); risk of severe hyponatremia, if there has been overtreatment in previous phase
     • Diabetes insipidus of long duration

c. *CSF leak* (may also be the result of medical treatment of prolactinoma)

Tumor	Presentation/ demographics	Imaging/other diagnostics	Other	Treatment
	2. Pituitary adenomas may **secret two different hormones** (frequently PRL and GH) 3. They may rarely be **invasive** (usually prolactino- mas) 4. There is **association with MEN syndromes**	*For all the above adenomas*		3. **Radiation therapy** (40–50 Gy in 4–6wks): • Consider when medical and surgical options have been exhausted.[32] • Response evolves slowly. • *Complications include* pituitary insufficiency and vision worsening (progressively in years)

- **Empty sella syndrome:**
  - a. *Primary* (diaphragma sella is incompletely developed andarachnoid expands into the sella)
  - b. *Secondary* (after surgery, radiation, intrapartum is chemicnecrosis: Sheehan's syndrome)
  - *If symptomatic*, usually visual deficit due to chiasmatic herniation, consider surgical correction by "pushing up" chiasm with fat graft
- **Rathke's cleft cyst:** Remnant of craniopharyngeal duct in females aged 30–40 y with frequent suprasellar expansion. May present rim enhancement on MRI
- **Pituitary carcinoma:**
  - a rare entity that may secrete various hormones (most frequently ACTH, PRL) and metastasize
  - ~35% survival at 1 y even with surgery, radiation therapy, and chemotherapy

4.14 Craniopharyngioma (Table 4.14) G

Presentation/ demographics	Imaging other diagnostics	Other	Treatment
1. **Grade I:** a benign tumor with aggressive behavior 2. 4% of brain tumors 3. Typically pediatric patients (5–15 y) and a second peak for adults at 50 y of age 4. **Presenting with:** • Headache • Visual field defect • *Panhypopituitarism:* – GH deficiency (frequently short stature in children) – Hypothyroidism – Adrenal insufficiency – Diabetes insipidus	1. **MRI:** • Usually suprasellar (in 70% of cases) lesion • Solid and cystic part • Hyperintense on T1WI (if high cholesterol content in cyst) and on T2WI • Contrast enhancement • Edema may be present along the optic tracts. 2. **CT:** calcification (almost always in children and less frequently in adults) 3. **Differentiate from Rathke's cleft cyst,** which has only a thin rim of enhancement around cyst wall without solid component 4. **Endocrinologic evaluation** similar to pituitary adenomas 5. **Histology subtypes:** a. Adamantinomatous (cystic: children) b. Papillary (solid: adults)	Derives from Rathke's pouch epithelium	1. **Preoperative endocrinologic evaluation** 2. **Surgical resection** is the treatment of choice when safely possible a. *Approaches:* • Transsphenoidal (*not* if the tumor is lateral to the carotid) • Transcallosal • Pterional • Subfrontal b. *Be careful of* intraoperative hypothalamic injury, optic chiasm ischemia (major blood supply is from below) and postoperative diabetes insipidus. 3. ***Stereotactic biopsy and cyst aspiration*** has also been applied instead of surgery for lesions with significant hypo-thalamic involvement and large cystic part. This also allows for a higher prescription dose on subsequent radiation therapy because it reduces the lesion dimension.[33] 4. **Radiation therapy** for residual tumor (postpone in children) 5. **Intratumoral bleomycin** for cystic craniopharyngiomas has been tried but there are no definitive conclusions about the effectiveness.[34] **Prognosis:** • 5-y survival rate of 75%. • *Recurrence is:* – 20% for tumor <5 cm – 85% for >5 cm – MIB-1 >7% is predictive of recurrence

4.15 Cerebral Metastases (Table 4.15) G

Primary tumor	Presentation/demographics	Imaging/other diagnostics	Treatment
Lung (45% of cerebral metastases, most frequent): a. Small cell ("oat cell") b. Non-small-cell (adenocarcinoma, squamous cell, bronchoalveolar and large cell)	1. **Small cell:** • Younger patients (compared to non-small-cell). Typically with history of cigarette smoking • The tumor most commonly associated with Lambert–Eaton myasthenic syndrome (frequently precedes the diagnosis of cancer) 2. Frequently the primary lung tumor is discovered after the metastasis 3. Commonly metastases are multiple		a. **Small cell:** • is very radiosensitive. ***Whole brain radiation*** is administered prophylactically even in absence of visible lesion to reduce disease relapses in the brain • ***Prognosis:*** survival is 6–10 mo b. **Non-small-cell:** • ***Prognosis:*** slightly better than small cell cancer
Breast (10% of cerebral metastases, 2nd in frequency)	1. **Increased risk for brain metastases in**[35]**:** a. Younger age b. High-grade lesions c. Hormone receptor negative d. >4 metastatic lymph nodes e. Human epidermal growth factor (HER-2) positive f. Triple-negative breast cancer (estrogen receptors + progesterone receptors + HER-2 negative) 2. **REMEMBER:** a brain metastasis from breast cancer can occur even several years after successful treatment of primary lesion		Prognosis: • Depends on the breast cancer subtype (triple-negative breast cancer having the worst). • ***Survival*** is approximately 12–18 mo

(Continued) ▲

Primary tumor	Presentation/demographics	Imaging/other diagnostics	Treatment

Melanoma	1. Invades pia/arachnoid
	2. Typically hemorrhagic
	3. Most commonly, metastases are multiple
		1. **CT brain:** hyperdense lesion
		2. **Positive for:**
		  • S-100
		  • HMB-45
		  • Microphthalmia transcription factor
			1. **Radiation therapy** is part of the treatment although melanoma is a radioresistant tumor
			2. **Chemotherapy** (dacarbazine, temozolomide)
			3. **Immunotherapy** (ipilimumab)
			
			Prognosis: survival of 3–4 mo

Renal cell (hypernephroma)			**Radiation therapy** has poor results (radioresistant tumor) **Prognosis:** survival of 6–9 mo
Gastrointestinal carcinoma (esophageal, gastric, liver, pancreatic, colorectal)	Rare		**Prognosis:** survival of 6–12 mo

For all of the above metastases

Primary tumor	Presentation/demographics	Imaging/other diagnostics	Treatment
	1. Cerebral metastases are the most common brain tumors in clinical practice and may be the presenting symptom in 15% of cancer patients.	**Workup**	1. **Medical treatment:**
	2. When neurological symptoms are present, 70% of patients will be diagnosed with multiple lesions on MRI brain	1. **MRI brain with contrast:**	a. *Dexamethasone* for symptomatic cerebral edema
	3. A solitary posterior fossa lesion in an adult is considered metastasis until proven otherwise	• Multiple lesions may be revealed in 20% of patients with single lesion on CT brain.	b. *Anticonvulsants* for:
	4. **Carcinomatous meningitis:**	• Lesion is typically in gray-white matter junction (supratentorial frontal or parietal)	• Supratentorial lesions in patients with history of seizures
	• Patient with history of cancer and onset of multiple cranial nerve dysfunction or/and hydrocephalus (most frequently associated with breast cancer, lung cancer melanoma).	• significant edema (disproportionate to size of lesion)	• First postoperative week after craniotomy
	• Lumbar puncture aids diagnosis when there is no contraindication.	2. Consider **MRS** (↓ creatinine, ↑ lipid and lactate)	2. Consider **surgical resection** for:
	• *Treatment:*	3. **CT chest-abdomen and pelvis** for identification of primary lesion and staging	a. Patients with Karnofsky's Performance Scale >70 and controlled systemic disease
	a. Radiation therapy	4. **PET scan or bone scan** may also be needed.	b. Up to three intracranial accessible and symptomatic lesions
	b. Chemotherapy	Tumors with predilection for bone:	c. Life-threatening lesion
	Prognosis is poor: < 6 mo survival	a. Prostate	*Surgical resection provides tissue for biopsy and immediate resolution of mass effect symptoms.*
		b. Breast	3. **Biopsy** for:
		c. Thyroid	a. Lesion with no indication for surgical resection AND
		d. Kidney	b. Unknown primary tumor
		e. Lung	4. **Radiation therapy options:**
		5. PSA (men)	a. Whole brain radiation (30 Gy in 10 fractions over 2 wks)
		6. Mammogram (women)	b. Stereotactic radiosurgery
			c. Local fractionated

(Continued) ▲

Primary tumor	Presentation/demographics	Imaging/other diagnostics	Treatment

		(For all of the above metastases)	• Radiation therapy in one of above forms is practically always indicated[36,37]
			• ***Very radiosensitive tumors:*** small cell lung cancer, germ cell tumors, lymphoma, multiple myeloma
			a. ***Whole brain radiation:***
			   • After surgical resection of single lesion (prevents recurrence and patients are less likely to die from neurological causes)
			   • For multiple lesions (independently of surgery)
			     There are significant neurocognitive side effects.
			b. ***Stereotactic radiosurgery*** is an option instead of surgical resection in case of:
			   • Up to 4 asymptomatic or non accessible lesions
			   • Lesions size <3 cm
			   • In radioresistant tumors
			It may be used combined with surgical resection to the postsurgical resection margin to reduce local recurrence or avoid the use of whole brain radiation.
			Contraindications:
			   a. Hemorrhage
			   b. Significant edema
			2. **Chemotherapy:** usually no indication except for small cell lung cancer, breast cancer, melanoma, choriocarcinoma
			
			REMEMBER: Surgical resection + whole brain radiation is superior to stereotactic biopsy + whole brain radiation regarding recurrence, survival and functional status.[38] Consequently, surgically resect single accessible metastases. Consider the alternative or addition of stereotactic radiosurgery.
			Average median survival:
			   a. With corticosteroids only: 1–2 mo
			   b. With whole brain radiation only: 6 mo

4.16 Other Lesions (Table 4.16) G

Lesion	Presentation/ demographics	Imaging/other diagnostics	Other	Treatment

Colloid cyst or neuroepithelial cyst	1. Adult presenting with **obstructive hydrocephalus** (dilation of lateral ventricles because of periodic obstruction of foramina of Monro)
	2. **Symptomatic acute raise of ICP** (due to the movement of the cyst and ball-valve mechanism):
	• Headache
	• Gait disturbance
	• Nausea/vomit
	• Vision disturbance
	• Papilledema
	3. Sudden death has been described
		1. **MRI brain:**
		• No significant enhancement
		• Lesion in anterior roof of third ventricle (between the columns of the fornices) blocking foramina of Monro.
		• *T1WI:* hyperintense
		• *T2WI:* hypointense
		2. **CT brain:** 2/3 are hyperdense
		3. May present in other locations
			Benign	**Surgery** for patients with dilation of ventricular system and symptoms (usually cysts > 7 mm).
				
				Approaches:
				• Transcallosal
				• Transcortical/ transventricular:
				  – consider when there is hydrocephalus
				  – higher morbidity (particularly relating to post-op seizures) when compared to transcallosal.[39]
				• Endoscopic
				
				Surgical technique: open microsurgery (superior extent of resection and decreased rate of recurrence) vs. *endoscopic resection* (lower complication rate). Similar results for both regarding mortality and shunt dependency.[39]

(Continued) ▲

219

Lesion	Presentation/ demographics	Imaging/other diagnostics	Other	Treatment

Epidermoid cyst	1. 1% of tumors
	2. Intracranial or intraspinal (may follow lumbar puncture)
	3. *Anatomic location:*
	  a. CPA (50%)
	  b. Suprasellar
	  c. Intraventricular
	  d. Thalamic
	  e. Intradiploic (extradural)
	4. Recurrent episodes of aseptic meningitis (Mollaret's)
		1. **MRI brain:**
		  • No enhancement
		  • Same intensity as CSF on T1WI and T2WI
		  • *DWI:* restricted diffusion
		  • *FLAIR:* hyperintense to CSF (allows for differential diagnosis from arachnoid cysts that follow CSF in all sequences)
		2. **Histology:** stratified squamous epithelium + keratin + cholesterol
			Both epidermoid and dermoid cysts are:
			1. Benign (but may rarely transform to squamous cell carcinoma)
			2. Formed by inclusion of ectodermal elements during neural tube closure
			3. Present linear growth
				Surgical resection:
				  a. Pursue gross total resection but do not try to remove the capsule if it adheres to critical structures such as the brainstem
				  b. The contents of the cyst should not be released in CSF intraoperatively to avoid meningitis
				  c. Perioperative steroids may reduce the incidence of meningitis.

Dermoid cyst	1. 0.3% of brain tumors
	2. Intracranial or intraspinal (there is association with dermal sinus tract). May also be acquired (due to lumbar puncture, trauma)
	3. **Anatomic location:** midline (fourth ventricle, parasellar, interhemispheric)
	4. Associated with bacteria (septic)
		1. **MRI brain:**
		  • typically hyperintense on T1WI and generally similar to fat
		  • No contrast enhancement
		2. **Histology:** Sebaceous or sweat glands, hair follicles, teeth and cholesterol may be included in the lesion
			1. Arises from remnants of notochord along neuraxis
			2. Locally aggressive
				Surgical resection: see epirdemoid cyst treatment (Table 4.16: epidermoid cyst treatment)

Chordoma	Adult presenting with painful osteolytic lesion:
	  a. **40% in clivus** (cranial nerve palsies)
	  b. **60% in sacrum** (presents with pain, sphincter or nerve roots dysfunction)
		1. **MRI:** typically hyperintense on T2WI (because of the cartilaginous component)
		2. **Histology:** physaliphorous cells surrounded by mucin
				1. **Surgical resection:** en block removal (to prevent metastases)
				2. **Proton beam radiation or high-dose radiation therapy** (it is radioresistant)
				
				Prognosis:
				  • Recurrence rate of 85% and metastases in approximately 15%
				  • median survival of 6 y

4.17 General Medical Treatment for Brain Tumors (Table 4.17 🔊) ⏎ G

Medication	To remember

Dexamethasone[40]	1. **Indicated** in patients with:
	• Symptomatic peritumoral edema
	• CNS lymphoma
	• Carcinomatous meningitis
	• Tumor-associated pain
	2. **Dosage:**
	  a. *Acute clinical deterioration:*
	    • *Adults:* 10 mg IV loading followed by 6–10 mg every 6 h (can also be administered every 4 h if needed). If a patient is already receiving steroid treatment, then consider increasing the dose ×2 (double dose)
	    • *Children:* 0.5–1 mg/kg IV loading, followed by 0.25–0.5 mg/kg/d every 6 h (prolonged treatment should be avoided)
	  b. *Maintenance (adults):* 4–24 mg/d in divided doses
	3. Improvement in 24–48 h
	4. **Side effects** correlate with dosage and duration of treatment (most common is myopathy after 9-12th week of treatment. Persistent hiccups may also develop and are treated with chlorpromazine.
	5. Coadministration of common anticonvulsants (phenytoin, carbamazepine, phenobarbital) induces the hepatic metabolism of dexamethasone (higher doses of steroids may be needed)

Anticonvulsants	1. Do not administer[41]: • If there is no history of seizures • For posterior fossa lesions 2. In case of surgery, give prophylaxis, but discontinue 1 wk after the craniotomy, if no seizures occurred 3. Consider levetiracetam followed by lacosamide or valproic acid (they can also be combined with levetiracetam if monotherapy is insufficient) 4. Anticonvulsants may interact with steroids, chemotherapy, tyrosine-kinase inhibitors

4.18 Magnetic Resonance Spectroscopy (Table 4.18)

Disease	Choline (Cho): elevated in increased cell membrane turnover	NAA (N-acetylaspartate): diminished in neuronal, axonal dysfunction	Lactate (lac): not present in normal brain (indicates hypoxia)	Creatinine (Cr): useful as reference for choline	Lipid (lip)	Remember
Primary tumor *Ratios:* a. *Elevated:* • Cho/NAA • Cho/Cr b. *Decreased* NAA/Cr (except for low-grade gliomas)	↑		↑		↑	Gliomas: Cho is progressively higher with increasing grade but in grade IV may appear lower than expected (because of necrosis)
Metastasis *MRI:* lesions in gray-white matter, frequently multiple		↓	↑	↓	↑	
Radiation necrosis *Differential diagnosis* **with tumor recurrence**						
Demyelinating disease *Ratio:* decreased NAA/Cr		↓	↑			Bland pattern
Stroke	↓		↑	↓	↑	Lactate peak is the most typical finding
Abscess *MRI:* • Ring enhancement • Diffusion restriction	↓	↓	↑	↓		Atypical peaks (e.g., succinate)

1. All ratios are decreased (in radiation necrosis): Cho/Cr, NAA/Cr, Cho/Cho-n (Cho-n: choline peak in contralateral normal brain)
2. Radiation necrosis presents with low choline while tumor presents with high choline
3. Also consider *PET* (positron emission tomography): using [18F]-fluorodeoxyglucose, decreased glucose metabolism is expected in radiation necrosis as opposed to increased metabolism in tumor recurrence
4. Consider *SPECT* if PET is not available: decreased radiolabeled amphetamine uptake in radiation necrosis as opposed to tumor

4.19 Differential Diagnosis (Based on Anatomic Location of Lesion) (Table 4.19) G

Anatomic location	Mnemonic	Lesion
Single enhancing (supratentorial lesion)		1. **Tumor:** <ul><li>Primary</li><li>Metastasis</li></ul> 2. **Tumor like:** <ul><li>Abscess or cerebritis</li><li>Radiation necrosis</li><li>Subacute hematoma</li><li>Subacute infarct</li><li>Contusion</li><li>Tumefactive demyelination</li><li>Thrombosed giant aneurysm</li></ul> **Ring-enhancing (most common):** <ul><li>Metastasis</li><li>High grade glioma</li><li>Abscess</li><li>Lymphoma</li></ul> **Cystic with enhancing mural nodule:** <ul><li>Pilocytic astrocytoma</li><li>Hemangioblastoma (typically infratentorial)</li><li>Ganglioglioma</li><li>Neurocysticercosis</li></ul>
Intraventricular	C E N T R A L M S	• Choroid plexus papilloma • Ependymoma • Neurocytoma • Tuberous sclerosis/ Teratoma • Rule out infection • Astrocytoma (giant) • Lymphoma • Meningioma • Subependymoma
Suprasellar	S A T C H M O	• Suprasellar extension of pituitary lesion • Aneurysm • Teratoma/ Germinoma • Craniopharyngioma/ Cyst (Rathke's) • Hamartoma • Meningioma • Optic glioma
Corpus callosum		• Tumefactive multiple sclerosis • Lipoma • Lymphoma • Metastasis
Posterior fossa		1. **Adult:** <ul><li>Metastasis</li><li>Hemangioblastoma</li></ul> 2. **Children:** <ul><li>Ependymoma</li><li>Medulloblastoma</li><li>Pilocytic astrocytoma</li><li>Choroid plexus papilloma</li><li>Brainstem glioma</li></ul>

4.20 Various Things to Remember (Table 4.20)

Highly radiosensitive tumors	1. Small cell lung cancer 2. Lymphoma 3. Germinoma 4. Ependymoma
Hemorrhagic tumors	Choriocarcinoma > Renal Cancer > Melanoma
Tumors of temporal lobe frequently associated with seizures	1. DNET 2. Ganglioglioma 3. Pilocytic astrocytoma
Meningeal carcinomatosis	**Presentation:** 1. Patient with history of cancer presenting with hydrocephalus nonattributable to the anatomic location of tumor 2. Meningismus 3. Sciatica 4. Multiple cranial nerve palsy **Diagnosis:** 1. First lumbar puncture has a 50% sensitivity 2. Second has a 70% sensitivity 3. Third has a 90% sensitivity **Treatment:** 1. *Methotrexate* (can also be used prophylactically in lymphoma/leukemia) 2. *Radiation therapy* (specific sites may be radiated for symptom relief) **Prognosis:** Survival < 4 mo

4.21 Tumors and Syndromes (Table 4.21) ᴳ

Syndrome	Presentation/tumors	Imaging/other diagnostics	Other	Treatment

Neurofibromatosis type I (NF1)
 	
AKA von Recklinghausen's disease
	1. First degree relative suffering from the syndrome
	2. Two **Lisch nodules** (pigmented iris hamartomas)
	3. 6 **café au lait spots** (> 0.5 cm in children and > 1.5 cm in adults)
	4. Inguinal, axillary **freckling**
	5. 2 **neurofibromas** (grade I tumor). Usually presents as cutaneous nodule
	6. One **plexiform neurofibroma** (pathognomonic variant with malignant potential)
	7. **Bony dysplasia**
	8. **Optic glioma**
	NF1 **is associated with:**
	• Spinal astrocytoma
	• Kyphoscoliosis
	• Malignant tumors and pheochromocytoma
		See "presentation/ tumors": 2 out of 8 are necessary for diagnosis	1. **Autosomal dominant** but can also be sporadic (chromosome 17).
			2. **Responsible gene:** neurofibromin
			3. 1:3,000 births (it is the most common neurocutaneous disorder)
				1. **Surgery** for symptomatic, accessible lesions
				2. Consider **radiation therapy** when an intracranial lesion cannot be resected
				3. When a plexiform neurofibroma transforms to **malignant peripheral sheath tumor:**
				  a. Surgery
				  b. Radiation therapy to operative site
				  c. Chemotherapy for metastases

Syndrome	Presentation/tumors	Imaging/other diagnostics	Other	Treatment

Neurofibromatosis type 2 (NF2)
 	
AKA Multiple Inherited Schwannoma Meningioma Ependymoma ("MISME")
	1. Bilateral **vestibular schwannomas**
	2. Diagnosed relative + one Schwannoma
	3. First-degree relative PLUS:
	  a. Unilateral vestibular schwannoma at age < 30 y
	    OR
	  b. 2 out of following 5:
	    • Schwannoma
	    • Meningioma
	    • Neurofibroma
	    • Glioma
	    • Juvenile posterior subcapsular lenticular opacity
	
	NF2 **is associated with:**
	  a. *Neoplastic lesions:*
	    • Spinal Schwannoma
	    • Ependymoma
	  b. *Non neoplastic lesions:*
	    • Meningioangiomatosis
	    • Glial hamartoma
		1. See "Presentation / tumors": (1) OR (2) OR (3) are necessary for **diagnosis**
		2. **Screening process:**
		  a. *Ophthalmologic* evaluation (annually)
		  b. *Neurologic* evaluation (annually)
		  c. *Skin* inspection
		  d. *Brain MRI* every 2 y (age 10–20 y) and every 3 y (age 20–40 y)
		  e. Spine MRI every 3 y
			1. **Autosomal dominant** but can also be sporadic (chromosome 22).
			2. **Responsible gene:** schwannomin
			3. 1:40,000 births
			4. Consider the syndrome in a patient diagnosed at young age with vestibular schwannoma
			5. Neurofibromas are rare compared to NF1
				1. **Surgery** for symptomatic, accessible lesions
				2. Consider **early surgery** for a vestibular schwannoma in order to preserve hearing *unless* hearing is already unilaterally lost. In this case be more conservative with removing the contralateral lesion on the side with intact hearing.
				3. Consider *radiosurgery* when indicated
				
				REMEMBER: Growth of vestibular schwannomas may be accelerated in pregnancy

Syndrome	Presentation/tumors	Imaging/other diagnostics	Other	Treatment
von HippelLindau (VHL)	1. Relative with disease 2. **Hemangioblastoma** (usually multiple: cerebellum and retina are the most frequent locations) 3. **Optic angioma** 4. **Pheochromocytoma** 5. **Renal carcinoma** (the most common malignant tumor in the syndrome and the most common cause of death) VHL is **associated with:** • Endolymphatic sac tumors • Epididymal and broad ligament cystadenomas • Pancreatic neuroendocrine tumors	1. See "Presentation/ tumors": 2 out of 5 are necessary for **diagnosis** 2. **Screening:** a. *Pediatric patients:* • Ophthalmological evaluation • Catecholamine levels (24 h urine test) b. *Adolescents:* the above AND: • CT abdomen • MRI brain + spine c. *Adults:* the above AND ENT evaluation	1. Autosomal dominant (chromosome 3) 2. **Responsible gene:** pVHL	1. **Surgery** for symptomatic, accessible lesions 2. For retinal angiomas, early diagnosis and treatment with **laser photocoagulation and cryotherapy** may allow the patient to maintain vision (retinal angiomas carry the risk of retinal detachment, glaucoma, blindness) 3. **Radiation therapy** when indicated

(Continued) ▲

Syndrome	Presentation/tumors	Imaging/other diagnostics	Other	Treatment

Tuberous sclerosis
 	
AKA Bourneville's disease
	1. Three or more **ash - leaf spots** (hypomelanotic macules seen with Wood's lamp)
	2. **Subependymal giant cell astrocytomas** (usually in proximity to foramen of Monro)
	3. **Cortical/subcortical tubers** (hamartomatous lesions that can be epileptogenic foci)
	4. **Facial angiofibroma**
	5. **Ungual fibroma**
	6. **Shagreen patch** (connective tissue nevi usually on lower back)
	7. Multiple retinal nodular **hamartomas**
	8. **Heart** (rhabdomyomas) / kidney (angiomyolipoma)
	9. **Lymphangioleiomyomatosis Vogt triad:**
	  a. Mental retardation
	  b. Adenoma sebaceum
	  c. Seizures
		1. See "Presentation / tumours": 2 out of 8 are necessary for diagnosis
		2. **Intracerebral calcifications are common**
			1. **Autosomal dominant or sporadic**
			2. **Responsible genes:**
			  a. TSC1 (hamartin on chromosome 9)
			  b. TSC2 (tuberin on chro mosome 16).
			
			One gene mutation is enough.
			
			3. 1:6,000 births
				1. **Anticonvulsant medication**
				2. **Surgery for:**
				  a. symptomatic subependymal giant cell astrocytomas
				  b. pharmacoresistant epilepsy and identifiable seizure focus (usually cortical tubers)

Syndrome	Presentation/tumors	Imaging/other diagnostics	Other	Treatment

Sturge – Weber
 	
AKA encephalotrigeminal angiomatosis
	1. **Seizures** (usually initially partial motor, but they tend to progress to generalized)
	2. **Facial angioma** in V1 > V2 distribution (port-wine stain)
	3. **Eye involvement:**
	  a. Glaucoma
	  b. Iris heterochromia
	  c. Strabismus
	  d. Visual field defect
	  e. Episcleral, conjunctival angiomas
	  f. Retinal detachment
	4. **Mental retardation**
	5. **Neurological deficits**
	6. **Vein abnormalities:**
	  a. Reduced cortical veins
	  b. Large deep cerebral veins
	  c. Parieto-occipital leptomeningeal venous angiomatosis
		1. **Tram-track sign** of cortical and subcortical calcification.
		2. **Cortical atrophy** (usually occipital lobes)
			1. Vast majority is **sporadic**. May be associated with recessive inheritance on chromosome 3
			2. **Facial angioma:**
			  a. When in upper and lower eyelids, it is associated with parieto-occipital leptomeningeal venous angiomatosis
			  b. When bilateral, it is associated with seizures
				1. **Anticonvulsants**
				2. **Surgery** for pharmaco-resistant epilepsy
				3. Avoid laser surgery for facial nevus (consider skin colored tattoo)

Wyburn–Mason
 	
AKA Bonnet–Dechaume–Blanc
	1. **AVMs:**
	  • intracranially (mid-brain)
	  • in visual pathways (retina)
	  • face
	2. Facial vascular nevus
	3. Association with SAH
	4. Headache, seizures, visual disturbance
			Rare neurocutaneous disorder	Consider on an individual basis:
				1. **Surgery**
				2. **Embolization**
				3. **Radiation therapy**

4.22 Cases

4.22.1 Glioblastoma

Chief complaint/History of present illness	• A 60 y/o man presents to the ER with a 4-week history of worsening headaches and difficulty with speech.
	• His past medical history is remarkable only for lupus erythematosus.
Physical examination	• Unremarkable except for difficulty with speech.

Imaging

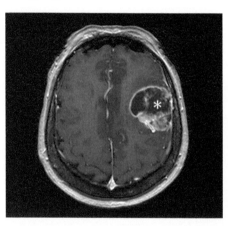

MRI brain (T1 with gadolinium) shows an intra- axial brain lesion (*asterisk*) located in the left frontal lobe with inhomogeneous enhancement with cystic and solid component.

1. **What is your differential diagnosis based on the MRI appearance?**
   Metastasis, high-grade glioma, abscess, lymphoma, tumor-like (radiation necrosis, hematoma, infarct, contusion, tumefactive demyelination, thrombosed giant aneurysm. (See Table 4.19).

2. **What further imaging studies would you like to obtain?**
   • MR spectroscopy (MRS) of brain (assesses the chemical composition of the lesion and can help narrow the differential diagnosis).
   • Metastatic workup (CT chest, abdomen and pelvis).
   • Functional MRI (fMRI, to assess the proximity of speech and motor areas to the tumor).
   • DTI (to assess the relation of the tumor with the white matter tracts).

3. **If this is a primary high-grade glioma, what do you expect to find on MRS?**
   MRS findings for high-grade glioma are: ↑ Choline (Cho), ↓ N-acetyl aspartate (NAA), ↑ Cho/NAA, ↑ Cho/Cr, ↓ NAA/Cr, ↑ lactate, ↑ lipid. (See Table 4.18).

4. **MRS is consistent with high-grade glioma. What is your surgical plan?**
   Given the tumor's location in the left frontal lobe near the inferior frontal gyrus patient should undergo a left awake frontal craniotomy with direct cortical stimulation for language mapping.

5. **What is your plan for preoperative and postoperative seizure prophylaxis?**
   Do not administer anticonvulsants if there is no history of seizures. In case of surgery administer anticonvulsants for prophylaxis, but discontinue one week after surgery, if no seizures occurred. (See Table 4.17)

6. During tumor resection the patient has what appears to be a generalized seizure. What is your plan?
   (See Table 11.1b).

7. Postoperatively, the patient is nonfocal neurologically, but slow to wake up. A postoperative CT scan shows the following. What is your management?

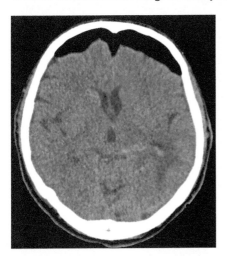

CT revealed tension pneumocephalus (Mt Fuji sign). This is an emergency situation and patient should undergo immediate decompression with needle placement through existing burr hole. Afterward 100% O_2 mask for 24 to 48 hours will help faster absorption of pneumocephalus. (See Table 5.17).

8. The patient does well and is discharged home on postop day 5. The patient returns to your office on postop day 10 with complaints of progressive difficulty climbing stairs. Clinical examination shows symmetrical proximal weakness affecting the lower extremities more than upper extremities. He is also noted to be diffusely hyporeflexive.
   All imaging studies are unremarkable and consistent with expected postoperative findings. What are you concerned about? What is your treatment plan?
   Patient might suffer from Guillain-Barré syndrome. He should undergo lumbar puncture and EMG/NCV tests to confirm diagnosis. Treatment options are IV immunoglobulin or plasmapheresis. (See Table 12.2: Guillain—Barré).

9. The patient returns to the office 4 weeks later with purulent drainage from his craniotomy wound. His laboratory values are: white blood cell (WBC) 15.400, CRP 43 mg/dL, ESR 89 mm. His MRI brain is the following. What is your plan?

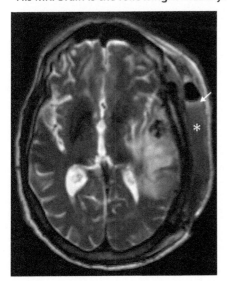

T2-weighted image (T2WI) MRI shows subcutaneous collection (*asterisk*) with air-fluid level (*arrow*) over craniotomy flap, which represents a subcutaneous pus collection. Patient should undergo removal of infected bone flap. After intraoperative cultures are obtained, empirical antibiotic treatment should be started. Antibiotic treatment should be adjusted later according to sensitivity results. Generally, antibiotics should be administered IV for 6 weeks followed by 6 weeks of p.o. antibiotics. (See Table 11.3c: Craniotomy infection).

10. **What is the typical treatment for glioblastomas?**
    Current treatment for glioblastoma is open surgery with the aim of gross total resection followed by radiation of tumor bed and margin (60 Gy administered as 2 Gy in 30 fractions) and chemotherapy (temozolomide). (See Table 4.1a: Gioblastoma, treatment).

11. **What is methylation of MGMT (O6-methylguanine-DNA-methyltransferase) predictive of?**
    Methylation of *MGMT* gene is a good predictor for tumor response to temozolomide. (See Table 4.1a: Anaplastic astrocytoma, treatment, chemotherapy).

4.22.2 Pituitary Apoplexy

Chief complaint/History of present illness	• A 42 y/o gentleman presents to the emergency room with the onset of acute headache, double vision, and blurry vision. His past medical history is significant for decreased libido and impotence over the past 12 months and gynecomastia.
Physical examination	• His neurological examination is consistent with CN VI palsy on the right side and decreased visual acuity especially on the right.

Imaging

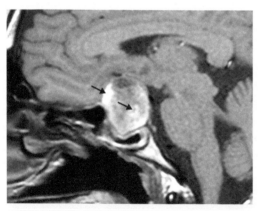

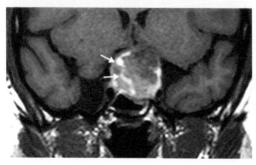

MRI of sella turcica (T1WI without gadolinium: top and middle images, T2WI: image on next page) shows mass in the area of sella turcica extending to the suprachiasmatic cistern and compressing the optic chiasm (left > right). The mass infiltrates the left cavernous sinus. Furthermore, the mass is inhomogeneous with areas of increased signal (*arrows*), which are compatible with hemorrhage.

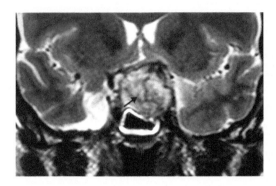

1. **What is your plan?**
   Patient has suffered pituitary apoplexy.
   - Rapid administration of corticosteroids.
   - Early transsphenoidal decompression of optic chasm.
     (See Table 4.13: Pituitary apoplexy).

2. **What laboratory tests do you want to order?**
   Sodium, potassium, glucose, thyroid stimulating hormone (TSH), free thyroxine (T4), adreno-corticotropic hormone (ACTH), 8 am cortisol, follicle-stimulating hormone (FSH), luteinizing hormone (LH), prolactin, growth hormone, insulin-like growth factor 1 (IGF1). (See Table 4.13: "Pituitary adenomas, for all the above adenomas")

3. **Describe your surgical approach?**
   Transnasal transsphenoidal approach. (See Table 10.8b).

4. **The mass initially is very fluid-like and can be easily suctioned but you are having difficulty resecting the lateral aspect of the mass. You decide to expand your exposure laterally with the high-speed drill. Suddenly, the field is filled with bright-red blood. What is your plan?**
   Internal carotid artery (ICA) injury. (See Table 11.1h and Table 10.8d).

5. **How would you monitor the patient postoperatively for diabetes insipidus (DI) and what is the triphasic response?**
   We should check urine output, urine specific gravity, and serum sodium. Diagnosis of DI can be made based on urine output more than 250 mL for 1 or 2 hours and urine specific gravity less than 1.005. Frequently serum sodium is elevated. The triphasic response constitutes of DI of short duration followed by normalization or syndrome of inappropriate antidiuretic hormone secretion (SIADH) followed by DI of long duration. (See Table 4.13: Treatment).

6. **Following removal of nasal packings on the third postoperative day your ENT colleague notes clear fluid dripping from the patient's nose. What is your plan?**
   A lumbar drain should be placed for 3 to 7 days. If CSF leak persists after clamping of drain, primary repair should be attempted and lumbar drainage should be continued for another 3 to 7 days. (See Table 11.1g and Table 10.8d).

7. **When you see the patient in follow-up, how would you determine the patient's steroid reserve and need for oral steroid supplementation?**
   - Cosyntropin stimulation test.
   - Discontinue p.o. hydrocortisone for 24 hours and check 6-am serum cortisol level.
     (See Table 4.13: Treatment).

4.22.3 Solitary Brain Metastasis

Chief complaint/History of present illness

- A 45 y/o man presents with 1-month history of visual disturbances, dizziness, and slight balance problems.
- The patient was diagnosed with esophageal carcinoma one year ago and underwent neoadjuvant chemotherapy pre- and postoperatively and resection.

Physical examination

- The neurological examination revealed only left homonymous hemianopsia.
- Tandem walking was possible without difficulty.

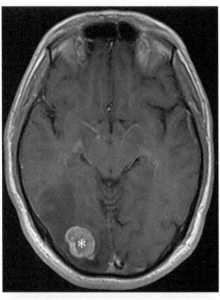

MRI brain (enhanced T1WI, axial) shows an intra-axial tumor (*asterisk*) with inhomogeneous contrast enhancement located in the right occipital pole. There is also significant perifocal edema (best seen in the following T2 image)

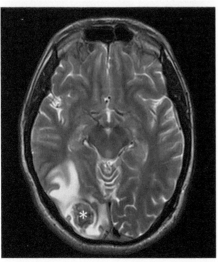

MRI brain (T2WI, axial) shows the intra-axial tumor (*asterisk*) with significant vasogenic perifocal edema (hyperintense signal).

1. **Which are the typical imaging findings that favor the diagnosis of a brain metastasis?**
   Small size of lesion vs. significant edema, located in grey-white matter junction. (See Table 4.15: Imaging/other diagnostics).

2. **What is the most probable diagnosis? What is the differential diagnosis of a single enhancing supratentorial intra-axial space occupying lesion?**
   Metastasis. (See Table 4.19).

3. **Which are the most common primary tumors causing brain metastases?**
   (See Table 4.15).

4. **What metastatic tumors have the highest tendency to bleed?**
   (See Table 4.20).

5. **What further workup is required?**
   - A full body positron emission tomography (PET)-CT should be done for preop staging. If there was no previous malignancy history, a full workup should be done to confirm the diagnosis of a metastasis and to find the primary tumor. (See Table 4.15: Imaging/other diagnostics).

6. **The preop whole body PET-CT revealed no other metastasis and no recurrence of the primary tumor. What is your treatment plan?**
   Although the tumor size is less than 3 cm stereotactic radiosurgery should not be offered to this patient due to significant perifocal edema, which will worsen after the radiation. Surgery should be offered to this patient for the following reasons:
   - Young age.
   - Good performance status.
   - Single symptomatic metastasis and controlled systemic disease.
   - Easily accessed lesion.
   - Gross total resection is possible.

   Patient should also receive some type of radiotherapy postoperatively (whole brain or local).(See Table 4.15: Treatment).

7. **What is the medical treatment of cerebral metastases?**
   (See Table 4.15: Treatment).

8. **What are the indications for surgical resection of brain metastases? What are the indications for biopsy of brain metastases?**
   (See Table 4.15: Treatment).

9. **What types of radiotherapy are used to treat brain metastases? What are the indications of whole brain radiation and stereotactic radiosurgery? Which tumors are radiosensitive?**
   (See Table 4.15: Treatment).

References

[1] Jakola AS, Myrmel KS, Kloster R, et al. Comparison of a strategy favoring early surgical resection vs a strategy favoring watchful waiting in low-grade gliomas. JAMA 2012;308(18):1881–1888

[2] Potts MB, Smith JS, Molinaro AM, Berger MS. Natural history and surgical management of incidentally discovered low-grade gliomas. J Neurosurg 2012;116(2):365–372

[3] van den Bent MJ, Afra D, de Witte O, et al; EORTC Radiotherapy and Brain Tumor Groups and the UK Medical Research Council. Long-term efficacy of early versus delayed radiotherapy for low-grade astrocytoma and oligodendroglioma in adults: the EORTC 22845 randomised trial. Lancet 2005;366(9490):985–990

[4] Chang EF, Smith JS, Chang SM, et al. Preoperative prognostic classification system for hemispheric low-grade gliomas in adults. J Neurosurg 2008;109(5):817–824

[5] Kreth FW, Thon N, Simon M, et al. German Glioma Network: "gross total but not incomplete resection of glioblastoma prolongs survival in the era of radiochemotherapy. Ann Oncol 2013;24(12):3117–3123

[6] McGirt MJ, Chaichana KL, Gathinji M, et al. Independent association of extent of resection with survival in patients with malignant brain astrocytoma. J Neurosurg 2009;110(1):156–162

[7] Curran WJ Jr, Scott CB, Horton J, et al. Recursive partitioning analysis of prognostic factors in three Radiation Therapy Oncology Group malignant glioma trials. J Natl Cancer Inst 1993;85(9):704–710

[8]   Stupp R, Hegi ME, Mason WP, et al; European Organisation for Research and Treatment of Cancer Brain Tumour and Radiation Oncology Groups. National Cancer Institute of Canada Clinical Trials Group. Effects of radiotherapy with concomitant and adjuvant temozolo- mide versus radiotherapy alone on survival in glioblastoma in a randomised phase III study: 5-year analysis of the EORTC-NCIC trial. Lancet Oncol 2009;10(5):459–466

[9]   Ryken TC, Kalkanis SN, Buatti JM, et al. The role of cytoreductive surgery in the management of progressive glioblastoma: a systematic review and evidence-based clinical practice guideline. J Neurooncol. 2014;118(3):479-88

[10]   Louis DN, Perry A, Reifenberger G, et al. The 2016 World Health Organization Classification of Tumors of the Central Nervous System: a summary. Acta Neuropathol 2016;131(6):803–820

[11]   Buckner JC, Shaw EG, Pugh SL, et al. Radiation plus Procarbazine, CCNU, and Vincristine in low-grade glioma N Engl J Med 2016;374(14):1344–1355

[12]   Cohen AL, Holmen SL, Colman H. IDH1 and IDH2 mutations in gliomas. Curr Neurol Neurosci Rep 2013;13(5):345

[13]   Cage TA, Clark AJ, Aranda D, et al. A systematic review of treatment outcomes in pediatric patients with intracranial ependymomas. J Neurosurg Pediatr 2013;11(6):673–681

[14]   Merchant TE, Haida T, Wang MH, Finlay JL, Leibel SA. Anaplastic ependymoma: treatment of pediatric patients with or without cranio-spinal radiation therapy. J Neurosurg 1997;86(6):943–949

[15]   Duffner PK, Horowitz ME, Krischer JP, et al. Postoperative chemotherapy and delayed radiation in children less than three years of age with malignant brain tumors. N Engl J Med 1993;328(24):1725–1731

[16]   Cappelli C, Grill J, Raquin M, et al. Long-term follow up of 69 patients treated for optic pathway tumors before the chemotherapy era. Arch Dis Child 1998;79(4):334–338

[17]   Bettegowda C, Adogwa O, Mehta V, et al. Treatment of choroid plexus tumors: a 20-year single institutional experience. J Neurosurg Pediatr 2012;10(5):398–405

[18]   Wolff JE, Sajedi M, Brant R, Coppes MJ, Egeler RM. Choroid plexus tumours. Br J Cancer 2002;87(10):1086–1091

[19]   Wrede B, Liu P, Wolff JE. Chemotherapy improves the survival of patients with choroid plexus carcinoma: a meta-analysis of individual cases with choroid plexus tumors. J Neurooncol 2007;85(3):345–351

[20]   Thompson EM, Hielscher T, Bouffet E, et al. Prognostic value of medulloblastoma extent of resection after accounting for molecular subgroup: a retrospective integrated clinical and molecular analysis. Lancet Oncol 2016;17(4):484–495

[21]   Rothenberg AB, Berdon WE, D'Angio GJ, Yamashiro DJ, Cowles RA. The association between neuroblastoma and opsoclonus-myoclo-nus syndrome: a historical review. Pediatr Radiol 2009;39(7):723–726

[22]   Sindou MP, Alvernia JE. Results of attempted radical tumor removal and venous repair in 100 consecutive meningiomas involving the major dural sinuses. J Neurosurg 2006;105(4):514–525

[23]   Pannullo SC, Fraser JF, Moliterno J, Cobb W, Stieg PE. Stereotactic radiosurgery: a meta-analysis of current therapeutic applications in neuro-oncologic disease. J Neurooncol 2011;103(1):1–17

[24]   Simpson D. The recurrence of intracranial meningiomas after surgical treatment. J Neurol Neurosurg Psychiatry 1957;20(1):22–39

[25]   Modha A, Gutin PH. Diagnosis and treatment of atypical and anaplastic meningiomas: a review. Neurosurgery 2005;57(3):538–550, discussion 538–550

[26]   Moliterno J, Cope WP, Vartanian ED, et al. Survival in patients treated for anaplastic meningioma. J Neurosurg 2015;123(1):23–30

[27]   Dunger DB, Broadbent V, Yeoman E, et al. The frequency and natural history of diabetes insipidus in children with Langerhans-cell histiocytosis. N Engl J Med 1989;321(17):1157–1162

[28]   Fernández-Latorre F, Menor-Serrano F, Alonso-Charterina S, Arenas-Jiménez J. Langerhans' cell histiocytosis of the temporal bone in pediatric patients: imaging and follow-up. AJR Am J Roentgenol 2000;174(1):217–221

[29]   Bamberg M, Kortmann RD, Calaminus G, et al. Radiation therapy for intracranial germinoma: results of the German cooperative pro-spective trials MAKEI 83/86/89. J Clin Oncol 1999;17(8):2585–2592

[30]   Singh TD, Valizadeh N, Meyer FB, Atkinson JL, Erickson D, Rabinstein AA. Management and outcomes of pituitary apoplexy. J Neurosurg 2015;122(6):1450–1457

[31]   Gao Y, Zhong C, Wang Y, et al. Endoscopic versus microscopic transsphenoidal pituitary adenoma surgery: a meta-analysis. World J Surg Oncol 2014;12:94

[32]   Loeffler JS, Shih HA. Radiation therapy in the management of pituitary adenomas. J Clin Endocrinol Metab 2011;96(7):1992–2003

[33]   Liu X, Yu Q, Zhang Z, et al. Same-day stereotactic aspiration and Gamma Knife surgery for cystic intracranial tumors. J Neurosurg 2012;117(Suppl):45–48

[34]   Fang Y, Cai BW, Zhang H, et al. Intracystic bleomycin for cystic craniopharyngiomas in children. Cochrane Database Syst Rev 2012;(4):CD008890

[35]   Tabouret E, Chinot O, Metellus P, Tallet A, Viens P, Gonçalves A. Recent trends in epidemiology of brain metastases: an overview. Anti-cancer Res 2012;32(11):4655–4662

[36]   Gaspar L, Scott C, Rotman M, et al. Recursive partitioning analysis (RPA) of prognostic factors in three Radiation Therapy Oncology Group (RTOG) brain metastases trials. Int J Radiat Oncol Biol Phys 1997;37(4):745–751

[37]   Gaspar LE, Scott C, Murray K, Curran W. Validation of the RTOG recursive partitioning analysis (RPA) classification for brain metastases. Int J Radiat Oncol Biol Phys 2000;47(4):1001–1006

[38]   Patchell RA, Tibbs PA, Walsh JW, et al. A randomized trial of surgery in the treatment of single metastases to the brain. N Engl J Med 1990;322(8):494–500

[39]   Sheikh AB, Mendelson ZS, Liu JK. Endoscopic versus microsurgical resection of colloid cysts: a systematic review and meta-analysis of 1,278 patients. World Neurosurg 2014;82(6):1187–1197

[40]   Dietrich J, Rao K, Pastorino S, Kesari S. Corticosteroids in brain cancer patients: benefits and pitfalls. Expert Rev Clin Pharmacol 2011;4(2):233–242

[41]   Glantz MJ, Cole BF, Forsyth PA, et al. Practice parameter: anticonvulsant prophylaxis in patients with newly diagnosed brain tumors. Report of the Quality Standards Subcommittee of the American Academy of Neurology. Neurology 2000;54(10):1886–1893

5 Head Injury and ICU

5.1 Head Injury

5.1.1 Definitions (Table 5.1)   G

Concussion	Definition	Immediate and transient alteration in brain function including mental status and level of consciousness
	Differences from mild traumatic brain injury (TBI)	• Imaging studies are normal • Onset of symptoms is immediate (in mild TBI may be hours after trauma)
Contusion	• "Bruise" of the brain • Associated with multiple microhemorrhages, vascular disruption and perifocal edema	
Coup/countercoup injury	Location of brain injury may be the same as impact (coup) or opposite to impact (countercoup)	
Malignant cerebral edema	• Rapid hyperemia with loss of autoregulation after trauma resulting in severe brain swelling • Edema of second-impact injury • Very high mortality	
Diffuse axonal injury (DAI)	• **Mechanism of injury:** acceleration/deceleration injury • **MRI/CT findings:** hemorrhagic foci in corpus callosum and brain stem primarily • **Histopathology:** microscopic axonal damage • **Possible presentation:** posttraumatic coma for greater than 6 h without mass lesions or ischemia	

5.1.2 Glasgow Coma Scale (GCS)[1] (Table 5.2)   G

Score	BEST eye opening	BEST verbal	BEST motor in ANY limb
6			Spontaneous movement, following commands
5		Oriented, conversant	Localizes pain
4	Spontaneously	Confused	Withdrawal to pain
3	To sound	Inappropriate words	Flexion posturing: decorticate
2	To pressure/pain	Inappropriate sounds	Extension posturing: decerebrate
1	None	None	None

5.1.3 TBI Classification Based on GCS Score (Table 5.3) G

Classification	GCS score
Minor	15
Mild	13–14
Moderate	9–12
Severe	3–8

5.1.4 Cerebral Edema (Table 5.4a) G

Type	Cellular level	Blood–brain barrier	Location	Causes	Comments
Cytotoxic	Intra	Intact	Gray and white matter	• Posttraumatic • Hypothermia • Intoxication	Not steroid responsive
Vasogenic	Extra	Disrupted	White matter	• Tumors • Inflammation • High-altitude edema[a]	Steroid responsive
Delayed ischemic	Extra	Disrupted	Gray and white matter	• Post SAH or stroke • Toxin-mediated	May be a type of vasogenic edema
Interstitial (Hydrocephalic)	Extra	Intact	White matter	Hydrocephalus	• Transependymal CSF flow • Responds to CSF reduction
Osmotic	Intra + extra	Intact	Gray and white matter	Reduced plasma oncotic pressure • Hyponatremia • SIADH	

High-altitude cerebral edema (Table 5.4b) G

Occurs with climbs above 2,000 meters in 50% of people

Symptoms	Ranging from headaches to paralysis and coma
Cause	Relative hypoxia
Treatment	• Immediate descent • Oxygen, steroids
Prevention	• Gradual ascent over 2–4 d • Avoidance of alcohol and hypnotics

Concussion[2-5] (Table 5.4c) G

Epidemiology	• Most common TBI (6 per 1,000/y) • Most common in young male adults

Characteristics	• **Mechanisms of injury:** direct OR indirect head trauma
	• **Symptoms:**
	  – ±Short loss of consciousness (LOC)
	  – Physical, cognitive, and emotional symptoms
	• GCS 13–15
	• **Imaging:** normal!!

Indications for CT/MRI	• Age > 65 y
	• Coagulopathy
	• **Symptoms:**
	  – Severe headache, vomiting
	  – Seizures
	• GCS < 15
	• Focal or worsening neurological examination

Second impact syndrome (Table 5. 4d) G

Definition	Second injury while still symptomatic from first
Epidemiology	Rare condition primarily in athletes
Causes/Mechanisms	• Loss of autoregulation • Malignant edema from vascular engorgement and increased cerebral blood flow (CBF)
Presentation	• "Walks off field" after second injury • Collapses within 1–5 min, coma, death
Mortality	50–100%

5.1.5 Herniation Syndromes (Table 5.5a) G

Name (alternate name)	Description
Subfalcine (cingulate)	• **Definition:** lateral displacement of cingulum underneath falx cerebri • Can lead to compression of anterior cerebral artery (ACA) branches
Transtentorial (central)	• **Definition:** downward displacement of cerebrum (typical stage-by-stage progression; see Table 5.5b) • Eye movement difficulty
Uncal (lateral transtentorial)	• **Definition:** mesial temporal lobe compressed against ridge of the tentorium notch at the level of mesencephalon → causing midline shift resulting in anisocoria (typical "blown pupil") • Most common
Cerebellar (foramen magnum)	• **Definition:** compression of medulla from cerebellar tonsils • **Presentation:** fulminant heart rate and blood pressure (BP) changes; tetraparesis
External	• **Definition:** herniation through a skull defect • **Causes:** posttraumatic, postsurgical
Upward	• Usually iatrogenic • **Mechanisms:** extensive CSF drainage from ventriculostomy in the presence of posterior fossa mass

Stages of central herniation (Table 5.5b) G

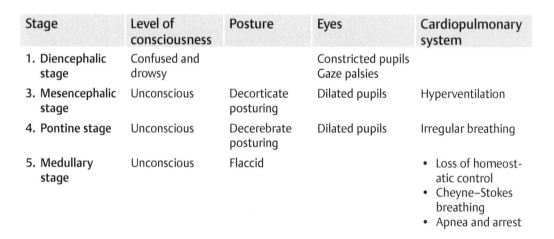

Stage	Level of consciousness	Posture	Eyes	Cardiopulmonary system
1. Diencephalic stage	Confused and drowsy		Constricted pupils Gaze palsies	
3. Mesencephalic stage	Unconscious	Decorticate posturing	Dilated pupils	Hyperventilation
4. Pontine stage	Unconscious	Decerebrate posturing	Dilated pupils	Irregular breathing
5. Medullary stage	Unconscious	Flaccid		• Loss of homeostatic control • Cheyne–Stokes breathing • Apnea and arrest

5.1.6 Brain Death (Table 5.6)

Definition of death (Uniform Determination of Death Act 1981 and Affirmation 2010)		• Irreversible cessation of circulatory and respiratory functions OR • Irreversible cessation of all functions of the entire brain and brainstem (brain death)
Brain death examination criteria		• Core temperature > 36°C (96.8°F) • Systolic BP (SBP) ≥ 100 mm Hg • No drugs that could influence examination, blood alcohol < 0.08%
	Reflexes	• Fixed pupils, no pupillary reaction to light • **No corneal reflex** (touching cornea with gauze or Q-tip) • **Absent vestibulo-ocular reflex:** no eye movement with ice water into external ear canal and head of bed (HOB) elevated to 30 degrees • **Absent oculocephalic reflex (Doll's eyes):** head turning does not cause contralateral eye deviation • **No gag reflex** (test by pulling on endotracheal tube [ET] tube) • **No cough reflex** (test with bronchial suctioning) • No response to deep central pain • **Failed apnea challenge:** no respirations with pCO_2 > 60 mm Hg
Ancillary tests (may vary between countries and states)	Electroencephalogram (EEG)	No electrical activity for 30 min
	Cerebral angiography	Absence of CBF at carotid bifurcation or circle of Willis
	Cerebral radionuclide angiogram	No radionuclide uptake in the brain parenchyma

5.1.7 Cerebral Blood Flow (Table 5.7a) G

Values of CBF (ml/100 g of tissue/ min)	Normal values	• **Average global CBF:** 50 • **Average CBF in gray matter:** 67–80 • **Average CBF in white matter:** 18–25
	Thresholds	• **30:** minimum CBF for normal neuronal function • **20–30:** neuronal dysfunction, EEG slowing • **10–20:** reversible neuronal dysfunction if CBF is restored, suppressed EEG • **<10:** irreversible neuronal dysfunction—cell death
Formulas/ relationship with other parameters	CPP = MAP – ICP	• **CPP:** cerebral perfusion pressure • **MAP:** mean arterial pressure • **ICP:** intracranial pressure
	CBF = CPP/CVR	**CVR:** cerebrovascular resistance (CVR is mainly dependent on the diameter of the arterioles, meaning when the smooth muscle of their wall contracts→ ↓ diameter → ↑ CVR → ↓ CBF and vice versa)

Factors regulating CBF (Table 5.7b)

Flow–metabolism coupling	• **Definition:**
	  – ↑ Metabolism (seizure, hyperthermia) leads to ↑ CBF
	  – ↓ Metabolism (anesthesia, sedation, hypothermia) leads to a ↓ to CBF
	• **Mediators:** via regional metabolic and neurogenic factors
	• **Response rate:** very fast (≈1 s)

Cerebral autoregulation

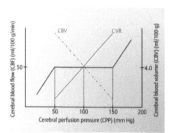

- **Definition:**
  - Between CPP values 50 and 150 mm Hg, autoregulation works and cerebral arterioles can maintain stable CBF regardless of CPP fluctuations via changes in CVR (↑ CPP → ↑ CVR, ↓ CPP → ↓ CVR)
  - When CPP < 50, ↓ CPP → ↓ CBF (linearly) → ischemia
  - When CPP > 150, ↑ CPP → ↑ CBF (linearly) → ↑ CBV (cerebral blood volume) → ↑ ICP → edema/disruption of blood–brain barrier
- **Mediator:** myogenic reflexes of smooth muscle in wall of arterioles and neurogenic factors
- **Response rate:** slower than flow–metabolism coupling

PaCO$_2$, PaO$_2$ (arterial carbon dioxide and oxygen tension)

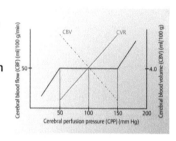

PaCO$_2$

- For PaCO$_2$ 20–80 mm Hg, CO$_2$ has a linear relationship with CBF:
  - ↑ PaCO$_2$ (hypercapnia) → ↓ CVR → ↑ CBF
  - ↓ PaCO$_2$ (hypocapnia) → ↑ CVR → ↓ CBF
- CO$_2$ is a very potent vasodilator
- Hyperventilation (↓ PaCO$_2$) can be used as a short-term measure for ↓ CBF and thus ↓ ICP

PaO$_2$

- For PaO$_2$ > 60 mm Hg, oxygen has almost no effect on CBF
- For PaO$_2$ < 60 mm Hg, ↓ PaO$_2$ → ↓ CVR → ↑ CBF
- The oxygen effect on CBF is not as significant as that of CO$_2$

5.1.8 Intracranial Pressure (Table 5.8a) G

ICP	• **Definition:** the pressure within intracranial space relative to atmospheric pressure • **Normal values:** 8–15 mm Hg
Intracranial volume	**The intracranial volume (V_{total}) within intact skull is fixed.** $V_{total} = V_{brain} + V_{blood} + V_{CSF}$ = constant • $V_{brain} \approx 1{,}400$ mL (80%) • $V_{blood} \approx 150$ mL (10%) • $V_{CSF} \approx 150$ mL (10%)
Monro–Kellie doctrine	An increase in the volume of one of the intracranial contents requires an equal reduction in the volume of the other intracranial contents, so that ICP within the fixed skull remains constant

Pressure–volume curve

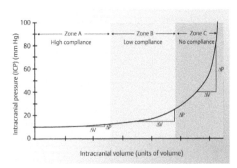

- **Zone A (high compliance vs. low elastance):** compensatory mechanisms (blood, CSF) are intact → large changes in volume cause little or no change in ICP
- **Zone B (↓ compliance, ↑ elastance):** compensatory mechanisms progressively decrease → for the same change in volume, the ICP starts to increase more
- **Zone C (decompensation point, almost no compliance vs. high elastance):** after a threshold, small increase in volume causes exponential increase in ICP → effects, if not treated: ischemia, herniation

- Compliance = ΔV/ΔP
- Elastance = ΔP/ΔV (differential change in pressure per unit volume)
- **Buffering mechanisms:** CSF displacement into lumbar subarachnoid spaces, ↑ venous outflow, ↓ CBF and CBV

Management algorithm of increased ICP (Table 5.8b 🔊)

GCS ≤ 8 in resuscitated patient

STAGE 1

- Surgery if indicated
- NO STEROIDS [H]
- ICP monitor if meeting criteria—external ventricular drain (EVD) with antimicrobial catheter preferred method [M]
- Seizure prophylaxis (phenytoin or divalproex preferred) [M]
- HOB elevated at 30 degrees
- Keep body temperature normal
- Keep SBP ≥ 110 mm Hg (for age 50–69: ≥100 mm Hg) [L]
- Keep CPP 60–70 mm Hg [L]
- Do NOT use prophylactic hyperventilation [M]

ICP > 22 mm Hg?

!! **Consider repeat CT**

STAGE 2

- ICP calibrated?
- Good waveform?
- Drain CSF if possible and leave EVD open [L]
- Sedation + analgesia (i.e., propofol + morphine; midazolam + fentanyl, etc.)[6]
- Neuromuscular blocking agents (NMBA)
- Mannitol 0.25–1.0 g/kg bolus administration if < 320 mOsm/L [M]
- Use 3% saline if mannitol contraindicated (hypotension)
- 24-h postinjury: consider mild hyperventilation (PaCO$_2$ of 30–35 mm Hg) with CAUTION (data suggest possible harmful effects).

ICP remains > 22 mm Hg?

!! **Consider repeat CT**

STAGE 3

- Decompressive craniectomy with large (>12 cm) uni- or bilateral decompression [H][7,8]
- High-dose barbiturates [M]
- Mild hypothermia 32–35°C [L]

Level of evidence: Level I: good-quality randomized controlled trial (RCT) = high[H], Level II—moderate-/poor-quality RCT OR good-quality cohort = medium [M], Level III: moderate-/poor-quality RCT or cohort OR moderate-/poor-quality case-control OR case series, databases, registries = low [L].

5.1.9 Admission and Discharge Management Algorithm for TBI[9] (Table. 5.9) ᴳ

Category	Criteria	Management
Low risk	a. Asymptomatic b. Nonprogressive headache c. Dizziness d. Scalp hematoma or wound e. No LOC	Observation at home with written head injury instructions

Moderate risk	**Any of the following:**
	a. Age < 2 y
	b. **Mechanism of injury:**
	  • Multiple trauma
	  • Suspected child abuse
	  • Unreliable or inadequate history
	  • Alcohol/drug intoxication
	c. **Types of head injury:**
	  • Serious facial injury
	  • Significant subgaleal swelling
	  • Possible penetrating skull injury OR depressed fracture
	  • Signs of skull base fracture
	d. **Symptoms:**
	  • Alteration/LOC on or after injury
	  • Posttraumatic amnesia
	  • Progressive headache
	  • Vomiting
	  • Posttraumatic seizure
		Get noncontrast head CT:
		a. If CT reveals findings of TBI →in-hospital observation
		b. If CT is normal→discharge only if:
		  • Patient is asymptomatic (except amnesia)
		  • GCS ≥ 14
		  • No domestic abuse
		  • Patient has access to hospital
		  • Responsible competent adult can stay with patient at home

High risk	a. Penetrating injury/depressed skull fracture b. Decreased OR decreasing level of consciousness not due to other causes (drugs, alcohol, postictal, metabolic, etc.) c. Focal neurological deficit	1. STAT noncontrast head CT 2. Admission to ICU

5.1.10 Monitors Used in Traumatic Brain Injury

ICP monitors (Table 5.10a ◀))   G

Type of ICP monitor	Risk of hemorrhage	Bacterial colonization or infection	Malfunction	Comments
Intraventricular catheter (EVD)	1%	15%	5%	• Preferred method!! • Most accurate • Most reliable • Least expensive • Allows CSF drainage • May be difficult to place
Intraparenchymal monitor	2%	15%	20%	Drift over time
Subarachnoid bolt	0	5%	15%	Lumen can occlude at high ICP and show false readings
Subdural sensor	0	5%	10%	

Indications for ICP monitor placement	Salvageable patient with GCS 3–8 and either:		
	a. Abnormal CT		• Hematoma • Contusions • Swelling • Herniation • Compressed basal cisterns
	b. Normal CT + 2 of the following:		• Age > 40 y • Uni- or bilateral motor posturing • SBP < 90 mm Hg

ICP values

Normal ICP values	• Preterm infants: 0–3 mm Hg • Term infants: 1.5–6 mm Hg • Children: 3–7 mm Hg • Adults: 10–15 mm Hg
Treatment threshold	• Children: 20 mm Hg • Adults: 22 mm Hg

CBF monitor (Table 5.10b) G

Devices	Laser Doppler flow	• Continuous • Non-invasive • Only regional
	Thermal diffusion flowm-etry probe	Invasive bedside monitor using thermal diffusion flowmetry probe inserted into white matter
CBF values	Normal values	• Gray matter: 67–80 mL/100 g/min • White matter: 18–25 mL/100 g/min
	Abnormal values	• < 15 mL: may indicated vasospasm or ischemia • < 10 mL: may indicate infarction

Microdialysis probe (Table 5.10c) G

Device	• Invasive bedside monitor • Probe inserted into white matter, connected to micro-pump • Obtains extracellular fluid micro-samples
Measured substances	• Glucose → ↓ extracellular glucose associated with ↑ mortality • Lactate → may ↑ in SJVO$_2$ (jugular venous oxygen saturation) desaturation • Pyruvate • Lactate/pyruvate ratio

5.1.11 ICP Waveforms (Table 5.11)

Name	Interpretation	Waveform	Characteristics
A wave	Physiologic		A-wave with 3 peaks: • P1: percussion wave = arterial pulsation • P2: tidal wave = intracranial compliance • P3: dicrotic wave = aortic valve closure Physiologic condition: P1 > P2 > P3 Pathological condition: P2 > P1 indicates noncompliant brain = ↑ICP
Lundberg's A waves	Pathologic: indicative of neurological deterioration and possible herniation		Plateau waves: ICP ≥ 50 mm Hg for 5–20 min
Lundberg's B waves	Pathologic: probably related to change in vascular tone (vasospasm) and failing intracranial compensation		Oscillations at frequency 1–2/min ICP 20–30 mm Hg
Lundberg's C waves	Has been documented in healthy adults Significance unknown		Oscillations 4–8/min ICP >20 mm Hg

5.2 Traumatic Hemorrhagic Brain Injuries

5.2.1 Traumatic Intracerebral Hemorrhage (TICH)

TICH (AKA hemorrhagic contusions) (Table 5.12a)

Epidemiology	• Common (13–35% of severe TBI)[10] • More common in temporal lobe, frontal lobes (however, they occur anywhere)
Mechanism	Sudden deceleration with resultant impact of brain on skull in coup/contracoup fashion[11]
Presentation	Variable (from no level of consciousness alteration to coma)
CT appearance	• Areas of increased density • Areas of heterogeneous density due to hemorrhage, infarction /necrosis, edema

Management (level III)[10] (!! no firm surgical criteria have been established)	Nonsurgical	Recommendations (indications): • No evidence of neurological compromise • Controlled ICP • No significant mass effect on serial CT scans **Close observation with: ICP monitoring (see Table 5.10a) + serial CTs**	

	Surgical	Recommendations (indications)	• Clinical: progressive neurological deterioration referable to lesion
			 • ICP monitoring: medically refractory intracranial hypertension with large TICH lesion(S)
			 • CT findings:
			   – mass effect
			   – volume > 50 mL
			 • GCS 6–8 + all of the following CT findings:
			   – Volume > 20 mL
			   – Frontal OR temporal location
			   – Midline shift > 5 mm and/or cisternal compression

		Options	• For diffuse medically refractory post-traumatic cerebral edema → bifrontal craniectomy within 48 h from injury
			 • For diffuse medically refractory paren-chymal injury → decompression:
			   – Decompressive craniectomy
			   – Subtemporal resection
			   – Temporal lobectomy

Outcome[10]	Evidence suggests, but does not prove, that outcome is poor in patients with progressive neurological deterioration, medically refractory intracranial hypertension, and mass effect on CT, who are not treated surgically

Delayed Traumatic Intracerebral Hemorrhage (DTICH) (Table 5.12b) G

Definition[12]	Appearance of TICH (usually within 72 h of head trauma) in areas of the brain that were normal in appearance or nearly so on the initial CT scan
Epidemiology	3.3–7.4% in patients with moderate to severe TBI
Mechanism	Primary TICH progresses (microhematomas coalesce)
Factors[10,12]	Coagulation abnormalities Decompressive surgery for other intracranial hemorrhages Secondary systemic insults Dysautoregulation
Presentation	Patients are doing well initially after the injury and suddenly deteriorate (GCS < 8; most occur within 72 h)
CT appearance	Identical with TICH
Management	Treatment identical to primary TICH but higher mortality (50–75%)

5.2.2 Epidural Hematomas

Acute epidural hematoma (AEDH) (Table 5.13a) G

Definition	Bleeding occurs between: inner table of skull—dura
Epidemiology[11,13,14]	• 20% of severe TBIs • 10.6% of admissions for TBI • Usually male • Usually young (mean age: 20–30 y; rare < 2 y old or > 60 y old) • Usually laterally over hemispheres (70%; however, they occur anywhere)
Source of bleeding	• Arterial: 85% (usually middle meningeal artery after temporoparietal skull fracture) → symptoms present soon after injury • Venous: 15% (middle meningeal vein, diploic veins, sinus) → symptoms present hours/days after injury, more benign
Presentation	• Lucid interval[11,15] (<10–27%; definition: brief LOC just after head injury → transient complete recovery → followed by sudden neurological deterioration, hemiparesis, anisocoria, coma, death) • No posttraumatic LOC 60%
CT appearance[11]	• Classic appearance: uniformly high-density biconvex lesion adjacent to skull (84%) • However, in 10% it is crescent shaped (differential diagnosis [DDx] from subdural hematoma [SDH]) • Does not cross sutures → confined (vs. SDH) • May cross the falx (vs. SDH) • Usually associated with fracture of overlying skull • Associated underlying acute subdural hematoma (ASDH) in 20% → rule out (R/O) intraoperatively

Management (level III)[13]	Nonsurgical	GCS > 8 without focal deficit + all of the following CT findings • Volume < 30 mL • Thickness < 15 mm • Midline shift < 5 mm
		Close observation + serial CTs
	Surgical	**Recommendations (indications)** • Volume >30 mL regardless GCS score • Hematoma evacuation as soon as possible for AEDH in coma (GCS < 9) + anisocoria
		Technique • Craniotomy: hematoma evacuation • R/O underlying ASDH • Place multiple tack-up sutures + central tenting suture
Mortality[14]		• **With optimal treatment:** 10% (better outcome than with all other traumatic hemorrhagic brain injuries; factors affecting mortality rate: pre-op motor response, pupillary asymmetry, presence of other intracranial pathology) • **Overall:** 20–55% (increased mortality usually due to delay of diagnosis [Dx] + surgery)

Delayed Epidural Hematoma (DEDH)[11] (Table 5.13b)

Definition	An EDH not present on the initial CT
Epidemiology	10% of EDH
Risk factors	• Skull fracture (most common) • Coagulopathies • Rapid lowering of ICP (with medicines or surgery) • Rapid shock correction
CT appearance	Identical with AEDH
Management	Treatment identical to AEDH

5.2.3 Subdural Hematomas

ASDH (traumatic) (Table 5.14a) G

Definition	Hematoma is located between: dura and arachnoid layer (< 48 h from injury)
Epidemiology[16]	• 12–29% of severe TBI patients (more common than EDH) • Mechanism of injury: in younger patients, mainly due to motor vehicle accident (MVA) vs. in older patients mainly due to falls • Location: usually lateral hemispheric, but also interhemispheric, along tentorium, posterior cranial fossa • Delayed SDH (0.5% of operated ASDH) = SDH not present on initial CT (same treatment [Tx] as ASDH)[11]

(Continued) ▶

Source of bleeding[11]			• Subdural accumulation of blood around/from brain laceration (burst lobe) → more severe primary brain injury (usually) without lucid interval (usually) • Rupture of bridging or cortical veins due to brain acceleration–deceleration →less severe primary brain injury (usually) with lucid interval (usually)
Presentation[17]			• GCS < 8 (37–80%) • Lucid interval(may be present) • Worse vs. EDH
CT appearance[11]			• High-density crescentic lesion adjacent to skull • Associated brain edema and underlying brain injury (more often vs. EDH) • DDx from EDH: ASDH is less uniform, more diffuse, crescentic in shape
Management (level III)[17]	Nonsurgical		• All patients not fulfilling the surgical criteria should be closely observed with: intensive monitoring + serial CTs • Place ICP monitor in all SDH patients in coma (GCS < 9) **Small interhemispheric SDH: observe; surgery only for patients with neurological deterioration (high risk due to superior sagittal sinus, risk of venous infarct)**

	Surgical	Recom-mendations (indications)	Surgery ASAP for:
			a. CT criteria regardless of GCS (any one of the following criteria):
			  • Thickness > 10 mm
			  • Midline shift > 5 mm
			b. CT criteria (thickness < 10 mm + midline shift < 5 mm) + comatose patient (GCS < 9) → operate ASAP if any of the following criteria is fulfilled:
			  • ↓ GCS by 2 point between injury and admission and/or
			  • Pupils: asymmetric OR fixed dilated and/or
			  • ICP > 20 mm Hg
			
			Caution: due to the association of ASDH with TICH, take into consideration the recommendations for management of both lesions

		Technique	a. Large craniotomy
			b. Hematoma evacuation
			  • If severe brain swelling, consider:
			    – Duraplasty
			    – Leave bone flap off

Mortality[11]			• Overall mortality:
			  – 50–90% (high mortality mainly due to underlying brain parenchymal injury; much worse than EDH)
			  – Lower when surgery occurs < 4 h after injury[18]
			• Factors for poor outcome: ↓ GCS of admission, ↑ age, postop ↑ ICP, associated TICH[14]

Spontaneous SDH[11,19] (Table 5.14b)   G

Source of bleeding	Depending on cause: • Bleeding site is usually arterial (cortical MCA branch in area of Sylvian fissure)[a] • Venous (from bridging vein rupture)
Risk factors/causes	• Hypertension • Intracranial hypotension (spinal tap) • Coagulopathies (including iatrogenic) • Substance abuse • Vascular malformations (arteriovenous malformation [AVM], aneurysm) • *Ginkgo biloba* extract • Infection • Tumor [a]Minor trauma: rarely a seemingly harmless head trauma or even a whiplash neck injury without direct head injury can be the cause particularly in the presence of pre-existing sylvian arachnoid cyst
Presentation	Usual presentation: sudden severe headache (without history of trauma) → level of consciousness alterations + variable focal neurological deficits
CT appearance	• SDH of different density (hyper-, iso-, hypodense) depending on elapsed time from initial bleeding • Consider CTA to R/O AVM or aneurysm
Management	Same as traumatic ASDH + treat/address underlying cause: • AVM, aneurysm: take into consideration/treat first—can complicate SDH removal • Intracranial hypotension: identify site of CSF leak in spine → blood patch • Coagulopathies → treat OR reverse if iatrogenic • Treat infection • Treat tumor • Stop substances

Chronic subdural hematoma (CSDH) (Table 5.14c)   G

Definition[11]	SDH of with low density in CT (around 2–3 wk since initial bleeding) → contains dark "motor oil," which does not clot
Epidemiology[11]	• Typical age: usually in older patients (average age: 63) → with age brain volume ↓ → vs. subdural space ↑ • 20% bilateral
Mechanism[20,21]	Initially small ASDH → causes inflammation → fibroblasts form neomembranes (about 4 d after injury) on both hematoma surfaces (cortical, dural) → angiogenesis in membranes bleeding → enzymatic fibrinolysis of blood clot → liquefaction of blood clot + fibrin degradation products inhibit hemostasis after rebleeding **Loss of balance between plasma effusion and/or rebleeding from neomembranes vs. fluid absorption**

Risk factors	• Trauma <50% (usually trauma is so minor, it cannot be recalled) • Alcohol abuse • Seizures • Coagulopathies • CSF shunts • Patients at risk of falls

Presentation[11]	• Very slow worsening of neurological status
	• Variable:
	  – (20–30%) → incidental finding[14]
	  – Minor symptoms (headache, confusion, speech difficulties, walking difficulties) or transient ischemic attack (TIA) like symptoms
	  – Major symptoms: alterations of level of consciousness (even coma), hemiparesis, seizures

CT appearance	• Low-density collection of crescentic shape over lateral surface of hemisphere (variable extent) ± diaphragms (see Table 5.14e) • Subacute SDH (4 d to 2–3 wk since initial bleeding) isodense → may be missed → look for midline shift, ask for enhanced CT

Management[11]

Nonsurgical measures	• Seizure prophylaxis • Treat coagulopathies (reversal if iatrogenic anticoagulation) • Steroids (controversial)	
Surgical	**Indications**	• Symptomatic CSDH • CT findings: thickness > 1 cm
	Surgical options	• Twist drill hole • Single burr hole • Two burr holes (recommended) • Craniotomy + excision of superficial CSDH membrane only (indications: multiloculated CSDH, persistent CSDH recurrences after above options have been used)
		Placement of subdural drain for 24–48 h + patient flat in bed reduces rate of recurrence by 50%[22]

Outcome of surgical management	• Clinical improvement (>80% of patients) can be achieved by removal of >20% of CSDH[23] • 90% resolution with one or two procedures (with twist drill hole + subdural drain) • CSDH recurrence in 10% (even with subdural drain left for 24–48 h) • 78% show residual fluid on post-op CT, which may take 6 mo to resolve • Overall surgical mortality: 0–8%[11,14]

Traumatic subdural hygroma (Table 5.14d) G

Definition	Subdural collection of CSF
Types	• Simple hygroma: only CSF • Complex hygroma: CSF + EDH or SDH or ICH
Mechanism	Possible arachnoid tear
Risk factors/causes	• Almost always trauma (alcoholic falls, assaults, skull fractures) • Cerebral atrophy • CSF shunts • Intracranial hypotension
Presentation	Variable: from disorientation to comatose
CT appearance	Crescentic collection of fluid with density similar to CSF over lateral surface of hemisphere (variable extent)
Management	**Nonsurgical measures** — Observe patients with asymptomatic hygromas with serial neurologic examination + serial CTs
	Surgical — Surgery with burr hole + drain or craniotomy especially for symptomatic complex hygromas High recurrence rate with burr hole alone Subdural-peritoneal shunt may be required

SDH appearance on CT depending on elapsed time from injury (Table 5.14e) G

Type of SDH	Elapsed time from injury	Density in CT
Acute	< 48 h	Hyperdense
Subacute	From 48 h until 2 – 3 wks	Isodense
Chronic	Around 2 – 3 wks	Hypodense

Posterior fossa mass lesions (including EDH) (Table 5.15) G

Surgical management	**Surgery ASAP for:** • Mass effect on CT (pressure on fourth ventricle) OR • Neurological dysfunction or deterioration referable to the lesion
Non Surgical management	• No significant mass effect on CT • No signs of neurological dysfunction ↓ Close observation and serial imaging

5.2.4 Surgical Management of Skull Fractures (Table 5.16)

Lesion	Surgical management	Nonsurgical management	Comments
Linear convexity skull fracture	Surgery if fracture is growing	Typically treated with observation	• Best seen on skull X-ray as dark, nonbranching line • 90% of pediatric skull fractures
Depressed skull fracture	Early surgery (to reduce infection) with elevation and debridement for open (compound) fractures IF: • Depression >1 cm or > thickness of skull bone • Significant intracranial hematoma • Dural penetration • Intradural pneumocephalus • CSF leak • Frontal sinus involvement • Gross contamination or wound infection • Gross cosmetic deformity	• Open compound fractures not meeting surgical criteria • Closed fractures	Use antibiotics for all open skull fractures
Temporal fractures	• Immediate-onset cranial nerve (CN) VII palsy: if no improvement while on steroids, consider surgical CN VII decompression • Delayed onset CN VII palsy: – Follow with serial facial EMG – If deterioration to <10% activity compared to contralateral side, then consider surgical CN VII decompression	Steroids (unproven)	• **Longitudinal fractures:** – Common – Parallel to ear canal – Do not cause CN VII and VIII injury – May cause ossicular injury • **Transverse fractures:** – Perpendicular to ear canal – Cause CN VII and VIII injury
Clival fractures	Surgery rarely needed for cranial nerve or vascular repair	Treat associated head injury	• **Associated with:** – CN III to VIII deficits – CSF leak – vascular injury • High mortality
Frontal sinus fracture	**Posterior wall fracture:** consider surgery for possible dural repair, cranialization of frontal sinus, frontal sinus exenteration, stripping of mucosa	**Anterior wall ONLY fractures:** observation	• Intracranial air = dural laceration • Complications of posterior wall frontal sinus fracture (CSF leak, abscess, mucocele) may be delayed by years

Pneumocephalus (Table 5.17)

| Pneumocephalus | • **Pneumocephalus + persistent CSF leak:** locate and repair CSF leak
• **Tension pneumocephalus:** emergency like any other space occupying lesion, must be immediately decompressed (burr holes, needle through existing burr hole) | • **Simple pneumocephalus:** no infection and no CSF leak—gets absorbed over time
• **Pneumocephalus from gas-producing organisms:** treat infection | 100% O_2 mask for 24–48 h helps absorb pneumocephalus faster |

Gunshot wound to the head (Table 5.18)

| Gunshot wound to the head | • **For salvageable patients:** debridement of devitalized tissue → evacuation of hematoma → removal of accessible bullet fragments and bone fragments ("don't go fishing") → hemostasis watertight closure
• **For nonsalvageable patients:** simple debridement and wound closure | When poor prognostic factors exist:
• Track crosses midline
• Track crosses ventricle
• Track crosses center of brain
• Comatose on arrival
• Hematoma on CT
• Suicide attempt | • **Mortality:** 90%
• **Impact velocity >100 m/s:** uniformly fatal |

Nonmissile penetrating injuries (Table 5.19)

Lesion	Surgical management	Nonsurgical management	Comment
Nonmissile penetrating injuries (arrows, knives, darts, etc.)	Do not remove the object until patient is in surgery and dura is open		Consider pre-op angiogram if larger vessels are in track

5.2.5 TBI Parameters Estimated from CT[24] (Table 5.20)

Evaluation of basal cisterns	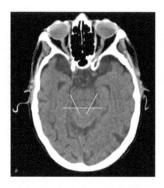	Evaluated cisterns (@ midbrain)	• Two lateral limbs = posterior portion of ambient cistern • One posterior limb: quadrigeminal cistern
		Findings	a. Open: all three limbs open b. Partially closed: one or two limbs open c. Completely closed: all limbs obliterated
		Value	Compression or absence of basal cisterns correlates with ICP and poor outcome
Midline shift estimation	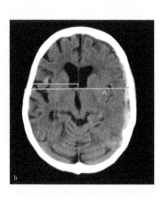	Formula	a. Measure biparietal diameter @ the level of foramen of Monro b. Measure the distance from inner table of skull to septum pellucidum on side of shift midline shift = (A/2) – B
		Value	Midline shift correlates with worse outcome

Estimation of volume of mass lesion on CT	1. Find scan with largest extent of mass lesion = slice 1
	2. At slice1 measure anteroposterior extent = A
	3. At slice 1 measure thickness at 90-degree angle to A = B
	4. Identify every 10-mm slice showing mass lesion and compare it to slice 1:
	  • Each 10-mm slice with mass lesion >75% of size of slice 1, count as 1
	  • Each 10-mm slice with mass lesion 25–75% of size of slice 1, count as 0.5
	  • Each 10-mm slice with mass lesion <25% of size slice 1, count as 0
	  • Add up corresponding assigned values of each 10-mm slice showing mass lesion = C
	Estimated volume = (A × B × C)/2

5.2.6 Blunt Cerebrovascular Injuries (BCVI; Traumatic Dissections)[25,26] (Table 5.21a) G

Epidemiology	• 1–2% of blunt trauma patients • Internal carotid artery (ICA) dissection in 62% vs. vertebral artery (VA) dissection in 38% of BCVI cases
Causes	• MVA (most common for carotid injuries) • Attempted strangulation • Spinal (chiropractic) manipulation (mostly VA)

Risk factors	a. Head injuries:
	  • Closed head injury consistent with DAI + GCS < 6
	  • Basilar skull fracture with carotid canal involvement
	  • Displaced midface fracture
	b. C-spine/neck injury:
	  • Mechanism of injury:
	    – Near hanging with anoxia
	    – Seat belt/other clothesline-type injury + significant cervical pain/swelling OR altered mental status
	  • C-spine injuries:
	    – Levels C1–C3: any fracture
	    – All C-spine levels:
	1. Vertebral body or transverse foramen fracture
	2. Subluxation
	3. Ligamentous injury

Symptoms and signs	• Arterial hemorrhage from neck/nose/mouth
	• Expanding cervical hematoma
	• Cervical bruit in patient <50 y old
	• Focal neurological deficit:
	  – TIA
	  – Hemiparesis
	  – Vertebrobasilar symptoms
	  – Horner's syndrome
	• Imaging:
	  – Stroke on CT/MRI
	  – Neurological deficit inconsistent with head CT

Diagnostic tests	a. CTA = test of choice (if equivocal finding OR high clinical suspicion → angiogram) b. Four-vessel cerebral angiogram = gold standard (use if CTA not possible or endovascular procedure planned) c. MRA: recommended for Dx of VA injury after blunt cervical trauma in complete spinal cord injury (SCI) or vertebral subluxation (level III) (see Table 5.21d)
Mortality	a. For unilateral blunt ICA injuries: 17–40% b. For unilateral blunt VA injuries: 8–18%

5.2.7 Blunt Cerebrovascular Grading Scale (Denver's Grading Scale) and Treatment Recommendations[25,26] (Table 5.21b) G

Denver's grading scale[27]	Vessel abnormality	Treatment	Follow-up CTA and further management (grades I–IV)	Prognosis
I	< 25% stenosis	Aspirin or heparin	Follow-up CTA in 7–10 d:	Most resolve spontaneously
II	≥ 25% stenosis OR intraluminal thrombus OR raised intimal flap	Aspirin or heparin	a. If lesion is healed, stop antithrombotics b. If lesion not healed:	Most resolve spontaneously
III	Pseudoaneurysm	Heparin preferred over aspirin	• Consider stenting for severe laminar stenosis or expanding pseudoa-neurysm (with caution[a])	
IV	Occlusion	Endovascular occlusion with the aim to prevent embolization	• Otherwise antiplatelet for 3 mo and reimage → if lesion persists, consider lifelong antip-latelet therapy	
V	Transection with free extravasation	a. Incomplete transection: endovascular stenting OR surgical repair b. Complete transection: endovascular occlusion OR surgical ligation [a]Surgical ligation/occlusion for accessible lesions only		High mortality

5.2.8 Blunt ICA Injury[27] (Table 5.21c) G

Denver's grading scale	Vessel abnormality	Tx	Stroke risk	Progression risk
I	<25% stenosis	See Table 5.21b	3%	• 70% heal • 25% persist • 5% progress
II	≥25% stenosis OR intraluminal thrombus OR raised intimal flap		11%	70% progress to higher level despite anticoagulation
III	Pseudoaneurysm		33%	Most progress
IV	Occlusion		44%	
V	Transection with free extravasation		100%	

Note: Most ICA dissections start 2 cm from ICA origin.

5.2.9 Blunt VA Injury[28] (Table 5.21d) G

Diagnostic tests	a. CTA: recommended as a screening tool for patients after blunt cervical trauma with suspected VA injury (level I data) b. Conventional angiography: recommended for Dx of VA injury for selected patients after blunt cervical trauma if concurrent endovascular Tx is considered OR when CTA is not available (level III data) c. MRA: recommended for Dx of VA injury after blunt cervical trauma in complete SCI or vertebral subluxation (level III data)
Treatment (level III data)	• Treatment for VA injury should be individualized depending on VA injury, associated injuries, and bleeding risk • Treatment options are antiplatelet OR anticoagulation OR no Tx (observation) • Role of endovascular therapy for VA injuries remains to be defined; there are no recommendations
Mortality, stroke risk	Denver grading scale does not correlate with stroke risk or mortality for blunt VA injuries (unlike ICA injuries) Mortality: a. Unilateral dissection: 8–18% b. Bilateral: usually fatal

5.2.10 Outcome Scales[29]

Glasgow Outcome scale (GOS) (Table 5.22a)

5	Good recovery, resumption of normal life despite minor deficits
4	Moderate disability but independent
3	Severe disability, dependent for daily support
2	Persistent vegetative state
1	Dead

Modified Rankin Scale [30] (Table 5.22b)

0	No symptoms
1	No significant disability, despite some symptoms; able to perform all usual duties and activities
2	Slight disability; able to look after own affairs without assistance, but unable to carry out previous activities
3	Moderate disability; requires some help, but able to walk unassisted
4	Moderately severe disability; unable to attend to own bodily needs without assistance, unable to walk unassisted
5	Severe disability; requires constant nursing care and attention, bedridden, incontinent

WHO Performance Scale (Table 5.22c)

0	Fully active, no restrictions
1	Restricted in strenuous activities, ambulatory, able to do light work
2	Unable to work, ambulatory
3	Able to perform limited self-care, wheelchair 50% of time
4	Disabled, unable to perform self-care, wheelchair bound, or bedridden
5	Dead

5.3 Pediatric Head Injuries

5.3.1 Guidelines for the Acute Medical Management of Severe TBI in Infants, Children, and Adolescents[31] (Table 5.23) G

Topic		Recommendations	Comments	Level of evidence
Treatment thresholds	ICP threshold	20 mm Hg	• Sustained ICP > 20 mm Hg is associated with poor outcome • Optimal ICP treatment threshold may be age dependent	Low (III)
	CPP threshold	• In infants: ≥ 40 mm Hg • In adolescents: ≥ 40–50 mm Hg	There may be age-specific threshold with infants (at the lower end) and adolescents (at the upper end of this range)	Low (III)
Monitoring	ICP monitoring	May be considered in infants and children with severe TBI	There is evidence of improved outcome with successful ICP lowering therapies	Low (III)
	Neuroimaging	Routine repeat CT > 24 h after admission + initial follow-up study may not be indicated for decisions about neurosurgical intervention, if: • No neurological deterioration • No ICP increase	Role of acute MRI in TBI is not validated yet in large studies for influencing management decisions, although MRI sensitivity is superior to CT	Low (III)

Noninvasive measures	Hyperosmolar therapy	Hypertonic saline should be considered for Tx of severe pediatric TBI with ↑ ICP:
		• Effective doses of 3% saline for acute use: 6.5–10 mL/kg (level II)
		• Effective doses as a continuous infusion of 3% saline: 0.1–1 mL/kg/h on a sliding scale (level III)
		  – Use minimum dose needed to keep ICP < 20 mm Hg
		  – Keep serum osmolality <360 mOsm/L
			Mannitol, although commonly used for management of ↑ ICP in pediatric TBI, lacks literature support	• Medium (II; for acute use of 3% saline)
				• Low (III; for continuous infusion of 3% saline)

Hypothermia	• Moderate hypothermia (32–33°C):
	  – Beginning within 8 h after severe TBI for up to 48 h duration should be considered as needed to ↓ICP
	  – Beginning early after severe TBI and lasting for < 24 h should be avoided
	• Rewarming after induced hypothermia @ >0.5°C/h should be avoided
		• Unclear evidence regarding the efficacy of moderate hypothermia vs. others as either a first-line agent or to treat refractory intracranial hypertension
		• There is level II evidence that mild/moderate hypothermia can attenuate intracranial hypertension vs. normothermia
		• There are conflicting results concerning the effect of hypothermia on mortality and/or neurologic outcome
		• Short periods of hypothermia (< 24 h) and rapid rewarming were associated with most complications
		
		Medium (II)

Noninvasive measures **Barbiturates**	• High-dose barbiturate therapy may be considered in hemodynamically stable patients with refractory intracranial hypertension despite maximal medical–surgical Tx
	• *Take measures to maintain adequate CPP with high-dose barbiturate therapy:*
	  – Continuous arterial blood pressure monitoring
	  – Continuous cardiovascular support
		• Barbiturates ↓ICP effectively
		• No sufficient evidence of beneficial effect on survival or neurological outcome with high-dose barbiturate therapy
		• High-dose barbiturates is associated with hypotension → close arterial BP monitoring to avoid or treat promptly hemodynamic instability
		• No sufficient evidence for prophylactic use of barbiturates to prevent intracranial hypertension or for neuroprotective effects in children
		
		Low (III)

Noninvasive measures **Hyperventilation**	• Avoidance of prophylactic severe hyperventilation to a PaCO$_2$ < 30 mm Hg in initial 48 h after injury may be considered • *Caution with use of hyperventilation for refractory intracranial hypertension:* consider advanced neuromonitoring → evaluate cerebral ischemia	• Hyperventilation is commonly used in management of pediatric severe TBI despite the lack of adequate evidence • Prophylactic hyperventilation is associated with ↓CBF → use advanced neuromonitoring to prevent cerebral ischemia • Prolonged and/or significant hypocarbia is associated with poor outcome in pediatric severe TBI Low (III)

Steroids	Use of corticosteroids is not recommended to improve outcome OR ↓ICP for children with severe TBI	• Steroid Tx is not associated with: – Improved functional outcome – ↓Mortality – ↓ICP • Complications of steroid Tx: – ↓Endogenous cortisol (with dexamethasone) – ↑Incidence of pneumonia	Medium (II)
Analgesics, sedative, and muscle relaxation	• Medications that may be considered for control of intracranial hypertension: – Etomidate (*caution*: weigh risks resulting from adrenal suppression) – Thiopental (as a single dose) • *Continuous propofol infusion* for either sedation OR management of refractory intracranial hypertension in infants and children with severe TBI is not recommended by Food and Drug Administration (FDA)	There is no sufficient evidence for the use of analgesics, sedatives, and NMBA in pediatric severe TBI management, although they are commonly used	Low (III)
Noninvasive measures	Antiseizure prophylaxis	Prophylactic Tx with phenytoin may be considered to reduce incidence of early posttraumatic seizures in pediatric severe TBI	• Early posttraumatic seizures occur in 10% of pediatric TBI patients • *Caution*: monitor phenytoin levels • No sufficient data in pediatric TBI show ↓long-term posttraumatic seizures OR improvement of long-term neurological outcome with antiseizure prophylaxis	Low (III)

(Continued) ▲

| Invasive measures | CSF drainage | 1. CSF drainage through evd may be considered in the Mx of ↑ICP in children w/severe TBI
2. The addition of lumbar drain may be considered in the case of refractory intracranial hypertension w/ a functioning evd, if on imaging studies:
  • There is no mass lesion
  • There is no midline shift
  • Basal cisterns are open | No randomized controlled trial comparing efficacy of tx of ↑ICP in pediatric TBI with or w/o CSF drainage | Low (III) |
| | Decompressive craniectomy for increased ICP | Decompressive craniectomy (duraplasty, leave bone flap out) may be considered for pediatric pts w/ TBI:
• W/ early signs of neuro deterioration or herniation
• Intracranial hypertension refractory to medical Mx during the early stages of their Tx | • Surgical technique: large craniectomy, large duraplasty, leave bone flap out
• Possible effects of decompressive craniectomy:
  – Reversal of early signs of neuro deterioration/herniation
  – Tx of intracranial hypertension refractory to medical mx
  – There is correlation of above effects w/ improved outcomes | Low (iii) |

Note: Level of evidence—level I: good-quality RCT; level II: moderate-/poor-quality RCT OR good-quality cohort; level III: moderate-/poor-quality RCT or cohort OR moderate-/poor-quality case control OR case series, databases, registries.

5.3.2 Indications for CT in Children with GCS[14-15] After Head Trauma[32] (Table 5.24a) G

Recommendation	Child < 2 years of age	Child ≥ 2 years of age
CT recommended	• GCS = 14 or • Other signs of altered mental status[a] or • Palpable skull fracture (4.4% Risk of clinically important TBI)	• GCS =14 or • Other signs of altered mental status[a] or • Signs of basilar skull fracture (4.3% Risk of clinically important TBI)
Observation or CT Taking into account other clinical factors: • Physician experience • Multiple versus isolated findings • Worsening signs or symptoms after emergency department observation • Parental preference • Age < 3 mo	• Scalp hematoma occipital or parietal or temporal • History of LOC ≥ 5 seconds or • Severe mechanism of injury[b] or • Not acting normally per parent (0.9% Risk of clinically significant TBI)	• History of loc or • History of vomiting or • Severe mechanism of injury[b] or • Severe headaches (0.8% Risk of clinically significant TBI)
No CT recommended	Not meeting above criteria (<0.02% Risk of clinically significant TBI)	Not meeting above criteria (<0.05% Risk of clinically significant TBI)

[a]*Other signs of altered mental status:*
• Agitation, somnolence.
• Repetitive questioning.
• Slow response to verbal communication.

[b]*Severe mechanism of injury:*
• MVA with patient ejection.
• Death of another passenger.
• Rollover
• Pedestrian or bicyclist without helmet struck by a motorized vehicle.
• Falls > 0.9 M for age <2 y or >1.5 M for age ≥2 y.
• Head struck by high-impact object.

Radiation exposure from CT scans in pediatric patients[33-35] (Table 5.24b) G

• Estimated lifetime cancer mortality risk attributable to radiation in a 1-year-old from
  – Abdominal CT = 0.18%
  – Head CT = 0.07%
• An estimated 1 in 4000 brain CTs in children would be followed by a malignancy
• The estimated risk of cancer death from a single head CT is highest in the youngest patients (exponentially higher in age < 1 year)
• Estimated risk in the 10 years following CT for patients < 10 years of age is 1 brain tumor per 10,000 patients

5.4 Pediatric-Specific Head Injury

5.4.1 Cephalhematoma/Scalp Hematomas[11,36] (Table 5.25a)　G

Definition	Collection of blood under the scalp
Types	a. Subgaleal hematoma b. Subperiosteal hematoma

	Subgaleal hematoma	Subperiosteal hematoma
Definition	Blood collection between galea-periosteum	Blood collection under the periosteum (elevates periosteum)
Age	• Neonates during birth • Children of any age	• Usu. newborns during birth • Rarely in older children
Consistency	Soft, fluctuant, shifts with head repositioning	Firm, less fluctuant
Limitation by sutures	Crossing sutures	Limited by sutures
Scalp mobility		Scalp moves over the mass
Progression in size	May increase significantly in size (anemia, hypotension) and require blood transfusion (age <1 y) → potentially life–threatening (in neonates)	Very rarely increase in size so much as to cause hemoglobin decrease
Calcification	Does not calcify	Can calcify
Mx　Non surgical	• Close observation <1y, esp. Infants (resolution in 2 – 4 wks): – Serial blood exams for anemia – Watch for jaundice as blood absorbs (in infants, as late as 10 d after formation)	Observation (resolution in 2 – 4 wks)
Surgical	• Surgery may be required to control bleeding vessels (rarely)	• For persistent subperiosteal hematomas of >6 wks → obtain skull x-ray → if calcified: a. Surgical removal for cosmetic reasons or b. Observation → skull returns to normal contour in 3 – 6 mos w/o surgery

!! Caution: Avoid needle aspiration → risk of infection, risk of anemia (newborns)

5.4.2 Growing Skull Fracture (GSF; Posttraumatic Leptomeningeal Cyst)[11,36,37] (Table 5.25b) G

Definition	Fracture line that widens with time

Epidemiology	• 0.05–1.6% of pediatric skull fractures[38]
	• Age of injury[39]:
	  – Usually in children <1 y, >90% before age of 3 y (requires rapid brain growth)
	  – Rare adult cases reported
	• Location: >> parietal bone (but also elsewhere)

Mechanism[16]	• Trauma usually causes a widely separated bone fracture + dural tear (prerequisite) → brain + intact leptomeninges herniate through dural tear occupying fracture line → interference with bone healing (erosion/smoothing of bone edges) → bone defect expands • Caution: undiagnosed hydrocephalus can predispose to GSF
Elapsed time from injury	Median time: 18 mo postinjury May rarely occur within 6 mo postinjury
DDx	Pseudogrowing fractures: skull fracture lines that seem to initially grow without subgaleal mass without dural tear → heal spontaneously → follow-up skull X-ray within 1–2 mo to R/O
Presentation	• Soft pulsatile mass under the scalp • Head pain • Occasionally seizures, neurological deficit (mechanism: focal brain irritation/gliosis due to interaction between pulsatile brain and fracture edges)
Diagnosis	• Serial skull X-rays show progressive widening fracture and scalloping of edges • Head CT/MRI: more sensitive → also show herniated leptomeninges

Treatment[40]	a. **True growing skull fractures**	• Only surgical tx:
		  – Craniotomy surrounding fracture site exposing full extent of dural defect (dural defect> bone defect)
		  – Repair dural defect w/ pericranial / synthetic graft
		  – Repair bone defect (cranioplasty)
		• If hydrocephalus present → treat first w/ VP shunt and then repair fracture

	b. **Pseudo-growing fractures**	• F/U w/ x-rays
		• Surgery needed only if:
		  – Fracture line widening persists for months or
		  – Subgaleal mass develops

5.4.3 Depressed Skull Fractures (Table 5.25c)

Epidemiology	Location: most common in frontal and parietal bones

Most common types depending on age	a. Newborn: ping-pong ball fracture
	   • Definition: focal bone indentation like crushed ping-pong ball
	   • Usually temporal bone
	b. Children < 3.5 y: simple fractures from home accidents
	c. Older children: compound fractures from MVAs with dural laceration

Treatment	**Non surgical**	• Ping – pong • Simple depressed skull fractures !! In younger children remodelling of skull occurs with brain growth
	Surgery	**Indications**
		Technique

Surgery — Indications
- Dural laceration or underlying brain injury
- Focal neurological deficit related to fractures
- Persistent cosmetic defect in older child
- CSF leak
- Signs of increased ICP

Surgery — Technique
Fracture elevation can be attempted by pushing bone fragments back out with Penfield instrument

5.4.4 Non-accidental Trauma (Table 5.25d) [G]

Epidemiology	10% Of children < 10 y brought to ER are victims of child abuse
Mech of injury	Shaken baby syndrome: vigorous shaking of child causing acceleration-deceleration type brain injury
Associated findings	• Often associated with retinal hemorrhages, SDH, SAH • Often no signs of external trauma
Suspicion	Suspect child abuse if: • Retinal hemorrhages • Bilateral chronic SDH in child < 2 y • Multiple skull fractures • Skull fractures with associated intracranial injury • Significant neurological injury with minimal signs of external trauma !! Caution: retinal hemorrhages in traumatized child with multiple injuries and inconsistent history is pathognomonic of battering

5.4.5 Infantile Acute SDH (Table 5.25e) $\boxed{G}$

Mechanism of injury	From minor head trauma
Presentation	• Often also retinal hemorrhages • Often seizure lasting from minutes to 1 h after trauma
Treatment	If small may be treated with subdural tap

5.4.6 Benign Extra-axial Fluid Collections in Children[41] (Table 5.25f) $\boxed{G}$

Epidemiology	More common in term infants Mean age of presentation: 4 mo	
Fluid properties	Fluid is clear yellow xanthochromic with high protein	
Etiology	Unclear	
CT appearance	Hypodensities over frontal lobes, interhemispheric, sylvian fissure, sulci Ventricles may be slightly enlarged but no transependymal flow	
Presentation	May show: • Large or tense fontanelle, accelerated head growth • Developmental delay • Frontal bossing • Possible seizures	
Treatment	**Non-interventional**	Observation, most resolve within 8–9 mo
	Interventional	Single subdural tap may accelerate rate of resolution
Prognosis	Head growth usually approaches normal growth curve at age 1–2 years As head growth normalizes, development also normalizes	

5.4.7 Symptomatic Chronic Extra-axial Fluid Collections in Children (Table 5.25g) $\boxed{G}$

Difference from benign	Difference to "benign" collections is degree of clinical manifestation	
Etiology	Post-traumatic (child abuse) Post infections Post surgery Tumors	
CT appearance	Ventricular compression and obliteration of sulci	
Presentation	Large head, seizures, vomiting, lethargy Full fontanelle, macrocrania, retinal hemorrhages, coma	
Treatment	**Non interventional**	Observation (no symptoms, only large head)
	Interventional	• Serial subdural taps • Burr hole drainage • Subdural-peritoneal shunt (unilateral shunt for bilateral drainage is sufficient) with extremely low pressure valve; remove after 2–3 mo

5.5 Intensive Care Unit

5.5.1 Conditions Requiring ICU Care (Table 5.26)   G

Post-operative care	• Craniotomy • Transsphenoidal procedures • Neuro-endovascular procedures • Carotid surgery • Craniofacial surgery • Major spine surgery • Any surgery with risk of neurological deterioration
Risk of systemic complications	• Loss of airway • Respiratory failure • Significant hemorrhage
Related to anesthesia	• Residual effect of sedation • Muscle paralysis • High-dose analgesia • Pharmacological coma • Intraop hypothermia • Significant drug reaction (anaphylaxis, malignant hyperthermia)
Related to patient	• Unanticipated complication intraoperatively • Advanced age • Organ dysfunction (cardiac, pulmonary, kidney, liver) • Sepsis • Trauma • Requiring blood pressure augmentation • Coagulopathy • Post iv rtPA, intra-arterial rtpa or endovascular embolectomy • Large hemispheric stroke with impeding mental status decline • Loss of airway-protecting reflexes • Basilar artery involvement • Crescendo TIAs

5.5.2 Intubation

Criteria for intubation (Table 5.27a)

a. Inability to protect airway	• Comatose state • Patient combativeness requiring sedation • Loss of protective airway reflexes (stroke …) • Facial trauma • Laryngeal edema or injury
b. Failure to ventilate or oxygenate	• Cervical spinal cord injury • Neuromuscular disease (myasthenia gravis) • ARDS • Multi-traumatized patient with pulmonary or cardiac impairment
c. Anticipated deterioration	• Progressive neurological disorder (Guillain-Barre) • Transverse cervical myelitis • Vasospasm in SAH

Note: Clinical judgment is the best predictor for the need to intubate.

Intubation checklist (Table 5.27b) G

a. Oxygen	• Supply is available and tested • Oxygen delivery device is available
b. Airway equipment	• Face mask • Laryngoscope × 2 and blades, tested • Endotracheal tubes, different sizes • Tape or tie for endotracheal tube
c. Difficult airway equipment	• Video laryngoscope • Oro- and nasopharyngeal airways • Rescue airways (laryngeal mask) • Cricothyroidotomy or tracheostomy kit
d. Monitoring	• Pulse oximetry (continuous) • Blood pressure (at least every 2 min or arterial line) • Ekg monitoring • Capnography
Intubation procedure	1. Pre-oxygenate with 100% for at least 3–5 minutes 2. Administer anesthetic or sedative (not necessary in comatose patient) 3. Administer neuromuscular blocking agent (not necessary in comatose patient) 4. Administer adjunct medication 5. Verify successful intubation (capnography, end-tidal CO_2) 6. Post-intubation management (sedation, ventilator settings etc.)

Extubation checklist (Table 5.27c)   G

a. Neurological	• No increased ICP
	• No repeated seizures
	• Following simple commands
	• Intact gag and cough reflexes
b. Respiration	• No significant secretions
	• No increased work breathing
	• Oxygenation > 60 mm Hg on 40% fio$_2$
	• Peep < 10 mm Hg
c. Ventilation	• Paco$_2$ <50 mm hg on spontaneous ventilation
	• Ventilation per minute < 20 ml/kg
	• RR/VT < 100 breaths/min/l (RR = respiratory rate, VT = tidal volume)
d. Hemodynamic	• No resolving shock
	• No decompensated cardiac failure
	• No significant hemorrhage
	• No significant arrhythmias
e. Pharmacological and metabolic	• No residual narcotics
	• No residual muscle paralytics
	• No metabolic acidosis
	• Afebrile and body temperature > 36°c

5.5.3 Sodium, Osmolality and Electrolyte Balance (Table 5.28a)   G

	Normal values	SIADH	Cerebral salt wasting (CSW)	Diabetes insipidus DI
Definition		Increased ADH secretion in absence of osmotic stimulus (syndrome of inappropriate antidiuretic hormone secretion)	Renal sodium loss with decreased extracellular fluid	Free water loss due to lack of ADH secretion
Volume status		Normal	↓	↓
CVP	3–8 mm Hg	Normal	↓	↓
Serum sodium	135–145 mEq/L	↓	↓	↑
Serum osmolality	275–295 mosm/kg	↓	↓	↑
Urine sodium	20 mEq/L spot test	↑	↑	↓
Urine osmolality	500–800 mosm/kg	↑	↑	↓ < 150 mosm/kg
Urine output	1 ml/kg/h	↓ < 0.5 ml/kg/h	↑	↑ > 250 ml/h
Hematocrit	40–54% M; 36–48% F	Normal	↑	↑
ADH		↑	Normal	↓

(Continued) ►

	Normal values	SIADH	Cerebral salt wasting (CSW)	Diabetes insipidus DI
Treatment		• Fluid restriction • Give Na⁺ • Conivaptan (ADH receptor blocker) • Demeclocycline	• Give fluid • Give Na⁺ • Fludrocorti-sone	• Drink to thirst • 0.45% NaCl to balance input/output • DDAVP

5.5.4 Treatment of Hyponatremia in SIADH (Table 5.28b) 〔G〕

Indications	Treatment protocol
a. Non-severe hyponatremia + asymptomatic b. Severe hyponatremia of unknown or long (> 48 hours) duration + asymptomatic	• Fluid restriction 500–1000 ml/d • Dietary salt supplement • Consider conivaptan

a. Non-severe hyponatremia + symptomatic
b. Severe hyponatremia of unknown or long (> 48 hours) duration + moderate symptoms
	• NaCl 0.9% at 100 ml/hr + furosemide 20 mg qd
	• **Consider:**
	  – Conivaptan (ADH receptor antagonist)
	  – Demeclocycline

a. Severe hyponatremia + short (<48 hours) duration b. Hyponatremia with severe symptoms	• ICU care • NaCl 3% at 1–2 ml/kg/hr + furosemide 20 mg qd • Check Na⁺ q 2–3 hours
Definitions	Hyponatremia	• Mild to moderate hyponat-remia: Na⁺:125–135 mEq/L • Severe hyponatremia: Na+ < 125 mEq/L
	Symptoms	• Moderate symptoms: headaches, lethargy • Severe symptoms: coma, seizures
Rate of serum sodium correction	• 1 mEq/L per hour or • 8 mEq/L in 24 hours or • 18 mEq/L in 48 hours !! Caution: avoid rapid correction (risk of central pontine myelinolysis)	

5.5.5 Antithrombotic Reversal Guidelines for Intracranial Hemorrhage[42] (Table 5.29) G

Medication	Use for reversal (ICH or suspected ICH)	Comments
Vitamin k antagonist: (Coumadin®, warfarin)	1. Vitamin K 10 mg slow iv, repeat dose after 24 h, if INR still ≥ 1.4 2. If INR ≥ 1.4: Prothrombin complex concentrate (PCC) with weight-adjusted dosing 3. Repeat inr test within 1 hour and then q 6 h × 48 hours 4. If repeat INR still ≥ 1.4: Fresh frozen plasma (FFP) ! If PCC not available, use Vitamin K + FFP !! Target INR < 1.4	Caution: • Cerebral venous thrombosis: do not reverse anticoagulation (even if ICH is present) • Do not use recombinant factor VIIa (RF VIIa) – high thrombosis rate
Factor Xa inhibitors (apixaban, rivaroxaban, edoxaban)	1. 50G activated charcoal in intubated patients with enteral access within 2 hours of medication ingestion 2. PCC 50 u/kg iv	Do not use RF VIIa

Direct thrombin inhibitors (DTI) (dabigatran, argatroban, bivalirudin, desirudin, lepirudin)	1. For dabigatran:
	  a. 50g activated charcoal in intubated patients with enteral access within 2 hours of medication ingestion and
	  b. Idarucizumab 5 g iv in 2 doses iv
	  c. Consider hemodialysis or idarucizumab redosing for refractory cases
	2. For other DTIs: activated PCC 50 u/kg iv	

Heparin and heparinoids (heparin, enoxaparin, dalteparin, nadroparin, tinzaparin, danaparoid)	1. Unfractionated heparin: protamin 1 mg iv per 100 units heparin in the previous 2–3 h (max. 50 mg single dose)
	2. Enoxaparin: depending on enoxaprin last dose
	  a. Dose within 8 hours: protamine 1 mg iv per 1 mg enoxaparin (max. 50 mg in single dose)
	  b. Enoxaparin dose 8–12 hours: protamine 0.5 mg iv per 1 mg enoxaparin (max. 50 mg in single dose)
	  c. Dose > 12 hours: no therapy
	3. Dalteparin, nadroparin, tinzaparin: last dose within 3–5 half lives (~ 12 hours):
	  • Protamine 1 mg iv per 100 units or
	  • RF VIIa 90 mcg/kg iv if protamine contraindicated
	4. Danaparoid: RF VIIa 90 mcg/kg iv
		Do not use FFP or PPC

(Continued) ▶

Medication	Use for reversal (ICH or suspected ICH)	Comments
Pentasaccharides (fondaparinux)	• PCC 20 u/kg iv or • RF VIIa 90 mcg/kg iv	Do not use protamine

Thrombolytics (alteplase, reteplase, tenecteplase)	Received thrombolytics < 24 hours before:
	• Cryoprecipitate 10 units iv or
	• If cryoprecipitate is contraindicated:
	  – Tranexamic acid 10–15 mg/kg iv over 20 min or
	  – E-aminocaproic acid 4–5g iv
		Consider additional cryoprecipitate if fibrinogen < 150 mg/dL

Antiplatelets (aspirin, ibuprofen, naproxen, dipyridamole, clopidogrel, ticagrelor, ticlopidine, cilostazol, anagrelide)	• DDAVP 0.4 mcg/kg iv × 1 • Only if neurosurgical intervention: platelet transfusion (1 apheresis unit)	• Platelet function testing if available; if platelet function normal – no platelet transfusion • No platelet transfusion for NSAIDs or GP IIb/IIIa inhibitors even if undergoing neurosurgical intervention

5.5.6 Effect of Anesthesia Medications on Central Nervous System[6] (Table 5.30) G

Medication	ICP	CBF	CMRO$_2$	Exception
Volatile anesthetics	↑	↑ Halothane>desflurane>isoflurane>-sevoflurane (Vasodilation)	↓	Nitrous oxide: increases CBF and CMRO$_2$
IV anesthetics (thiopental, propofol, etomidate)	↓	↓	↓	Ketamine: increase CBF and CMRO$_2$
Benzodiazepines	No effect or ↓	No effect or ↓	↓	
Opioids	No effect or ↓	No effect	Minimal effect	
Non-depolarizing neuromuscular blocking agents	No effect	No effect	No effect	Occasional decrease of CBF (histamine release)
Succinylcholine	No effect	No effect	No effect	Controversial

5.5.7 Medications Commonly used in Neuro-ICU and Anesthesia

Sedatives and analgesics (Table 5.31a)

Name	Category	Onset	Duration	Dose	Comments
Propofol	GABA agonist, NMDA antagonist	1 min	15 min	1–3 mg/kg/hr Max: 5 mg/kg/hr	• Sedation • Mild analgesia • Respiratory depression • Hypotension • Propofol infusion syndrome • Hypertriglyceridemia
Midazolam	Benzodiazepine binding site on GABA-A receptor	5 min	4 h	0.02–0.1 mg/kg/h	• Drug of choice for short-term sedation • Lacks analgesic effect • Anterograde amnesia
Flumazenil	Benzodiazepine antagonist	1–2 min	50 min	0.2 mg × 1–5 doses Max: 3 mg/hr	Half-life shorter than many benzodiazepines
Morphine	Hydrophilic opioid	3 min	1–2 h	0.1 mg/kg iv q 1–2h PCA: Basal rate: 0.5–1.0 mg/hr Bolus: 0.5–1.0 mg q 10 min	Hydrophilic opioid
Fentanyl	Opioid	1 min	30 min	0.1 mcg/kg/min Max: 300 mcg/h PCA: Basal rate: 25–50 mcg/h Bolus: 10–50 mcg q 10 min	100 × Potency of morphine
Sufentanyl	Opioid	Immediate	10 min	0.01 mcg/kg/min	1000 × Potency of morphine
Remifentanil	Opioid	Immediate	10 min	0.1 mcg/kg/min	• Selective mu-receptor agonist • Potency like fentanyl
Thiopental	Barbiturate	20–30 sec	20 min	1.5–3.5 mg/kg iv bolus 0.3 mg/kg/min continuous	• Respiratory depression • Myocardial depression • Hypotension • Lowers ICP

Name	Category	Onset	Duration	Dose	Comments
Pentobarbital	Barbiturate	15 min	Variable (3–4 h) Half-life often 48 h	1. Loading dose: 10 mg/kg iv over 30 min 2. Then 5 mg/kg/hr × 3 hours 3. Then 1 mg/kg/hr	• Indication: barbiturate coma • Side effects: respiratory depression, hypotension • Burst suppression: occurs in most patients at serum level of 50 mcg/ml • Level valid **for brain death**: <10 mcg/ml
Dexmedetomidine	α$_2$ agonist	5 min	2–6 h	1. Loading dose: 0.1 mcg/kg iv for 10 min 2. Then 0.2–0.7 mcg/kg/h	• Sedative and analgesic • No amnesia • No respiratory depression • Hypotension and bradycardia
Haloperidol	Neuroleptic Butyrophe-non	10 min	12 h	1. 1–5 mg increments iv q h until sedation 2. 25% Of effective dose iv q 6 h Max: 300 mg/24 h	• Contraindications: in parkinson's disease, pregnancy and seizures • Does not cause respiratory depression !! Caution: extrapyramidal symptoms even after 1 Use, QT-prolongation
Ketamine	NMDA antagonist	10 min	1 h	1. 0.5–2.0 mg/kg iv bolus 2. Then 0.1–0.5 mg/min iv continuous	Anesthetic, hypnotic, analgesic, amnestic !! Caution: ICP increase, seizure risk
Etomidate	GABA-A modulator and agonist	30 sec	5 min	0.3 mg/kg iv bolus	• Sedative • Reduces ICP !! Caution: prolonged use causes suppression of Corticosteroid synthesis – increases mortality
Diphenhydramine	H1 receptor antagonist	1–5 min	6–8 h	25–50 mg iv q 6–8 h	• Sedation • Used to treat: – Extrapyramidal symptoms of neuroleptics – Pruritus – Antitussive

Medications to treat hypertension (Table 5.31b)

Name	Category	Onset	Duration	Dose	Comments
Labetolol	A, β₁, β₂, antagonist	5 min	6 h	• Bolus: 10 mg iv over 2 min • Continuous: 1–2 mg/min • Max: 300 mg in 24 h	!! Caution in patients with left ventricular Dysfunction and pulmonary disease
Nitroglycerine	Nitro-vasodilator	1 min	10 min	• Bolus:50 mcg iv • Continuous: 5 mcg/kg/min • Max: 100 mcg/kg/min	!! Caution: can increase ICP, methemoglobin Production
Nicardipine	Ca⁺⁺ channel blocker	5 min	4 h	1. Continuous: 5 mg/h 2. Once bp control is achie-ved decrease by 3 mg/h Max: 15 mg/h	• No effect on ICP • No bradycardia
Nitropruside	Vasodilator			• Continuous: 0.25 mcg/kg/min • Max: 5 mcg/kg/min	
Enalaprilat	ACE inhibitor	15 min	6 h	• 1 mg slow iv over 5 min • Max: 5 mg q 6 h	Can cause hyperkalemia !! Caution: contraindicated in preg-nancy and Bilateral renal artery stenosis
Esmolol	β₁ antagonist	1 min	30 min	• Bolus: 500 mcg/kg iv over 1 min • Continuous: 50 mcg/kg/min • Max: 300 mcg/kg/min	!! Caution: pulmonary disease, left ventricular Dysfunction
Hydralazine	Vasodilator Nitrate	10 min	6 h	• 5–10 mg iv over 2 min • Max: 40 mg	Cardiac ischemia

Neuromuscular blocking agents (NMBAs) (Table 5.31c)

Name	Category	Dose	Comments
Pancuronium	• Non-depolarizing • For icu care • Long-acting (1 bolus = 90 min)	• 0.1 mg/kg iv bolus • Adjust continuous dose prn	NMBA of choice for ICU care !! Caution: • Vagolytic → causing tachycardia • In renal and liver failure (prolonged half life)
Vecuronium	• Non-depolarizing • Intermediate-acting	1. 0.1 mg/kg bolus 2. Then 1 mcg/kg/min continuous	No histamine release !! Caution: liver and renal failure → recovery time may be 1–2 d
Rocuronium	• Non-depolarizing • Intermediate-acting	1. 0.5 mg/kg iv bolus 2. Then 10 mcg/kg/min continuous	NMBA of choice for rapid sequence intubation
Cisatracurium	• Non-depolarizing • Intermediate-acting	• 0.1 mg/kg bolus, • 3 mcg/kg/min continuous	• NMBA of choice for renal and liver failure • Temperature and ph-dependent spontaneous Hoffman degradation
Succinylcholine	• Depolarizing • Very short acting	1.0 mg/kg bolus	For anesthesia induction and emergencies

Medications for blood pressure regulation in ICU setting (Table 5.31d)

Name	Category	Effect	Onset (min)	Duration (min)	Dose	Side effects
Adrenaline (Epinephrine)	α and β agonist	Positive inotrope Vasoconstrictor	1–2	1–5	0.03–0.5 mcg/kg/min Max 20 mcg/kg/min	Tachyarrhythmia
Noradrenaline	α- and β agonist (α > β)	Vasoconstrictor	1–2	1–2	0.01–0.5 mcg/kg/min Max 30 mcg/kg/min	Renal and visceral hypoperfusion
Phenylephrine	Selective α-1 agonist	• Vasoconstrictor • Increases cardiac output	1	15–30	40 mcg/min, titrate Max: 200 mcg/min	!! Caution: avoid in spinal cord injury

Name	Category	Effect	Onset (min)	Duration (min)	Dose	Side effects
Dopamine	• Low dose: d1 • Medium dose: β_1, d1 • High dose: α, β_1, d1	• Low dose = renal dose: increases urine output • Medium dose: positive inotrope • High dose: vasoconstriction	5	10	1–20 mcg/kg/min Max 50 mcg/kg/min	Coronary ischemia
Dobutamine	$\beta_1 > \beta_2 > \alpha$	Positive inotrope	1–10	10–15	2.5–10 mcg/kg/min Max 40 mcg/kg/min	Tachyarrhythmia Platelet dysfunction
Vasopressin	V1 agonist	Increases BP and Peripheral vascular resistance	1	60		

Other medications (Table 5.31e)

Name	Category	Indication	Dose	Comments
Magnesium	Electrolyte		1. 4–6 G iv bolus in 5 min 2. Then 1–2 g/h iv for 48 h	• Seizures • Eclampsia
Lidocaine	Local anesthetic	• Adjunctive medication for intubation • Antiarrhythmic	• 1.5 mg/kg • Max: 300 mg	Reduces cough reflex and therefore ICP rise when intubating
Clonidine[43]	α_2 agonist	• Sedative • To treat withdrawal symptoms • Postoperative shivering, • Hypertension • As adjuvant to opioids	• 0.1mg iv q 8–12 h • Max: 0.8 mg/d	

5.6 Cases

5.6.1 Severe Head Injury with Diffuse Axonal Injury

Chief complaint/History of present illness	• A 23 y/o man involved in a rollover MVA is brought to the ER intubated, with hard cervical collar, on a back board.
Physical examination	• His Glasgow Coma Scale (GCS) is 6T without eye opening, intubated and withdrawal to pain (E:1, V:1, M:4).
	• The trauma team has cleared him from all other injuries including spinal and vascular trauma.

Imaging

1. Describe the imaging findings of head CT.

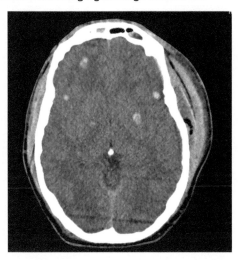

CT head without contrast shows diffuse swelling and multiple high-density foci in the white matter consistent with diffuse axonal injury (DAI) grade I; significant left extracranial swelling or fluid collection

2. How do you quantify midline shift and basal cistern compression?
   (See Table 5.20).

3. What are the three grades of DAI?
   • **Grade I (mild):** Coma 6 to 24 hours, hemorrhagic foci in grey-white matter interfaces.
   • **Grade II (moderate):** Coma >24 hours without abnormal posturing, hemorrhagic foci in corpus callosum.
   • **Grade III (severe):** Coma for months with abnormal posturing, hemorrhagic foci in dorsolateral quadrants of upper brainstem, superior cerebellar peduncles. (See Table 5.1: Diffuse axonal injury).

4. Management algorithm of increased ICP:
   a. **What is your plan?**
      Patient should be taken to ICU and an ICP monitor should be placed. (See Table 5.8b).

   b. **After placement of ICP monitor the patient's initial ICP is 30 mm Hg. What is your plan?**
      Take Stage 1 measures to lower ICP. Avoid prophylactic hyperventilation. (See Table 5.8b).

   c. **Despite your interventions the patient's ICP 2 hours later remains 30 mm Hg. What is your plan?**
      Take Stage 2 measures and if patient does not respond consider decompressive craniectomy. (See Table 5.8b).

d. **After initially responding to your treatment (decompressive craniectomy), 24 hours later the ICP has again increased to 35 mm Hg. What is your plan?**
Consider high-dose barbiturates. (See Table 5.8b).

5. **What kind of ICP monitor would you prefer and why?**
Intraventricular catheter (EVD) is the preferred method. It's the most accurate and reliable and allows CSF drainage. (See Table 5.10a).

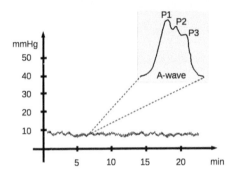

Physiologic waves. (See Table 5.11).

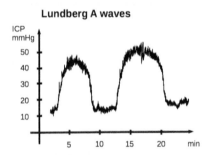

Lundberg A waves. (See Table 5.11).

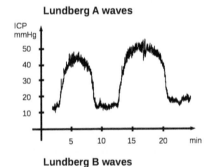

Lundberg B waves. (See Table 5.11).

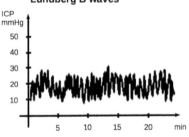

Lundberg C waves. (See Table 5.11).

5.6.2 Acute Subdural Hematoma

Chief complaint/History of present illness	• A 45 y/o man involved in a motorcycle accident is brought to the ER. • He wore no helmet.
Physical examination	• His GCS on arrival in ER is 7, without eye opening, without verbal response, and he localizes to pain with his left upper extremity and withdraws with his right upper extremity (E:1, V:1, M: 5). • His pupils are 4 mm and reactive bilaterally. • Trauma team resuscitated the patient (intubation, hemodynamic stabilization) and then cleared him from all other injuries.

Imaging

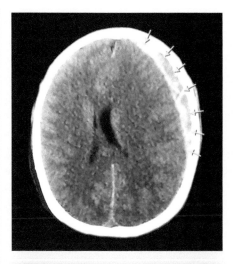

CT head shows an acute subdural hematoma (ASDH) (hyperdense, extra-axial collection, crescentic shape, *arrows*) extending from left frontal lobe to the parietal lobe (crossing sutures) resulting in marked midline shift.

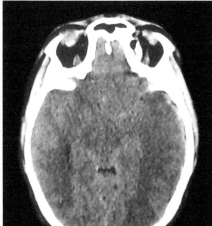

CT head shows complete effacement of basal cisterns.

1. How are the basal cisterns evaluated and what is the clinical value of this finding? (See Table 5.20).

2. **What is your plan?**
   STAT surgical evacuation of hematoma.

3. **What are the indications for surgical evacuation of an ASDH?**
   (See Table 5.14a: Management).

4. **Describe the craniotomy and the key procedural steps for the hematoma evacuation.**
   (See Table 5.14a: Management and Table 10.9b).

5. **After hematoma evacuation you notice acute brain swelling and herniation through craniotomy. What is your management?**
   (See Table 10.9d and Table 11.1a).

6. **What is the overall mortality and which are the poor prognostic factors of ASDH?**
   (See Table 5.14a: Mortality).

7. **What are the sources of bleeding in traumatic acute subdural hematomas?**
   (See Table 5.14a: Source of bleeding).

8. **What are the causes of spontaneous (acute) subdural hematomas? What is the management?**
   (See Table 5.14b).

5.6.3 Blunt Cerebrovascular Injury

Chief complaint/History of present illness	• You are called to the ER to evaluate a 62 y/o male s/p MVA because of fluctuating hemiparesis of the left upper and lower extremity.
Physical examination	• Patient appears to have 3+/5 strength in the left upper and lower extremity in an upper-motor neuron pattern • Small right pupil with decreased pupillary reaction to light.

1. **What is your plan? What condition do you suspect?**
   Patient should undergo CTA of neck and head to rule out blunt cerebrovascular injury.

2. **What are the indications to perform a CTA to rule out a blunt cerebrovascular injury? Why should the patient undergo a CTA of neck and head?**
   • To decide if a CTA of neck and head is indicated, look for:
   • Risk factors for cerebrovascular injury related to type of head injury and mechanism and type of neck/C-spine injury. (See Table 5.21a: Risk factors).
   • Symptoms and signs after examining the patient suggesting blunt cerebrovascular injury. (See Table 5.21a: Symptoms and signs).
   In this case the patient has developed Horner's syndrome and a left hemiparesis inconsistent with head injury.

3. **What is the Denver Grading Scale and what is its predictive value regarding stroke?**
   (See Table 5.21b and Table 5.21c).

4. **The patient underwent a CTA of neck and brain which revealed 20% stenosis of right ICA. What is your treatment plan for this patient (stenosis <25%)?**
   Patient should be treated either with aspirin or heparin for around 7 to 10 days. A repeat CTA should be performed then. (See Table 5.21b).

5. **The patient's symptoms have almost completely resolved 10 days later and a follow-up CTA shows no change. What is your plan?**
   We should consider treating patient with antiplatelet for 3 months and then repeat CTA. (See Table 5.21b).

References

[1] Teasdale G, Jennett B. Assessment of coma and impaired consciousness. A practical scale. Lancet 1974;2(7872):81–84

[2] Carney N, Ghajar J, Jagoda A, et al. Concussion guidelines step 1: systematic review of prevalent indicators Neurosurgery 2014;75:3–15

[3] Giza CC, Hovda DA. The new neurometabolic cascade of concussion. Neurosurgery 2014;75(Suppl 4):S24–S33

[4] McCrory P, Meeuwisse WH, Aubry M, et al. Consensus statement on concussion in sport: the 4th International Conference on Concussion in Sport held in Zurich, November 2012. PM R 2013;5(4):255–279

[5] Scorza KA, Raleigh MF, O'Connor FG. Current concepts in concussion: evaluation and management. Am Fam Physician 2012;85(2):123–132

[6] Oddo M, Crippa IA, Mehta S, et al. Optimizing sedation in patients with acute brain injury. Crit Care 2016;20(1):128

[7] Cooper DJ, Rosenfeld JV, Murray L, et al; DECRA Trial Investigators. Australian and New Zealand Intensive Care Society Clinical Trials Group. Decompressive craniectomy in diffuse traumatic brain injury. N Engl J Med 2011;364(16):1493–1502

[8] Hutchinson PJ, Kolias AG, Timofeev IS, et al; RESCUEicp Trial Collaborators. Trial of decompressive craniectomy for traumatic intracranial hypertension N Engl J Med 2016;375(12):1119–1130

[9] Arienta C, Caroli M, Balbi S. Management of head-injured patients in the emergency department: a practical protocol. Surg Neurol 1997;48(3):213–219

[10] Bullock MR, Chesnut R, Ghajar J, et al; Surgical Management of Traumatic Brain Injury Author Group. Surgical management of traumatic parenchymal lesions. Neurosurgery 2006;58(3, Suppl):S25–S46, discussion Si-iv

[11] Greenberg MS. Handbook of Neurosurgery. 8th ed. New York, NY: Thieme; 2016

[12] Cooper PR. Delayed traumatic intracerebral hemorrhage. Neurosurg Clin N Am 1992;3(3):659–665

[13] Bullock MR, Chesnut R, Ghajar J, et al; Surgical Management of Traumatic Brain Injury Author Group. Surgical management of acute epidural hematomas. Neurosurgery 2006;58(3, Suppl):S7–S15, discussion Si-iv

[14] Winn HR. Youmans and Winn Neurological Surgery. 7th ed. Philadelphia, PA: Elsevier; 2017

[15] Mckissock W, Taylor J, Bloom W, Till K. Extradural haematoma: observation on 125 cases Lancet 1960;276(7143):167–172

[16] Ellenbogen RG, Sekhar LN, Kitchen ND. Principles of Neurological Surgery. 4th ed. Philadelphia, PA: Elsevier; 2018

[17] Bullock MR, Chesnut R, Ghajar J, et al; Surgical Management of Traumatic Brain Injury Author Group. Surgical Management of acute subdural hematomas. Neurosurgery 2006;58(3, Suppl):S16–S24, discussion Si-Siv

[18] Seelig JM, Becker DP, Miller JD, Greenberg RP, Ward JD, Choi SC. Traumatic acute subdural hematoma: major mortality reduction in comatose patients treated within four hours. N Engl J Med 1981;304(25):1511–1518

[19] Hesselbrock R, Sawaya R, Means ED. Acute spontaneous subdural hematoma. Surg Neurol 1984;21(4):363–366

[20] Drapkin AJ. Chronic subdural hematoma: pathophysiological basis for treatment. Br J Neurosurg 1991;5(5):467–473

[21] Edlmann E, Giorgi-Coll S, Whitfield PC, Carpenter KLH, Hutchinson PJ. Pathophysiology of chronic subdural haematoma: inflammation, angiogenesis and implications for pharmacotherapy. J Neuroinflammation 2017;14(1):108

[22] Lind CRP, Lind CJ, Mee EW. Reduction in the number of repeated operations for the treatment of subacute and chronic subdural hematomas by placement of subdural drains. J Neurosurg 2003;99(1):44–46

[23] Tabaddor K, Shulman K. Definitive treatment of chronic subdural hematoma by twist-drill craniostomy and closed-system drainage. J Neurosurg 1977;46(2):220–226

[24] Bullock MR, Chesnut R, Ghajar J, et al. Appendix II: evaluation of relevant computed tomographic scan findings Neurosurgery 2006;58:62

[25] Biffl WL, Moore EE, Elliott JP, et al. The devastating potential of blunt vertebral arterial injuries. Ann Surg 2000;231(5):672–681

[26] Biffl WL, Cothren CC, Moore EE, et al. Western Trauma Association critical decisions in trauma: screening for and treatment of blunt cerebrovascular injuries. J Trauma 2009;67(6):1150–1153

[27] Biffl WL, Moore EE, Offner PJ, Brega KE, Franciose RJ, Burch JM. Blunt carotid arterial injuries: implications of a new grading scale. J Trauma 1999;47(5):845–853

[28] Harrigan MR, Hadley MN, Dhall SS, et al. Management of vertebral artery injuries following non-penetrating cervical trauma. Neurosurgery 2013;72(Suppl 2):234–243

[29] Jennett B, Bond M. Assessment of outcome after severe brain damage. Lancet 1975;1(7905):480–484

[30] Meyer BC, Lyden PD. The modified National Institutes of Health Stroke Scale: its time has come. Int J Stroke 2009;4(4):267–273

[31] Kochanek PM, et al. Guidelines for the acute medical management of severe traumatic brain injury in infants, children, and adolescents:second edition Pediatr Crit Care Med 2012;13(Suppl, 1):S1–S82

[32] Kuppermann N, Holmes JF, Dayan PS, et al; Pediatric Emergency Care Applied Research Network (PECARN). Identification of children at very low risk of clinically-important brain injuries after head trauma: a prospective cohort study. Lancet 2009;374(9696):1160–1170

[33] Brenner D, Elliston C, Hall E, Berdon W. Estimated risks of radiation-induced fatal cancer from pediatric CT. AJR Am J Roentgenol 2001;176(2):289–296

[34] Mathews JD, Forsythe AV, Brady Z, et al. Cancer risk in 680,000 people exposed to computed tomography scans in childhood or adolescence: data linkage study of 11 million Australians. BMJ 2013;346:f2360

[35] Pearce MS, Salotti JA, Little MP, et al. Radiation exposure from CT scans in childhood and subsequent risk of leukaemia and brain tumours: a retrospective cohort study. Lancet 2012;380(9840):499–505

[36] Albright AL, Pollack IF, Adelson PD. Principles and Practice of Pediatric Neurosurgery. 3rd ed. New York, NY: Thieme; 2015

[37] Ellenbogen RG, Winston KR, Kupsky WJ. Tumors of the choroid plexus in children. Neurosurgery 1989;25(3):327–335

[38] Ersahin Y, Gülmen V, Palali I, Mutluer S. Growing skull fractures (craniocerebral erosion). Neurosurg Rev 2000;23(3):139–144

[39]   Lende RA, Erickson TC. Growing skull fractures of childhood. J Neurosurg 1961;18(4):479–489

[40]   Iplikcioğlu AC, Kökes F, Bayar A, Buharali Z. Leptomeningeal cyst. Neurosurgery 1990;27(6):1027–1028

[41]   Carolan PL, McLaurin RL, Towbin RB, Towbin JA, Egelhoff JC. Benign extra-axial collections of infancy. Pediatr Neurosci 1985–1986;12(3):140–144

[42]   Frontera JA, Lewin JJ III, Rabinstein AA, et al. Guideline for Reversal of Antithrombotics in Intracranial Hemorrhage: A Statement for Healthcare Professionals from the Neurocritical Care Society and Society of Critical Care Medicine. Neurocrit Care 2016;24(1):6–46

[43]   Jamadarkhana S, Gopal S. Clonidine in adults as a sedative agent in the intensive care unit. J Anaesthesiol Clin Pharmacol 2010;26(4):439–445

6 Pediatric Neurosurgery

6.1 Craniosynostosis (Table 6.1) $\boxed{G}$

Type	Presentation	Diagnostics	Other	Treatment
Deformational plagiocephaly **AKA positional plagiocephaly** **CAUTION:** must be differentiated from true suture synostosis	 1. **Head** has a parallelogram shape (contralateral occipital bossing) 2. Ear may be anterior on symptomatic side **vs.** unilateral coronal suture synostosis **Unilateral coronal/lambdoid premature closure:** 1. **Head** has a trapezoid shape 2. Ear may be normal or in posterior/inferior position on symptomatic side	1. Imaging is rarely necessary. 2. **When needed** perform: a. Skull X-rays or b. Ultrasound of the suspected suture 3. **When above is not diagnostic, consider CT scan**[1,2]		• Usually **self-resolving** starting by 6 mo of age, which is when the child starts sitting up • **Six months of age** is also an important milestone because skull growth slows down and thus skull plasticity to reform diminishes • Always **rule out torticollis.** If present, start physical therapy • **Effectiveness of treatment options**[1]: 1. Repositioning < 2. Physical therapy < 3. Helmet • **Treatment options:** 1. *Positioning pillow:* equally effective as physical therapy but with significant compliance issues 2. *Physical therapy:* for children older than 7 wk 3. *Helmet:* preferred: a. in cases of poor response to repositioning/physical therapy b. in cases with severe deformity

The following craniosystosis types are treated surgically (craniosynostosis types are presented in order of frequency In the USA)

Type	Presentation	Diagnostics	Other	Treatment
Sagittal suture synostosis: a. *Dolichocephaly:* long and narrow head with cephalic index usually below 75 *OR* b. **Scaphocephaly:** *severely* long and narrow head (dolichocephalic) that presents as inverted boat with a keel. • So all scaphocephalic patients are also dolichocephalic but not the opposite[3] • **Cephalic index:** $\frac{max\ head\ width}{max\ head\ length} \times 100$	 a. Frontal/occipital/ (or both) bossing (depending of which part of suture has closed) b. Palpable sagittal ridge c. Reduced biparietal diameter d. No orbit or midface abnormalities	1. CT brain 2. MRI brain	• Most frequent nonsyndromic craniosynostosis in the United States (accounts for ~50% of cases) • Most frequent single suture craniosynostosis that may present with **increased ICP**[4]	**GOAL:** make head wider **Surgical technique:** 1. *Patient positioning:* a. *Supine* (allows access from orbital rim to behind lambdoid suture): consider if primarily anterior suture is involved requiring frontal bone remodeling. b. *Sphinx* (access from orbital rim to subocciput, but apply with caution because of extreme neck extension): consider if the entire suture is involved requiring frontal and occipital bone remodeling c. *Prone* (uncommon, access from subocciput to just anterior of coronal suture): consider if primarily posterior suture is involved[5] 2. *Zigzag incision* positioned between anterior and posterior fonta nelles. Leave temporalis muscle attached to skin 3. Leave *periosteum intact* 4. Use fontanelles to *strip dura* (otherwise perform burr holes on each side) 5. *Remove entire sagittal suture* along with 1 inch of bone on each side. Put patties on sinus (to reduce the risk of bleed and air embolism). 6. *Barrel stave osteotomies* between coronal and lambdoid sutures → bend outward. Head growth will also splay osteotomies open over time. ± **helmet** for 6 mos postop

Type	Presentation	Diagnostics	Other	Treatment

Coronal suture synostosis	A. Unilateral anterior plagiocephaly
	
	a. *Harlequin eye* (elevation of superolateral corner of the orbit on pathological side)
	b. *Strabismus*
	c. *Contralateral:*
	  i. *Frontal bossing* (secondary to open contralateral coronal suture and metopic suture)
	  ii. *Parietal bossing* (secondary to open contralateral coronal and sagittal sutures)
	d. *Nose deviation*
		1. CT
		2. MRI
		3. Depending on presentation, consider **genetic analysis**
			2nd most frequent synostosis in United States (accounts for ~25% of cases); metopic suture synostosis is a close 3rd	**GOAL:** make head longer
				
				Craniotomy for repair + orbital rim based on need (fronto-orbital advancement)
				
				Surgical technique
				
				Basics for both unilateral and bilateral:
				1. *Zigzag bicoronal skin incision* centered over middle of anterior fontanelle
				2. Leave *periosteum intact* (less bleeding)
				3. *Temporalis muscle* stays with skin
				4. Dissect *periorbita*
				5. Release lateral but not medial canthal ligament
				6. *Expose sphenoid* from frontozygomatic to posterior root of zygoma
				7. Use fontanelle to *strip dura* from bone
				
				A. **Unilateral**
				1. Patient *supine*
				2. *Bifrontal craniotomy* positioned behind coronal suture
				3. *Biorbital rim* ~1 inch wide + tenon extensions
				4. *Reshape* by drilling inner cortex and bend out recessed orbital rim (reconstruct this by superimposing parietal bone graft)
				5. *Reposition rim* by advancing ipsilateral tenon + recessing contralateral tenon
				6. *Drill part of hypertrophic ipsilateral sphenoid* to level of superior orbital fissure
				7. *Barrel stave osteotomies* to shape bifrontal bone, then replace it with absorbable plates or sutures

Type	Presentation	Diagnostics	Other	Treatment
	B. Bilateral (turribrachycephaly) Consider genetic syndromes: a. **Crouzon** = Cranial = bilateral closure of coronal suture + midface hypoplasia b. **Apert** = All over = bilateral closure of coronal suture + cleft palate + syndactyly c. **Pfeiffer** = craniosynostosis + broad/deviated thumbs and big toes + partial syndactyly + ocular proptosis/elbow ankylosis	1. CT 2. MRI 3. Depending on presentation, consider **genetic analysis**		B. **Bilateral** 1. Patient in supine or *sphinx position*: pre-op flexion/extension X-rays for stability 2. *Bifrontal craniotomy* to include both coronal sutures 3. *Biorbital rim* + tenon extensions 4. *Bend out both rims* and replace with tenons advanced (use absorbable mini plates) 5. *Biparietal craniotomy* with burr holes along sagittal sinus + transverse sinus → followed by *sagittal strip craniotomy* to include fontanelle (or the other way round: order is surgeon specific) 6. Dissect down to level of transverse sinus + *barrel stave osteotomies* on parietal and occipital bones 7. *Drill down bilateral–sphenoid ridges* to level of superior orbital fissure 8. *Replace all craniotomies* after barrel stave osteotomies (frontal bone may be rotated 180°, so previously bulging side is on previously recessed side) ± helmet for **4 wk postoperatively**
Metopic suture synostosis	a. **Trigonocephaly:** forehead is triangular with midline ridge b. ± hypertelorism	1. CT 2. MRI	• 19q chromosome is frequently involved • Metopic suture is the **first suture to close** physiologically at age 9 mo	**GOALs:** 1. Make head less pointy 2. Fix hypotelorism A. **If no hypotelorism:** craniotomy + fronto-orbital advancement similar to coronal synostosis B. **In case of hypotelorism:** craniotomy + address orbital rim similar to coronal synostosis, but first cut in half and place interposition graft in between the two pieces: 1. *Harvest* graft from temporal/parietal bone 2. *Plate on the inside* of rim to avoid cosmetic deformity

Type	Presentation	Diagnostics	Other	Treatment
Lambdoid suture synostosis	See Table 6.1: Positional plagiocephaly	When synostosis is suspected (such as cases of positional plagiocephaly with poor response to conservative treatment) perform: 1. CT brain 2. MRI brain	• The least frequently involved suture • Usually unilateral	Surgical technique 1. *Prone position* 2. *Bicoronal skin incision.* Dissect off muscle including occipital (leave attached to skin) 3. *Biparieto-occipital craniotomies* (both sides): start with burr holes near sagittal and transverse sinuses (a strip of bone may be left attached on sagittal sinus) 4. *Dissect dura* to below transverse sinus 5. *Barrel stave osteotomies* to include down into posterior fossa 6. *Flip bone flaps* 180° + barrel stave + reposition with absorbable plates 7. Even if frontal bossing exists, usually you don't have to surgically correct

For all craniosynostoses

Presentation	Diagnostics	Other	Treatment
Except for the typical skull and face deformities there may be accompanying: a. Cognitive deficits b. Visual impairment c. Hearing impairment d. Increased ICP (more frequently in multiple suture involvement but possibly even in single-suture involvement)[6,7] ↑ ICP *may present as:* • Papilledema • Suture diastasis (rare in synostosis) • Sellar erosion • Digital markings on inner calvarium (Luckenschadel skull)	1. Thin cut CT with reconstruction (diagnostic test of choice) *Be cautious* with the use of CT especially in young children. There is association with malignancies[8] 2. Technetium bone scan can clarify difficult cases: a. *The suture that prematurely tends to close* will have abnormally increased uptake (compared to the others) b. *The closed suture* will present with no uptake	• Focal brain hypoperfusion may also coexist[9] • Virchow's law: a. the *skull normally grows* perpendicular to the normal suture b. *Premature suture closure* will cause growth parallel to the suture	• Wait until 6 mo of age for surgery (more body weight and blood volume) • Be careful of blood loss during surgery; replace with 10 mL/kg matched blood • Consider absorbable plates (alternatives include nonabsorbable plates, sutures, wire) • Try to fill gaps with patient's own bone after the completion of surgical remodeling • Head of bed > 30° postoperatively (reduces swelling). • Expect swollen eyes for 3–4 d • If bones don't heal, redo surgery with rib grafts • Caution with air embolism during surgery (lower HOB and flood field with irrigation/wet sponges)

6.2 Encephalocele (Table 6.2)

For all encephalocele types[10]

Presentation	Diagnostics	Other	Treatment

a. CSF leak
b. Craniofacial deformities
	1. **MRI brain:**
	  a. Define *amount of brain herniation*
	  b. Rule out *hydrocephalus*
	  c. REMEMBER: rule out participation of *hypothalamus* in basal encephaloceles
	2. **MRV brain:** rule out vein/ sinus herniation
	3. **MRI spine** (15–20% of encephaloceles are associated with other neural tube defects)[11]
	4. **CT brain:** define bone defect
		• Prevalence of neural tube defects is reduced by folic **acid supplementation in pregnancy**[12]
		• Spinal myelomeningoceles are much more frequent than encephaloceles (ratio 5:1)
			• **Treatment is elective** unless CSF leak
			• **Included brain** is usually not viable so:
			  a. Reduce if possible
			  b. Otherwise amputate
			• Beware of **included blood vessels/sinuses**
			• **Dural defect** may be present depending on size of encephalocele: consider "vest over pants" closure
			• **Clean bone edges** so it can regrow together
			• Beware of **delayed onset of hydrocephalus.** Follow patient.
			
			Prognosis is related to amount of cerebral tissue herniating (since it is usually nonviable)

Type	Presentation	Diagnostics	Other	Treatment
Cranial vault	Protruding mass in convexity	See Table 6.2: For all encephalocele types	The most common in western world (~80%)	Use wedge osteotomies to expand the cranial cavity

Frontoethmoidal (sincipital): through foramen cecum	Protruding mass in face:
	 a. Nasofrontal
	 b. Nasoethmoidal
	 c. Naso-orbital
			2nd in frequency (~15%)	Usually **bifrontal craniotomy:**
				 1. Stem
				    a. *Small stem:*
				      i. Stay just extradural
				      ii. Tie off
				      iii. Amputate
				      iv. Pull it out of the nose or just let it shrivel up
				    b. *Large stem:*
				      • May have important structures
				      • Use combined extradural and intradural approach
				 2. **Multilayer repair**–use vascularized pericranial graft
				 3. If **bone defect is large:** reconstruct
				
				 CSF fistula is the most common complication

Basal: through cribriform plate or sphenoid bone	**Presentation:**
	 a. Protrusion mass through skull base into nasopharynx → **nonvisible**
	 b. **Recurrent meningitis**
	 c. **Obstructive airway**
	
	 Differential diagnosis
	 A. Encephalocele:
	    a. May be accompanied by *hypertelorism*
	    b. Mass medial to the middle turbinate
	    c. *Positive Furstenberg sign:* expansion/ pulsation with compression of jugular vein or anterior fontanelle and Valsalva maneuver
	          vs.
	 B. Midline nasal masses:
	    a. *Polyps:* pedunculated and lateral to middle turbinate, usually in adults
	    b. *Glioma:* no pulsation and no stem connection to brain)
	    c. Mucocele
	    d. Granuloma
	    e. Dermoid
			Rare (~1.5%)	

Note: Encephaloceles may also be secondary to trauma, tumor, surgery, inflammation

6.3 Chiari Malformations (Table 6.3) ⊡ G

(Left margin vertical text: LESS TO MORE SEVERE)

Type	Presentation	Diagnostics	Other	Treatment
0	**Syrinx** No descent/ no compression of neural structures	1. **MRI of brain** (T2WI is most useful) to ensure absence of supratentorial mass lesion or hydrocephalus[13] 2. **Cine MRI** to investigate CSF flow at level of foramen magnum in borderline cases		Regression of syrinx after posterior decompression has been described[14]
1	a. **Cerebellar tonsils descent** at least 5 mm below foramen magnum b. May be **asymptomatic**[15] c. **Presents with:** • *strain headache/ neck pain* (classic: tussive headache) • Signs and symptoms of *syrinx* • *Downbeat nystagmus* (pathognomonic of cervicomedullary compression) • *Other brainstem dysfunction* (drop attacks, other nystagmus, nausea, emesis, dizziness)		1. Usually in adults 2. Congenital or acquired 3. Rule out **pseudotumor cerebri** → fundoscopic examination to exclude papilledema	1. **Observation** for asymptomatic patients 2. **Surgery** for symptomatic patients in order to establish normal CSF flow through foramen magnum. a. *Primary Chiari 1:* • suboccipital craniectomy (3 × 3 cm) + C1 laminectomy • ± dural grafting • ± intradural dissection of adhesions[13] • ± dissection of tonsils with reduction of size *REMEMBER:* Always check position of transverse sinus preoperatively b. *Secondary/acquired Chiari 1* (such as in the presence of pseudotumor): first treat the cause, when possible (further treatment may not be needed) **Posttreatment results:** a. *Symptom relief:* • *Tussive pain* (80% will improve) > • *Motor* (usually not back to normal baseline) > • *Sensory* (usually no improvement particularly if long standing)[16,17] b. *Syrinx:* • Wait up to 1 y for improvement (85% will improve) • If syrinx persists and symptoms recur or persist after decompressive surgery, consider: i. *syringosubarachnoid shunt via laminectomy* at lowest level of syrinx ii. second decompression with reduction of cerebellar tonsils iii. occipitocervical fusion if there is coexisting basilar invagination

Type	Presentation	Diagnostics	Other	Treatment
L E S S **T O** **M O R E** **S E V E R E** 2	a. **Vermis–pons/ medulla–fourth ventricle: herniate below foramen magnum. Consequently:** • Apneic spells • Lower cranial nerve issues • Opisthotonos • Downbeat nystagmus b. Spina bifida/myelomeningocele c. Hydrocephalus	Most frequently associated **MRI brain findings:** a. Beaking of tectum b. Large massa intermedia c. Polymicrogyria d. Dysgenesis of corpus callosum e. Medullary kinking	Infants	• **Development of symptoms** dictates urgency of treatment[18]. Some recommend preventative intervention • **Surgery:** a. Cranial surgery is *similar to Chiari 1* b. Place *shunt first!!* *CAUTION:* Consider prophylactic or post-op *tracheostomy* for patients with cranial nerve issues • **Following closure of myelomeningocele:** 80% will develop hydrocephalus and require shunt • **Post-op results:** resolution of symptoms in 70% of patients
3	**Chiari 2 + encephalocele:** a. herniation of posterior fossa contents into C-spine + b. suboccipital encephalo-myelomeningocele		Rare	Poor prognosis

For all the above Chiari types

1. **Flexion–extension C-spine X-rays** to rule out instability 2. **MRI spine** to rule out syrinx 3. **CT myelography** in case of MRI contraindication				• Rule out and treat **hydrocephalus** • In patients with recurrent symptoms after repair and shunt, first exclude shunt malfunction • Close post-op respiratory monitoring

6.4 Dandy–Walker Malformation (Table 6.4) G

Presentation	Diagnostics	Treatment	Remember

a. **Hydrocephalus**[19,20]
b. 50% of patients have some degree of **mental retardation**
c. **Motor impairment**
d. **Systemic anomalies** may be present
Always obtain preoperative cardiac evaluation
	MRI brain
	1. Atresia of Magendie and Luschka
	2. Agenesis of cerebellar vermis
	3. Enlarged posterior fossa cyst that communicates with the 4th ventricle (tentorium and torcular herophili are usually elevated)
	4. Possible agenesis of corpus callosum
		Various therapeutic choices[21] that may be combined.
		1. **Shunt:**
		  a. Ventriculoperitoneal shunt
		    OR
		  b. Cystoperitoneal shunt
		    OR
		  c. Both
		2. **Endoscopic third ventriculostomy** possibly combined with aqueductal stent placement or fenestration of the occluding membrane
		3. **Posterior fossa craniotomy** for membrane excision
		What to shunt?
		• Because the 3rd and 4th ventricles may not communicate[22,23], shunting one of them may not be enough and above all may cause upward or downward herniation → Best option: **shunt lateral AND 4th ventricle and connect with "Y"**
		• *In infants*, use low-pressure valve and *in children* use medium pressure OR just use programmable valve
		Surgical technique:
		1. **Plan trajectories carefully on MRI!!!** → The large posterior fossa causes upward displacement of anatomic structures including sinuses.
		2. **Curvilinear incision** (of sufficient length)
		3. **Supratentorial shunt:**
		  i. *Burr hole* 4–6 cm above inion and 2–4 cm lateral
		  ii. *Trajectory* points to spot 1.5 cm above eyebrow along projection of the anterior fontanelle
		4. **Infratentorial shunt:**
		  i. *Dissect down suboccipital muscle* and identify occipital squama
		  ii. *Burr hole:* dura may be blue secondarily to cyst or venous lake
		  iii. *Aspirate* with 22-gauge needle to make sure it is not vein.
		  iv. *Dural opening should be small* because there is no brain mantle to seal CSF leak
		  v. Beware of the *catheter length* (risk of brainstem injury)
			Dandy–Walker variant: there is no enlargement of the posterior fossa[24]
			
			Blake's pouch cyst: a posterior fossa cyst (below and posterior to vermis) communicating with the 4th ventricle
			
			Mega cisterna magna: vermis and 4th ventricle are normal

6.5 Vein of Galen Malformation (Table 6.5)

Remember	Presentation	Diagnostics	Other	Treatment
There is shunting of arterial blood into the vein of Galen or its embryologic precursor:	**A. Neonates:** a. Congestive heart failure b. Cranial bruit c. Multiple organ failure	1. **Frequently diagnosed before birth with ultrasound** (usually 3rd trimester)	**Vein of Galen varix:** dilation of vein of Galen with no arteriovenous shunts	**A. Antenatal diagnosis:** Consider abortion when found in utero due to: a. Cardiac failure b. Cerebral damage[25]
A. Type 1: arterial blood shunts *into the embryologic precursor* of vein of Galen (median prosencephalic vein of Markowski, formed at age 6–11 wk). It is congenital and may be:	**B. Infancy and childhood:** a. Hydrocephalus b. Symptoms of increased ICP c. Developmental delay	2. **MRI/MRA/MRV brain** 3. **Cardiac ultrasound** 4. **Angiography if** embolization is contemplated[24]		**B. Postnatal diagnosis:** 1. *Therapeutic abstention* could be considered in selected cases based on clinical condition (e.g., in patients with encephalomalacia)
a. *Choroidal:* choroidal arteries shunt via a fine vascular network into the embryologic precursor	d. Neurological deficits e. Seizures f. Intracranial hemorrhage			2. *Transarterial glue embolization:* • Wait until age 5 mo if possible.[25] • Cardiac failure dictates immediate embolization
b. *Mural:* choroidal arteries shunt directly into the embryologic precursor. May be associated with distal venous sinus stenosis. It is better tolerated than choroidal type.				**C. Surgery** is high risk and for very limited cases
B. Type 2: parenchymal AVM shunts *into fully developed vein of Galen.* Older infants.				**D. Stereotactic radiosurgery** also has a very limited role and may be considered for asymptomatic patients. Time required for therapeutic effect is too long to consider stereotactic radiosurgery in symptomatic cases.
				E. *Treatment of hydrocephalus* (shunting): • In the setting of untreated fistula is associated with neurologic deficits, seizures, and increased hemorrhagic risk of fistula. • It may be considered in late referrals after lack of response of hydrocephalus to ≤ embolization

6.6 Spinal Defects (Table 6.6) [G]

	Dorsal bone defect	Herniation of dura and subarachnoid space through bone defect	Herniation of neural elements through bone defect
1. Spina bifida occulta	+	–	–
2. Meningocele	+	+	–
3. Myelomeningocele	+	+	+

6.7 Tethered Cord (Table 6.7) [G]

Presentation	Diagnostics	Other	Treatment

1. Pain
2. Sensory abnormalities
3. Lower extremities weakness
4. Bladder and bowel dysfunction
5. Growth spurt may precipitate the symptoms
	MRI brain and spine to exclude other pathology (e.g., Chiari syndrome, dermal sinus, etc.)	a. May be an isolated finding
		OR
		b. Presents in the context of other spinal developmental pathology (described in the following tables)
			Surgical technique: sectioning of filum terminale
			• *Filum terminale* is thicker and bluer than nerves
			• *Stimulate intraoperatively* at low setting so as to avoid current spread
			• Always pick it up and *check behind it for nerves* before sectioning
			• *Coagulate prior to cutting* (because it will retract out of site)
			Complications:
			a. Some children have *temporary urinary difficulty* secondary to nerve manipulation
			b. Possibly *meningismus* secondary to blood in subarachnoid space
			c. Sectioned filum may very rarely retether
			Prognosis:
			a. *If symptoms for < 6 mo*: good chance of improvement
			b. *If symptoms for > 1 y*: good chance of symptom stabilization
			c. *Outcome:*
			  • 90% have complete relief of *pain*
			  • 75% have *motor improvement*
			  • 50% have *bowel/bladder improvement*

6.8 Closed Defects (Table 6.8a) G

- They **include**:
  - a. Split cord malformation
  - b. Dermal sinus tract or dimple
  - c. Lipomyelomeningocele
- May be **asymptomatic or symptomatic** (usually presenting with tethered cord symptoms).
- Always **be suspicious of skin abnormalities** (hypertrichosis, hemangioma, skin appendage, dermal tract) **overlying spine**: perform ultrasound
- **Repair** is usually done at age 3 to 6 months unless there is neurological deficit or an open sinus tract

6.8.1 Split Cord Malformation[26,27] (Table 6.8b)

Disease	Presentation	Diagnostics	Treatment
Type 1 (or diastematomyelia): a. 2 dural sacs b. 2 subarachnoid spaces c. Bone septum in between	a. Conus terminalis tethering b. Myelomeningocele, sinus tract, dermoid c. Hypertrophically fused adjacent laminae d. Long buttock cleft e. Asymmetry of leg sizes f. Foot deformity	1. MRI brain and spine 2. CT myelogram	**Surgical technique:** 1. Use intraop monitoring 2. The **bony septum** is usually located at the level of densest fusion mass of lamina 3. After you **free it up**, you can usually **pull out the septum** because it is loosely attached ventrally 4. A **vessel is always associated with the septum**: bleeding is easily controlled with coagulation and wax 5. Following the removal of the bony spicule, **open the dura** and **dissect the fibrous sleeve** off the hemicords (caudally it is always more stuck) 6. **Paramedian nerve roots** are nonfunctional and should be cut to detether the cords from the dural sleeve 7. **Resect the dural sleeve** all the way anterior 8. Look for **myelomeningocele manqué** (fibroneurovascular stalk tethering hemicords dorsally): cut flush with the hemicords and untether 9. **Cut the filum terminale** and address any other malformation 10. **Close dura** **REMEMBER:** If bony band is slanted and the cord is not evenly divided, the smaller cord is very sensitive

Disease	Presentation	Diagnostics	Treatment
Type 2 (or diplomyelia): a. 1 dural sac b. 1 subarachnoid space c. Fibrous septum stuck to two hemicords **Variations:** 1. Complete septum (the least common) 2. Purely ventral 3. Purely dorsal (the most common)	As above, but: a. Bifid laminae b. Short buttock cleft	1. **MRI brain and spine** 2. **CT myelogram**	The point of dorsal dural attachment is always more caudal than the point of hemicord attachment so **fibrous band looks as if it is pointing upwards** (see image) **Surgical technique:** 1. Use intraop monitoring 2. The *location* is usually correlated with bifid lamina 3. Frequently, the *cleft is very tight*, so do not explore. You can reach the ventral attachment (if present) by rotating the cord, but it is highly risky 4. *Preserve the vessels*, that are almost always seen on the cord around the septum; unlike the ones seen in split cord type 1, these are intradural and might be feeding the spinal hemicords 5. Look for *myelomeningocele manqué* and detether. It is usually comprised of nonfunctioning dorsomedian roots and vessels. It always attaches more caudal on dorsal dura than on cord. Thus, just like the fibrous septum, it appears to be pointing upward. Trim down to the level of the cord. 6. *Reconstruct the dura*

Cephalad

Caudal

Fibrous band

Spinal cord

Dura mater

For both split cord malformation types

- **CHILDREN:** Usually *treated preventatively*, because they almost always deteriorate and they may not recuperate the lost function
- **ADULTS:** Asymptomatic adults *may be followed*, but there is controversy.
- Use intraoperative monitoring.
- **Bladder management:**
  1. *Keep the Foley* catheter for the first 2 postoperative days
  2. *Discontinue the Foley* on day 3 + ambulation → *in case of difficulty in urination or large postvoid residual volume*, try prazosin
  3. *If difficulty persists*, begin intermittent catheterization → *evaluate again* in 4–6 wk
- **Risk of neurological worsening:** Overall, there is 5% risk of neurological worsening and 3% risk of permanent bladder function worsening
- **Composite split cord malformation:** usually type 1–type 2–type 1 in sequence (one after the other) with no cord in between them. Stay extradural for the type 1 and then go intradural for the rest
- **Associated dermal sinus tract:**
  a. *in type 1:* more straightforward, as the tract is not adherent directly to the cord
  b. *in type 2:* more difficult, because the tract is intradural and often adherent to the cord caudal to split reunion

Note: Conus terminalis in children is located at L1–L2 disk space; conus lower than the midbody of L2 is considered abnormal.[27]

6.8.2 Dermal Sinus Tract or Dimple (Table 6.8c) G

Disease	Presentation	Diagnostics	Other	Treatment

Dermal sinus tract	a. **Location:**
	  i. Above gluteal fold
	  ii. Can also be located at the cephalic end of neural tube (be suspicious of dimples in nasal and occipital area)
	b. Points up
	c. **Possibly:**
	  i. CSF leak
	  ii. Infection[29]
	  iii. Tethered cord symptoms
	  iv. Intradural mass
	Differentiate from pilonidal cyst which is:
	a. Superficial to postsacral fascia on imaging
	b. *Contains* hair and skin debris
	c. *Can be infected* (then it should be treated)
		1. **Ultrasound:** initial examination
		2. **MRI brain and spine** (other anomalies of CNS can be found)[30]
		3. **Do not use a probe** to confirm diagnosis (risk of infection)
			Associated with other malformations along its tract:
			a. Epidermoid cyst
			b. Dermoid cyst
			c. Teratomas
				A. **Tracts ending on dura** should be operated:
				  a. *Operate soon* to avoid meningitis!
				  b. The *tract must be followed* throughout its entire course
				  c. In case of *intradural extension*, open dura and follow (intradural dermoid)
				  d. If an *associated cyst* is present, remove the entire cyst wall to avoid regrowth
				B. **Tracts ending at coccyx** (that do not reach the dura) should be treated only in case of infection

Dimple	a. Usually below gluteal fold b. Points down c. No CSF leak	**Ultrasound** in asymptomatic patient[30]		None

Skin moving test:
a. *Moving the skin downward* will appear to be pulling down and occlude a sinus tract
b. *Moving the skin upward* will appear to be pulling up and occlude a dimple

6.8.3 Lipomyelomeningocele (Table 6.8d) G

Type	Coronal plane	Nerves involved	Other	Treatment
Dorsal (originates cephalad to the conus)	Good	No	Usually extends to skin	**Indications:** a. Surgery for *all children* even if asymptomatic → treat at 3–6 mo of age b. If patient presents *symptomatic at later age* → treat immediately c. If patient presents asymptomatic at later age → may chose to closely observe d. Investigate for *subtle findings of bowel/bladder dysfunction* (enuresis, repeated urinary tract infections, etc.) **Surgical technique:** a. ALWAYS use *intraoperative monitoring* b. Always go high, low and wide with *exposure* c. *Find normal edges* and do not start by dissecting first through the lipoma d. *Beware of underlying compressed nerves* when opening dura. e. *Nerve roots may not be in usual location*, so be cautious when dissecting around lipoma prior to sectioning **Specifics** a. *Dorsal:* Debulk as much as safely possible opting to *leave part of the lipoma*, rather than violating the spinal cord b. *Caudal:* • Use *nerve stimulator* to differentiate normal nerves from fibrous bands • *Find plane and work it* c. *Transitional:* • Start at *cord–lipoma junction* • Constantly use neurostimulation *Consequently: increasing surgical difficulty from dorsal → caudal → transitional* **Goals:** a. Untether spinal cord. *Always cut the filum* b. Resect as much fat as safely possible c. *Avoid retethering* by creating space for CSF to circulate around neural elements. *Reapproximate the pial surfaces including closing myeloschisis, even if fat is still present and enveloped in the center of the recreated cord*
Caudal (originates from or caudal to the conus)	Pseudoplane/ dorsally	Yes, but **manageable**. Usually, the dorsal half of the lipoma can be removed	Usually intradural only (along filum)	
Transitional (originates proximal and distal to conus)	None	**Significant** nerve root involvement	Usually extends to skin	

Presentation[32]

1. **Associated skin findings:**
   a. Dimpling outside gluteal cleft
   b. Hypertrichosis
   c. Hemangiomas
   d. Skin tags
2. **Progressive cord tethering.** Causes neurologic deterioration including weakness and bowel/bladder problems Rapid growth and weight gain may precipitate acutely the symptoms
3. **Foot deformities**

REMEMBER:

1. Diagnose with **MRI** (fat: very high T1 signal and high T2 signal. May use fat suppression sequences)
2. Consider **pre-op urological evaluation** with urodynamic testing
3. In addition to lipomyelomeningoceles (by definition subcutaneous fat entering the canal through spina bifida), there are also **intradural lipomas and lipomas purely of the filum terminal**

6.9 Spinal Defects ɢ

6.9.1 Open Spinal Defects (Table 6.9a)

Disease	Presentation[33]	Diagnostics	Other	Treatment
Open Myelomeningocele	a. Prenatally[33]: elevated *alpha fetoprotein* and *acetylcholinesterase* in amniotic fluid and/or maternal blood b. Various degrees of **motor, sensory, bladder, and bowel dysfunction** c. **Orthopaedic** deformities d. **Skin abnormalities** e. Possibly signs of **hydrocephalus**	1. *Prenatal ultrasound* (axial imaging): a. *"Lemon" sign:* inward convexity of frontal bones b. *"Banana" sign:* reflecting the shape of the cerebellum, tightly around brainstem as a result of spinal cord tethering The above may be present in spina bifida and Chiari II syndrome 2. *MRI brain:* exclude *hydrocephalus* (observed in more than 70%)[34] and/or *Chiari II syndrome* 3. *MRI and X-ray of entire spine:* evaluate presence of syringomyelia, scoliosis, or other deformities 4. Possibly **urodynamic testing** later in life to evaluate bladder function	• Folate (vitamin B6, best started before conception) reduces the incidence of neural tube defects[35] *Dosage:* a. 0.4 mg/d if no history b. 4 mg/d in case of previous birth with spinal dysraphism • Most frequently, but not exclusively, in **lumbar/sacral spine** • Frequently associated with **latex allergy** • Increased incidence in family with previous child with myelomeningocele or with first-degree relative with myelomeningocele	• **Surgery as soon as possible.** But if the patient is critically ill and must be stabilized, it is **possible to wait up to 72 h without** significantly increasing the risks • **Antibiotic prophylaxis:** nafcillin + gentamicin • **Keep pathologic area wet** (covered with sterile saline gauze) and **patient prone in Trendelenburg** • **Latex precaution** • **Hydrocephalus:** a. *In case of preoperative hydrocephalus:* surgical closure and shunt placement should be done at the same time[36,37] b. *In case of no preoperative hydrocephalus,* follow very carefully after surgical closure for any postoperative suspicious signs (bulging fontanelle, splayed cranial sutures, CSF leak): perform brain ultrasound every 3 d (70% of patients will develop hydrocephalus and require shunt)!

Disease	Presentation	Diagnostics	Other	Treatment
				Surgical technique: ***Placode is functional tissue!*** Even if there are no responses with intraoperative stimulation of placode, it might gain function postoperatively, so try to preserve it 1. *Incise circumferentially* at the junction of epithelial covering/placode with normal skin 2. *Dissect and free placode* all around preserving dorsal roots 3. *Preserve vascular supply* coming in from laterally 4. Be careful *not to leave skin on the lateral edge of placode* (risk of dermoid inclusion)[38] 5. *Avoid ventral dura dissection* (it is very thin and tears). *Dissect dorsal dura* (enough to allow watertight tension-free closure, that does not constrict the underlying reconstructed placode) 6. Detether cord: *cut filum* 7. At the end, the *placode should be floating* on the loculated ventral subarachnoid space 8. *Close the placode* back into tube and *reconstruct the spinal canal* from top to bottom (this reduces the risk of tethering and allows for safer future re-detethering if needed) 9. *Reconstruct intact subarachnoid space* around (further reducing the risk of retethering) 10. *Inspect for other abnormalities* (split cord, etc.): if the preoperative clinical examination presents asymmetric findings, be suspicious of other coexisting defects 11. *Watertight dural closure* 12. If possible (frequently it is not): *suture muscle and fascia* 13. *Mobilize fat and skin as one* with blunt dissection at the base of the fat layer in order to avoid disrupting blood supply to skin 14. *In case of post-op CSF leak*, a shunt is probably needed

Note: Myelomeningocele can also present covered **with intact skin**. If no neural tissue is included in the protruding mass: *meningocele* (which is much less frequent [1:20]). It can also be *anterior or lateral* and in this case it is associated with generalized mesenchymal abnormalities.[39] Consider *elective treatment* at 6 months of age.

6.9.2 Retethered Old Myelomeningocele (Table 6.9b) G

Presentation	Diagnostics	Treatment

• Child with history of myelo-meningocele repair that presents with **new worsening neurologic deficits or pain**
 	
 • **More severe traction** is usually applied between the bottom dentate ligament (at T12) and tethered placode (because of spinal column growth)
 	
 • Always **rule out hydrocephalus or shunt malfunction** as cause of recurrent symptoms or as potential coexisting pathology
	1. **CT or MRI brain:** exclude hydro-cephalus/ shunt malfunction
	 2. Patients with **history of shunt placement:**
	  a. **X-rays** following the course of the shunt catheter
	  b. Consider *shunt tapping*
	 3. **MRI of the entire spine with contrast:** define retethering
		Treat retethering on MRI in:
		 a. Patient with previous myelomeningocele and *new symptoms*
		 b. Before *surgical correction of scoliosis* even in asymptomatic children
		 c. Asymptomatic children who have not reached growth spurt. This is controversial
		
		 Surgical technique
		 1. Start *skin incision above the first normal lamina.* Perform laminectomy and find *normal dura.* Only then *extend the incision over the area of tethering.*
		 2. *Open dura* rostral to caudal preserving the arachnoid and find the *junction of normal spinal cord and placode.* Then follow caudally. *Find the lowest functional level.*
		 3. Open arachnoid, dissect, and stimulate the nerves and placode.
		 4. *Try to detether.* If you cannot, then transect placode at the lowest functional level
		 5. *Spinal cord usually retracts up.* Findings of successful release:
		  a. Superficial vasculature becomes coiled (from linear)
		  b. Nerves point caudal instead of cephalad
		 6. *Try to close the arachnoid* (use 10/0 stich) to avoid retethering and consider *patching* for dural closure

6.10 Pediatric Skull Fractures (Table 6.10 🔊) G

Type	Presentation	Diagnostics	Other	Treatment
Nondepressed (linear)	May present with **subgaleal hematoma** (especially in children <1 y of age)	1. **CT brain** 2. **X-ray:** fracture line is black, straight, and thin *Differential diagnosis:* a. Vessel groove b. Suture	The most common[40]	Surgery only if there is underlying lesion (epidural hematoma, etc.)

Closed (simple) depressed	• Usually frontal or parietal bone
	• Usually **younger children** (in comparison to open depressed)
	• **"Ping-pong" fracture** usually in newborns
		CT brain	30% of depressed fractures are closed	**Surgery vs. observation**
				Indications for surgery may include:
				a. Significant intracranial hematoma
				b. Neurologic deficit related to pressure on brain from fracture
				c. Persistent cosmetic deformity
				d. Depression more than a full skull thickness
				e. Frontal sinus involvement
				f. Dural tear
				General guidelines for surgery:
				A. **< 1 y of age:** Observation for several weeks to see if the child starts to remold fracture. Most children will not need surgery (particularly if in temporoparietal region)
				B. **> 1 y of age:**
				  i. *If it is near a sinus,* perform surgery with wide exposure
				  ii. *If it is far from sinus:*
				    1. Identify the closest suture line to fracture (it is usually the coronal suture)
				    2. Make an incision 2–3 cm from midline along the suture
				    3. Open periosteum with the Bovie
				    4. Use periosteal elevator to get inside the suture and strip the dura from bone
				    5. Use periosteal elevator to elevate fragment

Type	Presentation	Diagnostics	Other	Treatment
Open (compound) depressed	• Usually frontal or parietal bone • The fracture is exposed due to overlying skin laceration	CT brain	• Worse prognosis • Elevating a depressed fracture (open or closed) in the presence of underlying brain injury does not reduce the risk of posttraumatic seizures	Early surgery to reduce infection risk **REMEMBER:** a. *Debridement* of skin and devitalized brain b. *Bone can be replaced* if there is no wound infection c. *Antibiotics* perioperatively[41]

Growing skull fracture (leptomeningeal cyst)	a. There is always an **associated dural laceration.** The fracture line progressively widens. It **takes months to develop.**
	b. Pulsatile/palpable mass
	c. Often associated **meningocerebral cicatrix**
	d. **May cause** neurologic deficit, headache, seizures, hydrocephalus
	e. Most commonly in **parietal** region
	f. **Risk factors:**
	  i. *age* < 3 y
	  ii. *severe head injury* with hemorrhage and fracture
	  iii. *diastasis* of fracture > 4 mm on initial X-ray
		1. **CT brain**
		2. **MRI brain**
			• Rare[42]
			• **"Pseudogrowing fracture"** is a different entity: fracture line widens but with no mass and usually has spontaneous healing[43]
				Treatment:
				a. *No treatment* in asymptomatic adolescents/adults–but close observation for progression
				b. *Surgery:*
				  i. In children
				  ii. If it is a seizure focus
				Surgical technique:
				1. *Wide craniotomy far from fracture and dural laceration:* remember risk of dural tear and brain herniation
				2. *Save periosteum* to repair dura defect (or use graft)
				3. Make *burr holes* around the bony defect, dissect dura inward, and then remove the bony fragments
				4. Depending on brain eloquence, *debride gliotic brain and brain cyst* until there is a clear dural margin and normal brain tissue
				5. *Repair dural defect* with harvested pericranium
				6. *Repair craniotomy site:* if needed, you can split the craniotomy bone in inner and outer table
				7. Use sutures or absorbable plates. Do not use methylmethacrylate

Type	Presentation	Diagnostics	Other	Treatment
Basilar	a. CSF leak (rhinorrhea or otorrhea) b. Battle's sign c. Raccoon eyes d. Cranial nerve palsy e. Hemotympanum/deafness f. Always remember the major vessels based on anatomic location of fracture	1. CT brain 2. MRI brain 3. **Radioisotope cisternography** (CSF leak identification)		1. **If leak persists after 2–3 d,** use a lumbar drain if there is no other contraindication; frequent CSF cultures 2. **No antibiotic prophylaxis**[44] 3. **Surgery** if leak persists

Also remember

Cephalhematoma:

A. Subgaleal hematoma:
a. may be associated with linear non depressed fracture
b. *may cross sutures* and be of significant quantity
c. it does *not calcify*

B. Subperiosteal hematoma:
a. usually newborns
b. *limited by sutures*
c. *may calcify*

Treatment:
a. *Close follow-up of hematocrit and bilirubin* in children < 1 y of age (especially for subgaleal hematoma). Jaundice may present even 10 d later
b. *Do not aspirate* (risk of infection and anemia)
c. *Order an X-ray,* if a subperiosteal hematoma persists more than 6 wk and
d. *Consider surgery* for calcified lesions that persist after 6 mo and cause cosmetic deformity

6.11 Intracranial Hemorrhage in Neonates (Table 6.11) G

Papile's scale[45]	Presentation	Diagnostics	Other	Treatment
I subependymal blood (most frequent)	• **In order of increasing severity** (increasing grade): a. Asymptomatic b. decreased hematocrit and irritability c. symptoms of increased intracranial pressure (tense fontanelle, split sutures, increased occipitofrontal circumference, apnea and bradycardia, seizures, abnormal posturing) • Mostly presents in **first 12 h** of life with a **2nd peak** on days 3–4	1. **Ultrasound brain:** initial test and follow-up test 2. **MRI brain** before intervention (also clarifies if there is obstructive component in hydrocephalus)	• **Involution of germinal matrix is** completed at 35 wk of gestational age • Any factor that increases cerebral perfusion pressure, cerebral blood flow, or causes hypoxia can precipitate the hemorrhage	**Prevention:** a. One course of antenatal steroids 48 h before birth[47] b. Vitamin K > 4 h before birth **Treatment** a. Avoid diuretics and osmotic agents b. Surgical treatment of intracerebral hemorrhage is not advised c. **Close follow-up** to exclude progressive hydrocephalus. Treat hydrocephalus by CSF removal only when there are signs of increased intracranial pressure.[48] Treatment of hydrocephalus depends on body weight (see Table 6.12)
II subependymal blood + ventricular blood				
III subependymal blood + ventricular blood + hydrocephalus	• **Incidence increases inversely** with decreasing birth weight and estimated gestational age. • **Other risk factors:** a. high fraction of inspired oxygen in first 24 h b. pneumothorax c. fertility treatment (mostly IVF) d. early sepsis e. failure to provide antenatal steroid treatment[46]			**Prognosis** 1. *Grade of hemorrhage* is the most important variable in determining cognitive outcome, motor function, presence of seizures, survival[49] 2. 70% of newborns with **grade III and IV hemorrhage** will present with progressive dilation of the ventricles and 40% will need a shunt[50] 3. *Intraventricular hemorrhage without accompanying white matter lesion* is associated with no more than a mild increase (and possibly no increase) in the risk of adverse developmental outcome during infancy. 4. *White matter lesion is accompanied* by increased risk of cerebral palsy, low mental and motor scores, visual and hearing impairment[51]
IV brain parenchyma blood				

6.12 Treatment of Posthemorrhagic Hydrocephalus in Newborns (Table 6.12 🔊) G

Weight	When to treat	Treatment	Remember
< 800 gr	1. There is no evidence that repeated punctures produce any benefit over conservative management in neonates with or at risk of developing posthemorrhagic hydrocephalus in terms of reduction of disability, death, need for placement of a permanent shunt[1]	Tap fontanelle	Ventricular tap: 1. brain ultrasound (estimate depth of needle placement) 2. use a 23 gauge needle 3. sterile procedure under continuous cardiorespiratory monitoring 4. lateral angle of the anterior fontanelle (as lateral as possible to avoid sinus and venous lakes) 5. retract the skin (release it in the end): to avoid CSF leak 6. advance the needle towards the inner angle of ipsilateral eye without changing direction: to minimize brain injury 7. remove CSF slowly 8. apply pressure: to prevent CSF leak
800–1200 gr	So treat when…	a. Lumbar puncture (for non obstructive hydrocephalus) b. Tap fontanelle (for obstructive hydrocephalus)	
1200–2500 gr	2. There are clinical signs of raised intracranial pressure: a. Increasing head circumference (more than 1cm/week) b. Full/ tense anterior fontanelle c. Split sutures d. Lethargy e. Apnea/Bradycardia f. Poor feeding/Vomiting	a. Ventricular reservoir or b. Ventriculosubgaleal shunt (less CSF taps are usually required compared to reservoir[2])	1. For approximately 30 days before revising or placing a shunt[3] 2. Tap slowly with 25 gauge needle under continuous cardiorespiratory monitoring, avoiding previous sites of insertion
> 2,500 gr		Ventriculoperitoneal shunt: programmable	Rule out: 1. Enterocolitis (do not place shunt until resolved) 2. Protein > 150 mg/dL (in this case, use valveless shunt or wait) **For all punctures/taps:** 1. Remove 10ml/Kg CSF 2. Always check electrolytes in case of repeated punctures 3. Determine frequency based on clinical response

[1] Whitelaw A, Lee-Kelland R. "Repeated lumbar or ventricular punctures in newborns with intraventricular haemorrhage". Cochrane Database Syst Rev 2017;4:CD000216.

[2] Wang JY, Amin AG, Jallo GI, Ahn ES: "Ventricular reservoir versus ventriculosubgaleal shunt for posthemorrhagic hydrocephalus in preterm infants: infection risks and ventriculoperitoneal shunt rate". J Neurosurg Pediatr. 2014; 14(5): 447–454.

[3] Tubbs RS, Smyth MD, Wellons JC 3rd, Blount J, Grabb PA, Oakes WJ: "Life expectancy of ventriculosubgaleal shunt revisions". Pediatr Neurosurg 2003; 38(5): 244–246.

6.13 Cases

6.13.1 Germinal Matrix Hemorrhage in Premature Infant

Chief complaint/History of present illness

- You are called to the neonatal intensive care unit (NICU) to see a 29 wk/o baby because of concerns of a full anterior fontanelle.
- Past medical history:
    - The premature female is a twin delivered with C-section at age 29 weeks after pregnancy, complicated by hypertension of the mother.
    - In addition, the child has a patent ductus arteriosus and is being treated for enterocolitis.

Physical examination

- Anterior fontanelle is full but not tense.
- Sutures are not splayed.
- Head circumference is 40 percentile adjusted for age.
- Weight is 1000 g.
- Otherwise, the examination is normal, no episodes of apnea or radycardia.

1. Describe the findings of the imaging studies.

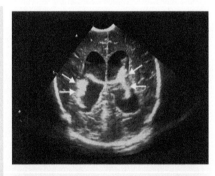

Ultrasound brain (axial section) shows echogenic blood clots (*arrows*) along bilateral choroid plexus. Ventricles are enlarged (Papile scale III).

 Imaging

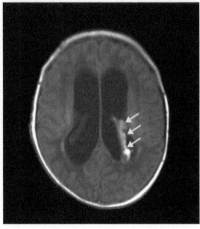

MRI brain (T1WI, axial) of the same patient (same date) shows high intensity signal along the left choroid plexus (*arrows*) indicative of hemorrhage. The right choroid plexus appears with higher intensity signal than CSF but with lower intensity compared with the left choroid plexus, probably due to different age of hemorrhage. Ventricles are dilated.

Imaging

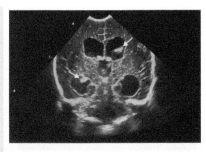

Ultrasound brain (coronal section) shows echogenic blood clots (*arrows*) along bilateral choroid plexus.

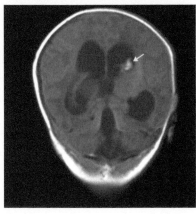

MRI brain (T1WI, coronal) of the same patient (same date) shows high intensity signal along the left choroid plexus (*arrow*) indicative of hemorrhage. The right choroid plexus in the right atrium coursing around the thalamus into the temporal horn appears with higher intensity signal than CSF but with lower intensity compared with the left choroid plexus, probably due to different age of hemorrhage. Ventricles are dilated.

2. **What is the predictive value of the Papile scale?**
   Grade of hemorrhage is the most important variable in determining cognitive outcome, motor function, presence of seizures, and survival. (See Table 6.11: Prognosis).

3. **What is your plan?**
   Patient should be followed with daily measurements of head circumference and daily neurological assessments. Special attention should be given to apnea or bradycardia. Sequential brain ultrasound studies should also be performed.

4. **On follow-up visit 4 days later the patient's neurological examination is unchanged with no reports of apnea or bradycardia but with the head circumference now at the 70 percentile adjusted for age, the anterior fontanelle full and now tense, and the sutures are splayed. Body weight is now 1100 g. Imaging studies are as follows. What is your plan?**

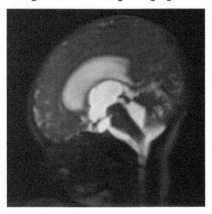

MRI brain (T2WI, sagittal) shows all ventricles enlarged. The aqueduct is also enlarged and patent. Since clinical examination revealed increased ICP signs (head circumference crosses percentiles, the anterior fontanelle is full and tense and sutures are splayed) CSF should be removed. Because body weight is between 800 and 1200 g only temporizing measures can be taken, such as ventricular tap or spinal tap. Since the hydrocephalus is nonobstructive, spinal taps can be performed as needed, hoping for the hydrocephalus to arrest or while waiting for body weight to increase and allow more permanent measures. (See Table 6.12).

5. Describe how to perform a ventricular tap.
   (See Table 6.12: Ventricular tap).

6. Assuming that the patient continues to show further ventricular enlargement and signs of increased ICP, what are your criteria for the placement of a ventriculoperitoneal (VP) shunt?
   - Body weight more than 2500 g.
   - CSF protein less than 150 mg/dL.
   - Rule out enterocolitis.
     (See Table 6.12).

7. Following placement of the shunt the patient develops a persistent visible subcutaneous CSF collection at the site of burr hole and valve. What is your plan?
   In case of a placement of a programmable VP shunt, the setting of the valve should be lowered, which would result in an increase in the CSF flow through the valve. An ultrasound of brain should be performed after some days to rule out subdural collections. Head of bed should be elevated.

6.13.2 Pediatric Skull Fracture with Epidural Hematoma

Chief complaint/History of present illness	• A 2 y/o boy presents to the ER after a fall from a height of 4 feet (1.2 m) striking his occiput on a hard tile floor.
Physical examination	• Neurological examination is normal.

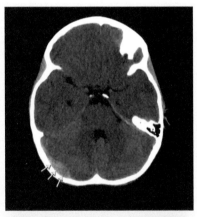

CT head shows small epidural hematoma (hyperdense, biconvex shape) in the right posterior fossa near the right transverse sinus.

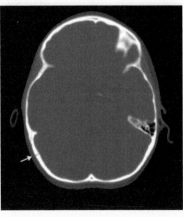

CT head (bone window) shows a fracture of the occipital bone in the area of the epidural hematoma on the right side.

1. **What is your plan?**
   Hematoma size is small with minimal mass effect on CT brain. Patient is asymptomatic. The patient should be followed closely with sequential neurological examinations. In case of neurological deterioration a CT brain should be performed immediately. (See Table 5.13a: Nonsurgical management).

2. **During the night the young patient becomes progressively more obtunded. STAT CT scan shows significant enlargement of the epidural hematoma. What is your plan?**
   Patient should undergo craniotomy and epidural hematoma evacuation as soon as possible. (See Table 5.13a: Surgical management).

3. **During craniotomy you notice that the cause of the hematoma is a 1-cm laceration along the transverse sinus. How would you treat this?**
   Depending on the size of the laceration either tamponade the sinus with Gelfoam/muscle patch etc., or directly suture the sinus. (See Table 11.1d: Treatment).

4. **During surgery the anesthesiologist notifies you of a sudden drop in blood pressure and a drop-in end-expiratory CO_2. What are you concerned about and how would you treat it?**
   There is concern about air embolism. (See Table 11.1e: Treatment).

6.13.3 Open Myelomeningocele

Chief complaint/History of present illness	• You are asked by the NICU to evaluate a lesion in the midline of the back of 1 h/o female neonate.
Physical examination	• She moves upper extremities normally.
	• Examination of lower extremities revealed no hip extension, moderate knee flexion, no foot dorsiflexion, and no foot plantarflexion bilaterally.
	• Hips are flexed and adducted, knees are extended and feet are flail.
	• Head circumference is normal and anterior fontanelle is not tense.
	• The inspection of her back revealed a ruptured myelomeningocele.

1. **What are the studies to diagnose this condition prenatally?**
   • Mother serum alpha-fetoprotein (aFP).
   • Amniotic fluid aFP and acetylcholinesterase blood sample.
   • Fetal ultrasound and MRI.
   (See Table 6.9a).

2. **What is the neurological level of involvement? What is the clinical presentation of a myelomeningocele? What other conditions are associated with myelomeningocele?**
   • The neurological levels below L3 are involved (i.e., last intact level is L3).
   • Clinical presentation depends on neurological level of involvement (various degrees of motor, sensory, bladder, and bowel dysfunction).
   • Skin abnormalities, orthopaedic deformities, hydrocephalus, Chiari II malformation. (See Table 6.9a: Presentation).

3. **What further imaging studies should be performed preoperatively?**
   MRI of brain and entire spine. (See Table 6.9a: Diagnostics).

4. **What are the first prophylactic measures to be taken?**
   Antibiotics, keep pathologic area moist, latex precautions, prone position. (See Table 6.9a: Treatment).

5. When should hydrocephalus be treated if present preoperatively? If there is no hydrocephalus preoperatively, should we follow-up the patient postoperatively for hydrocephalus and how? (See Table 6.9a: Treatment).

6. **When should the surgical repair take place?**
Earlier than 72 hours. (See Table 6.9a: Treatment).

7. **Describe the surgical technique.**
(See Table 6.9a: Treatment).

8. **Which layers should be closed in a myelomeningocele repair?**
Five layers: placode, dura, fascia, subcutaneous tissue, skin. (See Table 6.9a: Treatment).

9. How does retethering of an old myelomeningocele present? What other condition should be ruled out? What imaging studies are you going to order?
   • The child will present with new worsening of neurological deficits or pain. Hydrocephalus or shunt malfunction should be ruled out.
   • MRI of brain and entire spine should be performed.
   • Shunt series X-ray should also be performed in patients with shunt.
   (See Table 6.9b).

10. What are the indications for surgical treatment of retethered spinal cord?
   (see Table 6.9b: Treatment).

11. Describe the surgical technique for treating retethered cord.
   (see Table 6.9b: Treatment).

References

[1] Flannery AM, Tamber MS, Mazzola C, et al. Congress of Neurological Surgeons Systematic Review and Evidence-Based Guidelines for the Management of Patients with Positional Plagiocephaly: executive summary. Neurosurgery. 2016; 79(5):623–624

[2] Mazzola C, Baird LC, Bauer DF, et al. Guidelines: Congress of Neurological Surgeons Systematic Review and Evidence-Based Guideline for the Diagnosis of Patients with Positional Plagiocephaly: the role of imaging. Neurosurgery. 2016; 79(5):E625–E626

[3] Agrawal D, Steinbok P, Cochrane DD. Scaphocephaly or dolichocephaly? J Neurosurg. 2005; 102(2, Suppl):253–254, author reply 254

[4] Wall SA, Thomas GP, Johnson D, et al. The preoperative incidence of raised intracranial pressure in nonsyndromic sagittal craniosynostosis is underestimated in the literature. J Neurosurg Pediatr. 2014; 14(6):674–681

[5] Francel PC, Bell A, Jane JA. Operative positioning for patients undergoing repair of craniosynostosis. Neurosurgery. 1994; 35(2):304–306, discussion 306

[6] Cohen SR, Persing JA. Intracranial pressure in single-suture craniosynostosis. Cleft Palate Craniofac J. 1998; 35(3):194–196 [7] Renier D, Sainte-Rose C, Marchac D, Hirsch JF. Intracranial pressure in craniostenosis. J Neurosurg. 1982; 57(3):370–377

[8] Pearce MS, Salotti JA, Howe NL, et al. CT scans in young people in Great Britain: temporal and descriptive patterns, 1993–2002 Radiol Res Pract. 2012; 2012:594278

[9] David LR, Genecov DG, Camastra AA, Wilson JA, Argenta LC. Positron emission tomography studies confirm the need for early surgical intervention in patients with single-suture craniosynostosis. J Craniofac Surg. 1999; 10(1):38–42

[10] Suwanwela C, Suwanwela N. A morphological classification of sincipital encephalomeningoceles. J Neurosurg. 1972; 36(2):201–211

[11] Naidich TP, Altman NR, Braffman BH, McLone DG, Zimmerman RA. Cephaloceles and related malformations. AJNR Am J Neuroradiol. 1992; 13(2):655–690

[12] Milunsky A, Jick H, Jick SS,. Multivitamin / folic acid supplementation in early pregnancy reduces the prevalence of neural tube defects. JAMA 1989; 262(20):2847-2852

[13] Alden TD, Ojemann JG, Park TS. Surgical treatment of Chiari I malformation: indications and approaches. Neurosurg Focus. 2001; 11(1):E2

[14] Iskandar BJ, Hedlund GL, Grabb PA, Oakes WJ. The resolution of syringohydromyelia without hindbrain herniation after posterior fossa decompression. J Neurosurg. 1998; 89(2):212–216

[15] Bejjani GK. Definition of the adult Chiari malformation: a brief historical overview. Neurosurg Focus. 2001; 11(1):E1

[16] Dyste GN, Menezes AH, VanGilder JC. Symptomatic Chiari malformations. An analysis of presentation, management, and long-term outcome. J Neurosurg. 1989; 71(2):159–168

[17] Greenberg JK, Milner E, Yarbrough CK, et al. Outcome methods used in clinical studies of Chiari malformation type I: a systematic review. J Neurosurg. 2015; 122(2):262–272

[18] Pollack IF, Kinnunen D, Albright AL. The effect of early craniocervical decompression on functional outcome in neonates and young infants with myelodysplasia and symptomatic Chiari II malformations: results from a prospective series. Neurosurgery. 1996; 38(4):703–710, discussion 710

[19] Kumar R, Jain MK, Chhabra DK. Dandy-Walker syndrome: different modalities of treatment and outcome in 42 cases. Childs Nerv Syst. 2001; 17(6):348–352

[20] Patel S, Barkovich AJ. Analysis and classification of cerebellar malformations. AJNR Am J Neuroradiol. 2002; 23(7):1074–1087

[21] Mohanty A, Biswas A, Satish S, Praharaj SS, Sastry KV. Treatment options for Dandy-Walker malformation. J Neurosurg. 2006; 105 (5, Suppl):348–356

[22] Asai A, Hoffman HJ, Hendrick EB, Humphreys RP. Dandy-Walker syndrome: experience at the Hospital for Sick Children, Toronto. Pediatr Neurosci. 1989; 15(2):66–73

[23] Osenbach RK, Menezes AH. Diagnosis and management of the Dandy-Walker malformation: 30 years of experience. Pediatr Neurosurg. 1992; 18(4):179–189

[24] Barkovich AJ, Kjos BO, Norman D, Edwards MS. Revised classification of posterior fossa cysts and cystlike malformations based on the results of multiplanar MR imaging. AJR Am J Roentgenol. 1989; 153(6):1289–1300

[25] Lasjaunias PL, Chng SM, Sachet M, Alvarez H, Rodesch G, Garcia-Monaco R. The management of vein of Galen aneurysmal malformations. Neurosurgery. 2006; 59(5, Suppl 3):S184–S194, discussion S3–S13

[26] Pang D, Dias MS, Ahab-Barmada M. Split cord malformation: part I: a unified theory of embryogenesis for double spinal cord malformations. Neurosurgery. 1992; 31(3):451–480

[27] Pang D. Split cord malformation: part II: clinical syndrome. Neurosurgery. 1992; 31(3):481–500

[28] Kesler H, Dias MS, Kalapos P. Termination of the normal conus medullaris in children: a whole-spine magnetic resonance imaging study. Neurosurg Focus. 2007; 23(2):E7

[29] Rogg JM, Benzil DL, Haas RL, Knuckey NW. Intramedullary abscess, an unusual manifestation of a dermal sinus. AJNR Am J Neuroradiol. 1993; 14(6):1393–1395

[30] Ackerman LL, Menezes AH. Spinal congenital dermal sinuses: a 30-year experience. Pediatrics. 2003; 112(3, Pt 1):641–647

[31] Medina LS, Crone K, Kuntz KM. Newborns with suspected occult spinal dysraphism: a cost-effectiveness analysis of diagnostic strategies. Pediatrics. 2001; 108(6):E101

[32] Bruce DA, Schut L. Spinal lipomas in infancy and childhood. Childs Brain. 1979; 5(3):192–203

[33] Weiss RR, Macri JN, Elligers K, Princler GL, McIntire R, Waldman TA. Amniotic fluid alpha-fetoprotein as a marker in prenatal diagnosis of neural tube defects. Obstet Gynecol. 1976; 47(2):148–151

[34] Swank M, Dias L. Myelomeningocele: a review of the orthopaedic aspects of 206 patients treated from birth with no selection criteria. Dev Med Child Neurol. 1992; 34(12):1047–1052

[35] Wald N, Sneddon J; MRC Vitamin Study Research Group. Prevention of neural tube defects: results of the Medical Research Council Vitamin Study. Lancet. 1991; 338(8760):131–137

[36] Hubballah MY, Hoffman HJ. Early repair of myelomeningocele and simultaneous insertion of ventriculoperitoneal shunt: technique and results. Neurosurgery. 1987; 20(1):21–23

[37] Miller PD, Pollack IF, Pang D, Albright AL. Comparison of simultaneous versus delayed ventriculoperitoneal shunt insertion in children undergoing myelomeningocele repair. J Child Neurol. 1996; 11(5):370–372

[38] Scott RM, Wolpert SM, Bartoshesky LE, Zimbler S, Klauber GT. Dermoid tumors occurring at the site of previous myelomeningocele repair. J Neurosurg. 1986; 65(6):779–783

[39] Strahle J, Muraszko K. Spinal meningoceles. In: Albright AL, Pollack IF, Adelson PD. Principles and Practice of Pediatric Neurosurgery. New York, NY: Thieme Medical Publishers; 2015:286–293

[40] Greenes DS, Schutzman SA. Clinical indicators of intracranial injury in head-injured infants. Pediatrics. 1999; 104(4, Pt 1):861–867

[41] Al-Haddad SA, Kirollos R. A 5-year study of the outcome of surgically treated depressed skull fractures. Ann R Coll Surg Engl. 2002; 84(3):196–200

[42] Ersahin Y, Gülmen V. Growing skull fractures: a clinical study of 41 patients. Acta Neurochir (Wien). 1998; 140(5):519

[43] Sekhar LN, Scarff TB. Pseudogrowth in skull fractures of childhood. Neurosurgery. 1980; 6(3):285–289

[44] Ratilal BO, Costa J, Sampaio C, Pappamikail L. Antibiotic prophylaxis for preventing meningitis in patients with basilar skull fractures. Cochrane Database Syst Rev. 2011; 8(8):CD004884

[45] Papile LA, Burstein J, Burstein R, Koffler H. Incidence and evolution of subependymal and intraventricular hemorrhage: a study of infants with birth weights less than 1,500 gm. J Pediatr. 1978; 92(4):529–534

[46] Linder N, Haskin O, Levit O, et al. Risk factors for intraventricular hemorrhage in very low birth weight premature infants: a retrospective case-control study. Pediatrics. 2003; 111(5, Pt 1):e590–e595

[47] Wei JC, Catalano R, Profit J, Gould JB, Lee HC. Impact of antenatal steroids on intraventricular hemorrhage in very-low-birth weight infants. J Perinatol. 2016; 36(5):352–356

[48] Whitelaw A, Lee-Kelland R. Repeated lumbar or ventricular punctures in newborns with intraventricular haemorrhage. Cochrane Database Syst Rev. 2017; 4:CD000216

[49] Levy ML, Masri LS, McComb JG. Outcome for preterm infants with germinal matrix hemorrhage and progressive hydrocephalus. Neurosurgery. 1997; 41(5):1111–1117, discussion 1117–1118

[50] Murphy BP, Inder TE, Rooks V, et al. Posthaemorrhagic ventricular dilatation in the premature infant: natural history and predictors of outcome. Arch Dis Child Fetal Neonatal Ed. 2002; 87(1):F37–F41

[51] O'Shea TM, Allred EN, Kuban KC, et al; ELGAN Study Investigators. Intraventricular hemorrhage and developmental outcomes at 24 months of age in extremely preterm infants. J Child Neurol. 2012; 27(1):22–29

[52] Wang JY, Amin AG, Jallo GI, Ahn ES. Ventricular reservoir versus ventriculosubgaleal shunt for posthemorrhagic hydrocephalus in preterm infants: infection risks and ventriculoperitoneal shunt rate. J Neurosurg Pediatr. 2014; 14(5):447–454

[53] Tubbs RS, Smyth MD, Wellons JC, III, Blount J, Grabb PA, Oakes WJ. Life expectancy of ventriculosubgaleal shunt revisions. Pediatr Neurosurg. 2003; 38(5):244–246

Suggested Readings

Albright AL., Pollack IF., Adelson PD. Principles and practice of pediatric neurosurgery. 3rd ed. New York, Thieme; 2014

Goodrich JT. Neurosurgical Operative Atlas. Pediatric Neurosurgery. 2nd ed. New York, NY: Thieme Medical Publishers; 2008

Kuppermann N, Holmes JF, Dayan PS, et al; Pediatric Emergency Care Applied Research Network (PECARN). Identification of children at very low risk of clinically-important brain injuries after head trauma: a prospective cohort study. Lancet. 2009; 374(9696):1160–1170

7 Functional Neurosurgery

7.1 Pain

7.1.1 Neuralgia (Table 7.1a) ⬢ G

Disease	Presentation	Diagnostics	Other	Treatment
Trigeminal neuralgia AKA Tic Douloureux	• Paroxysmal, electric shooting character • **Triggers:** eating, talking, brushing teeth, touching nose, wind blowing on face • **Most frequent:** V2 + V3, followed by V2 • Right > left • Almost always **unilateral,** only 1% bilateral (more common in multiple sclerosis [MS]) • No neurologic deficit • Burning dysesthesia indicates permanent nerve injury	**MRI/MRA brain** to exclude tumor and MS **Causes:** • Microvascular compression at trigeminal nerve root entry zone by: a. Superior cerebellar artery b. Branch of petrosal vein c. Ectatic basilar artery d. Persistent trigeminal artery • MS plaque • Tumor • Idiopathic	Trigeminal nuclei: **a. Midbrain:** proprioception **b. Pons:** – motor – discriminative sensation – light touch **c. Medulla and upper cervical:** – pain – temperature – deep touch **REMEMBER:** • V1: superior orbital fissure • V2: foramen rotundum • V3: foramen ovale	1. **Medication:** a. *Carbamazepine:* progressive increase to maximum dose of 400 mg TID CAUTION: monitor levels + complete blood count b. *Gabapentin:* progressive increase to maximum 1,200 mg TID c. *Baclofen:* progressive increase to 20 mg QID d. *Phenytoin:* IV in crisis or oral CAUTION: monitor levels + blood tests 2. **Surgical procedure:** Consider when medications are no longer effective OR significant medication side effects occur: A. Percutaneous procedures a. Balloon compression b. Glycerol injection c. Radiofrequency (RF) rhizotomy *FOR ALL PERCUTANEOUS PROCEDURES:* Performed with monitored anesthesia care (MAC; i.e., propofol + fentanyl or similar) and local anesthesia injected at entry point

Disease	Presentation	Diagnostics	Other	Treatment

Treatment

Indications:

- Elderly patients
- Contraindication to craniotomy
- Immediate pain relief required

Technique:

- C-arm guidance: true lateral fluoroscopy (acoustic meatus from both sides MUST align)
- Coordinates:
  a. *ENTRY POINT:* Mark point 3 cm lateral to the angle of mouth
  b. Mark point 3 cm anterior to tragus
  c. Mark point at medial ipsilateral pupil

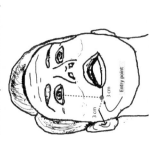

- Insert needle at *ENTRY POINT*
- Advance needle toward *TARGET POINT* (foramen ovale) at intersection of petrous bone with clivus line on lateral X-ray

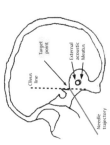

Disease	Presentation	Diagnostics	Other	Treatment

				• When needle passes into foramen ovale:
				  – wincing, tear drops, and masseter contraction are often observed
				  – change in resistance of needle is noted (cartilage)
				  – Possible CSF return

V1	V2	V3
Just above clival line	At clival line	Just below clival line

a. *Balloon compression:*
  • Attach external pacemaker (risk of bradycardia)
  • Patient in supine position
  • C-arm guidance
  • Place needle (14 gauge) into foramen ovale and advance balloon through the needle
  • Always place blocking device to avoid movement of balloon during inflation
  • Fill balloon with contrast dye and confirm position on lateral X-ray (pear shape appearance of balloon)
  • Inflate balloon at 1.5 atmospheric pressure for 60–90 s
  • Watch for bradycardia (consider atropine before inflation)
  • Balloon may rupture (not dangerous)

b. *Glycerol injection:*
  • Performed with patient in sitting position, head slightly flexed
  • Place 25-gauge spinal needle not beyond clival line on lateral X-ray
  • Inject up to 0.5-mL dye into trigeminal cistern until the dye starts to "run off" toward posterior fossa and note injected amount
  • Inject equal amount of 99.9% anhydrous glycerol + tantalum powder

Disease	Presentation	Diagnostics	Other	Treatment

Treatment

c. *RF rhizotomy:*
- Patient in supine position
- Place RF needle with 5 mm exposed tip into foramen ovale to target location
- Perform MANDATORY electrical stimulation:
  a. SENSORY HIGH frequency (50 Hz) 0.1–0.2 V (max 0.5 V) reproduces pain with facial flushing in corresponding trigeminal branch
  b. MOTOR LOW frequency (2 Hz) MUST produce visible masseter contraction (from motor fibers of V3)

Producing RF lesion:
- 70°C
- 70 s
- For redo procedures and high voltage (0.5 V) on sensory stimulation: choose 80°C for 80 s

CAUTION:
i. Needle tip in RF rhizotomy MUST NEVER be >5 mm beyond clival line
ii. DO NOT PROCEED with RF lesioning if electrical stimulation results are not clear
- No masseter contraction: electrode not in foramen ovale
- Eye deviation: the electrode is too deep (CN III, IV, or VI)
- Face grimacing: the electrode is in posterior fossa (CN VII)
- Visual disturbance: electrode is touching optic nerve (superior orbital fissure)

Complications of ALL percutaneous procedures:
- Numbness (extremely common)
- Loss of corneal reflex, keratitis (rare)
- Anesthesia dolorosa (very rare)
- Masseter weakness
- Arterial bleeding (Tx: retropharyngeal compression + ICU + delayed angiogram)
- Meningitis (including aseptic meningitis)

Disease	Presentation	Diagnostics	Other	Treatment

Treatment

REMEMBER:

- *V1:* difficult with RF
- Glycerol: highest recurrence rate
- Balloon: lowest corneal numbness rate
- Percutaneous procedures can be repeated multiple times

B. Microvascular decompression

Indications:

- Expected survival is more than 5 y
- Age < 65 y
- V1 distribution

Technique:

- Park-bench position
  - Painful side up
  - Head flexed
  - Head turned 15 degrees to the floor
  - No lateral tilt
- Consider neuromonitoring (BAEP)
- Retrosigmoid craniotomy
- Retract superolateral cerebellum to inferior-medial direction with small blade
- Open subarachnoid space at petrosal vein and release CSF
- Identify trigeminal nerve root entry zone: usually much more superior than expected
- Dissect arachnoid around nerve root and place small Teflon piece between nerve and compressing vessel

Complications:

- Hearing loss (VIII)
- facial dysesthesia (V)
- facial weakness (VII)
- craniotomy complications

Disease	Presentation	Diagnostics	Other	Treatment

Treatment

REMEMBER:
- The Most effective procedure for trigeminal neuralgia
- Not indicated for MS patients (percutaneous rhizotomy preferred).

C. <u>Stereotactic radiosurgery of nerve root entry zone</u>

Indications:
- Elderly patients who don't require immediate pain relief
- Patients on anticoagulation
- Recurrent pain after previous procedure
- Patient preference

Technique:
- Single isocenter 70–90 Gy treatment dose
- Procedure can be repeated ONCE (with cumulative radiation dose of 140 Gy)

Complications:
- Facial hypesthesia in 20% (30% with retreatment)
- NO severe morbidity
- NO mortality

Comments:
- Well tolerated
- Does not offer immediate relief (latency 1–3 mo)

Rate of success of all procedures:

	BC	GL	RF	MV	SR
I	90%	90%	95%	95%	80%
M	70%	50%	70%	80%	60%
L	50%		20%	65%	45%

I: immediate
M: medium term 1–5 y
L: long term >5 y
BC: balloon compression
GL: glycerol
RF: radiofrequency
MV: microvascular decompression
SR: stereotactic radiosurgery

Disease	Presentation	Diagnostics	Other	Treatment
Glossopharyngeal neuralgia	• Paroxysmal unilateral stabbing pain in: – tonsils – base of tongue – external auditory meatus – angle of mandible • Possibly hypotension • Syncopal episodes • **Triggers:** – talking – chewing – swallowing – coughing • No neurological deficit	**MRI and MRA brain**	Application of 10% cocaine on pharynx reduces pain significantly (may help in differential diagnosis)	1. **Medication:** low response rate • Antiepileptics (topiramate) • Antidepressants 2. **Surgery:** a. *Microvascular decompression:* – Follow sigmoid sinus to the jugular foramen where CN X and XI separate from CN IX – Vessel compression typically from posteroinferior cerebellar artery (PICA) b. *Rhizotomy:* – It is usually safe to section all of CN IX and upper 1/6 of CN X – avoid in case of contralateral pathology of CN X or gag dysfunction *Complications:* • Permanent dysphagia • Vocal cord paralysis • Intraoperative and immediate postoperative cardiac complications 3. **Stereotactic radiosurgery** • CN IX is targeted at glossopharyngeal meatus of jugular foramen • 80- to 90-Gy single isocenter

Disease	Presentation	Diagnostics	Other	Treatment
Geniculate neuralgia AKA Hunt's neuralgia AKA Neuralgia of the nervus intermedius (nerve of Wrisberg)	• Very intense pain deep inside the ear on one side that may be accompanied by burning sensation in part of ipsilateral face • Pain may coexist with: – bitter taste – salivation – tinnitus – Vertigo	• Exclude herpes infection • MRI/MRA brain • ENT evaluation	Hemifacial spasm may coexist (convulsive tic)	1. **Medication:** a. Antiepileptics 2. **Surgery:** a. Microvascular decompression (cutting the nervus intermedius) b. Section of geniculate ganglion
Postherpetic neuralgia	• **Most common:** thoracic roots (2/3 of cases) • **Second most common:** V1 distribution (20% of cases) • Continuous causalgia often leads to allodynia (even the light touch of clothes is perceived as painful)	• Diagnosis is based on history and clinical findings • **REMEMBER:** zoster "sine herpete" is just like normal herpes zoster BUT without vesicles	Varicella zoster AKA herpes zoster AKA human herpes virus type 3 lies dormant in cranial nerves, dorsal and autonomic ganglia until reactivation	1. **Antiherpetic medication** (acyclovir, famciclovir, valacyclovir) • Reduce the risk of postherpetic neuralgia (especially if given in first 72 h) • Corticosteroids given acutely during zoster infection are ineffective in preventing postherpetic neuralgia 2. **Pain medication:** • Antiepileptics (especially gabapentin) • Tricyclic antidepressants • Opioids: oxycodone (preferred); tramadol • Lidocaine patch • Capsaicin (patch or cream) 3. **Pain management procedures (for drug resistant cases):** a. Intrathecal methylprednisolone + lidocaine: effective long term (but not studied for V1 postherpetic neuralgia) b. Nerve blocks (only temporary relief) c. Dorsal column stimulation > intrathecal pump > DREZ (Dorsal Root Entry Zone) lesion

Disease	Presentation	Diagnostics	Other	Treatment
				a. Nucleus caudalis DREZ lesion: • Suboccipital craniotomy • Lesion in the trigeminal nucleus that extends from C2 DREZ to obex (2 mm dorsal to CN XI exit) • Distance between C2 DREZ and obex is ~ 2 cm • Entry of DREZ lesioning probe is at 45 degrees • Lesions every 1 mm for 15 sec at 80°C • DREZ electrode length is 1.2–2.0 mm *Prognosis:* 70% of patients have significant improvement *Complications:* – A\taxia (spinocerebellar tract) – Weakness (pyramidal tract)

Other facial pain conditions

Disease	Presentation	Diagnostics	Other	Treatment
Trigeminal neuropathic pain	• Burning constant pain • Numbness is common	MRI	After *accidental* trauma to trigeminal nerve system	Motor cortex stimulation
Trigeminal deafferentation pain (including anesthesia dolorosa)	Very similar to trigeminal neuropathic pain	Diagnosis based on history	After *intentional* trauma to trigeminal system (i.e., previous rhizotomies, DREZ lesions)	Motor cortex stimulation
Atypical facial pain	Constant or paroxysmal with long duration	MRI (to rule out tumors, MS, etc.)	Term often used for facial pain that does not fit other categories	• Often psychogenic • DO NOT offer surgical treatment options

Note: Medications to be considered in facial neuralgias: carbamazepine, gabapentin, valproic acid, pregabalin, topiramate, phenytoin, amitriptyline, duloxetine.

7.1.2 Motor Cortex Stimulation (Table 7.1b)w

Indications	Other	Surgical technique
• Neuropathic pain of face and limbs • **Best indication is:** a. neuropathic facial pain (pain after injury to CN V) OR b. trigeminal deafferentation pain (facial pain resulting from surgery to treat trigeminal neuralgia) • Central pain from thalamic, putaminal, lateral medullary stroke • **Less experience in:** a. Phantom limb pain b. Spinal cord injury pain c. Postherpetic neuralgia	• Stimulation increases cerebral blood flow in: a. Ipsilateral thalamus b. Cingulate gyrus c. Brainstem • Stimulation is not perceived as paresthesia • There is no reliable way to predict response • Generally **expected response:** – 50% pain relief – 50% of patients	1. Total intravenous general anesthesia (TIVA) like awake craniotomy 2. **Target** is the primary motor cortex corresponding to pain area (i.e., face area of motor cortex for facial pain, etc.) 3. **Craniotomy** over central sulcus 4. **Electrodes are placed epidurally** PERPENDICULAR to central sulcus spanning motor and somatosensory cortex (subdural placement has been described) 5. Median nerve somatosensory evoked potentials (SSEPs) are recorded while moving the electrode from cranially to caudally until **identification of hand region** is achieved 6. Identify the region of **phase reversal** by moving paddle electrode (phase reversal means one electrode is on motor cortex and one is on somatosensory cortex) 7. **Identify the threshold** for contralateral motor response (200-µs pulse width, up to 20 mA). CAUTION: be prepared for seizures 8. **Final four-plate electrode** is placed over identified area of motor cortex (PARALLEL to central sulcus). 9. **Electrode is sutured** to the dura. 10. **Repeated programming of electrode** is performed in postoperative phase 11. **Postoperative stimulation parameters:** • Voltage: 2–5 V • Pulse width: 50–450 µs • Frequency: 50 Hz 12. **Activate** in the first 24 h from surgery, but it may take weeks to have results 13. Some contacts may not be activated 14. Settings are progressively adjusted 15. **Goal:** maximal pain relief without seizures **Complications:** • Seizures (usually during titration programming) → iced saline should be available intraoperatively • Infection • Failure to relieve pain • Hemorrhage • Device malfunction

7.1.3 Dorsal Root Entry Zone Lesioning Procedure (Table 7.1c)

Indications: deafferentation pain	Target	Localization	Results	Treatment
Postherpetic facial neuralgia	Nucleus caudalis of CN V		Excellent	Administer intraoperatively iv 1–2 mg/kg/h methylprednisolone throughout the procedure **Depending on level:** a. *Cervical* • Laminectomy: start one level above level of pain • Entry into spinal cord: at highest dermatomal level of pain • Inter-root distance: close • Rootlets: 5–8 b. *Thoracic* • Laminectomy: start at least two levels above highest level of pain • Entry into cord: two levels above highest dermatome of pain • Inter-root distance: far (5 mm between) • Rootlets: 2–4 c. *Lumbar/sacral* • Laminectomy: start at conus • Entry into cord: conus • Inter-root distance: very close • Nerve roots at higher levels are more dorsal and hide the lower ones
Cervical avulsion (brachial plexus) injury	Cervical	**Localization:** • Find the unaffected root on top and the unaffected root on bottom • Draw an imaginary line and compare to contralateral side	Excellent	
Postherpetic thoracic neuralgia		Use SSEPs and electrodes on spinal cord to identify the largest amplitude	Mediocre	
Paraplegia pain (postspinal cord injury)	Thoracic	• Top of DREZ lesion should be at level of first unaffected root • Drain syrinx (shunt)	Good	
Phantom limb pain			Good	
Conus avulsion injury	Conus	**Localization for lumbosacral avulsion:** depends on exact level, but remember that avulsed level may be hidden by other more superior roots that have to be moved laterally to directly identify the affected root	Good	

Indications: deaf-ferentation pain	Target	Results	Treatment
			Surgical technique: • *The DREZ is located* at the intermediolateral sulcus (i.e., the sulcus lateral to the dorsal columns where sensory rootlets enter into spinal cord) and involves REXED laminae 1–4 • *Lesioning* performed caudal to rostral so as to identify upper most root of interest • *Lesions every 1 mm* (more lesions are associated with better results) • Enter at 45-degrees angle (similar to root) • Depth of 2 mm for spinal cord and 1.2 mm for nucleus caudalis DREZ • Duration of 15 s at 75°C • El-Naggar–Nashold DREZ electrode (Cosman Medical Inc, Burlington, MA) • Mobilize serpentine vessels so that they do not attach to electrode • Tack up stiches to dura to avoid epidural hematoma • Consider postoperative steroids **Main complications:** • CSF leakage • Epidural hematoma • Ipsilateral weakness (corticospinal tract): permanent in 5% of patients • Walking difficulty, ataxia **Prognosis:** • 75% of patients have a good response • Response rate decreases over time

7.1.4 Sympathectomy (Table 7.1d)

Indications	Presentation	Diagnostics	Treatment and others	Surgical technique

Raynaud's disease	• Digital arterial vasospasm triggered by cold or stress
	• Extremities (fingers and toes) feel cold, numb, progressively change color from white to blue to red
		Exclude secondary form:
		• Connective tissue disorders (in 50%)
		• Medications
		• Smoking
			• **Vasoconstriction** is caused by sympathetic input
			• **Vasodilation** caused by dysfunction of mast cells (releasing histamine)
			• **Histamine** release probably more responsible for disease
				A. Thoracic (upper extremities sympathectomy):
				  a. Supraclavicular
				  b. Posterior paravertebral costotransversectomy
				  c. Axillary transthoracic
				  d. Video-assisted thoracoscopic surgery (VATS)
				  e. CT-guided chemical sympathectomy
				REMEMBER: the sympathetic chain runs parallel to spine, each ganglion being a swelling within the chain, right under the rib head
				Target: sympathetic ganglia T2, T3, and T4 + *accessory nerve of Kuntz* (arises from ramus communicans of T2, conducts sympathetic signals)

Complex regional pain syndrome OR reflex sympathetic dystrophy syndrome	See Table 7.1e			• Never remove T1 stellate ganglion because of risk of Horner's syndrome • Remove T2, T3,–T4 • **Monitor palmar skin temperature** (unilateral increase of 1–3°C in 10–20 min predicts good results) • Sympathectomy T2, T3, T4, and T4 may also offer benefit in plantar hyperhidrosis

Hyperhidrosis	a. **Primary:** focal (palm, feet, face, axilla)
	b. **Secondary** (generalized)
	  • Sweating of palms is most prominent sign
	• Incidence: 1%
		Consider:
		• Hodgkin's lymphoma
		• Hyperthyroidism
		• Tumor of hypothalamus
		• Diabetes
		• Acromegaly
		• Parkinsonism
		• Pheochromocytoma
			• Sweating is sympathetically mediated
			• Neurotransmitter is acetylcholine
			• Nonsurgical treatment options:
			  a. Oral anticholinergic (glycopyrrolate, oxybutynin)
			  b. Iontophoresis
			  c. Botox injections (for underarms and hands)	

Indications	Presentation	Diagnostics	Treatment and others	Surgical technique

			Compensatory hyperhidrosis syndrome (increased sweating in nonaddressed areas) often occurs after sympathectomy and usually improves in 6 mo	B. Lumbar (lower extremities sympathectomy)
				• Retroperitoneal extreme lateral approach
				• Remove L2–L3 sympathetic ganglion
				• Lateral aspect of vertebral body:
				  a. Right side: vena cava
				  b. Left side: aorta (right side is more difficult)

Pancreatic carcinoma				Thoracic sympathectomy: T5–T11
Intractable angina			Rare indication	

7.1.5 Treatment Strategies for Various Pain Conditions (Table 7.1e) G

Disease	Presentation	Diagnostics	Other	Treatment

Dejerine–Roussy (thalamic pain syndrome)	Contralateral hypesthesia and paresthesia may progress in weeks or months to burning sensation, dysesthesia and allodynia	MRI brain: thalamic stroke		1. Medications:
				• Anticonvulsants (pregabalin, gabapentin)
				• Antidepressants (tricyclics and selective serotonin reuptake inhibitors [SSRIs])
				2. Surgery (from most to least effective):
				  a. Motor cortex stimulation
				  b. Deep brain stimulation
				  c. Dorsal column stimulation

Disease	Presentation	Diagnostics	Other	Treatment

Complex regional pain syndrome (reflex sympathetic dystrophy syndrome)	• Causalgia, allodynia
	• Autonomic nervous dysfunction (sweating, edema)
	• Trophic changes (skin, hair, nails)
	• Reduced range of motion and weakness
		No specific high-sensitivity diagnostic tests known	a. **Type I:** *without nerve injury*
			b. **Type II:** *after nerve injury* (median, ulnar and sciatic nerves are most commonly affected)
				1. Physical therapy
				2. Transcutaneous electrical nerve stimulation (TENS)
				3. Acupuncture
				4. **Medications**
				  a. Carbamazepine
				  b. Tricyclic antidepressants
				5. **Surgical options**
				  a. *Sympathectomy* (T2–T4 for arm and L2–L3 for leg)—see Table 7.1d
				  b. *Sympathetic block:* (use fluoroscopy or CT)
				    i. Stellate ganglion (for upper extremity):
				      • 22-gauge needle
				      • Patient is supine with head tilted backward
				      • *Target:* anterior tubercle of C6
				      • Withdraw 1–2 mm (and aspirate to avoid intravascular injection):
				      • 20-mL lidocaine 1%
				      • If the block is successful, Horner's syndrome will present
				      • NEVER perform bilateral block (risk of laryngeal paralysis)
				    ii. Lumbar (for lower extremity):
				      • Patient prone
				      • 22-gauge spinal needle
				      • Target: 4 cm deeper and cephalad to transverse process of L2–L3–L4
				      • 8-mL lidocaine 1% per level (aspirate before injection)
				      • CAUTION: transient orthostatic hypotension—bed rest for several hours
				  c. *Dorsal column stimulation* (electrodes ipsilateral to side of pain)
				  d. *Intrathecal medication pump*

Disease	Presentation	Diagnostics	Other	Treatment
Cancer pain in terminally ill patients	Pain below clavicle (C4/C5) that does not respond to medication in patient with life expectancy usually <12 mo	Diminishing response to strong opioids	• 10% of cancer patients will require interventional techniques for pain management • Excellent results in malignant pleural mesothelioma	**Percutaneous cervical chordotomy (anterolateral):** • *NEVER bilateral* (risk of central hypoventilation syndrome = Ondine's curse with no spontaneous breathing) • *ALWAYS* perform contralateral to pain • Performed at C2 level with CT (or fluoroscopic) guidance and patient supine *Target:* a. *In lateral projection:* midpoint between posterior limit of body of C2 and anterior of C2 spinous process (remaining on top level of lamina to avoid the exiting nerve) b. *In anteroposterior (AP) projection:* there is dura penetration when the needle is at the level of odontoid *Goal:* interruption of anterolateral spinothalamic tract: a. Cervical fibers anterior b. Sacral fibers posterior ***Dentate ligament:*** • First inject contrast to identify dentate ligament (= posterior limit of spinothalamic tract) • CAUTION: ALWAYS stay ANTERIOR to dentate ligament *Electrophysiology:* • Impedance increases upon entering spinal cord tissue • Motor stimulation at 2 Hz, 1–3 V should not cause any contralateral arm or leg contractions • *Sensory stimulation* at 100 Hz, <1 V SHOULD cause paresthesias in contralateral arm or leg • *Muscle tetany* indicates closeness to corticospinal tract (electrode is TOO POSTERIOR) • Lesion: 70°C for 30 s

Disease	Presentation	Diagnostics	Other	Treatment
				– Check on movement responses – Depth of RF lesion should be <5 mm (avoid lesion to reticulospinal tract to prevent respiratory complications) – Ipsilateral Horner's is to be expected with successful lesion *Success rate:* • 90% immediate relief • 60% at 1 y • 40% at 2 y *Complications:* ataxia, weakness, bladder dysfunction
Bilateral visceral pain below thoracic level	Patients with cancer pain of the abdomen, pelvis or lower extremities that do not respond to medication			**Commissural myelotomy:** Medial longitudinal spinal cord incision to interrupt pain fibers crossing in anterior commissure *Prognosis:* • 60% complete relief • 30% partial relief • 10% have no relief • Effect usually lasts <1 y *Complications:* • Bladder dysfunction • Sexual dysfunction • Weakness • Dysesthesias
Cancer pain from breast and prostate cancer	Terminally ill cancer patients with agonizing pain			• Surgical or radiosurgical hypophysectomy • Effectiveness reported also in tumors without hormone dependence • Pain relief in 70%

7.2 Movement Disorders

7.2.1 Parkinson's Disease (Table 7.2a)

Presentation	Diagnostics/demographics	Treatment

A. CARDINAL SYMPTOMS:
a. Asymmetric tremor at rest (frequency of 4–6 Hz) that disappears with sleep and movement
b. "Cogwheel rigidity" during passive movement
c. Bradykinesia
B. Additional or late symptoms:
a. Postural instability (later)
b. Autonomic dysfunction (bladder and bowel, sexual, orthostatic hypotension)
c. Depression
d. Progressive dementia
e. Hyposmia
	• **Onset** at age 60 y on average 1 in 100 people at age >60 y
	• **Cause:** degeneration of dopaminergic neurons of substantia nigra pars compacta reduces activity in supplemental motor cortex
	• CAUTION: PARKINSON PLUS syndrome is NOT PARKINSON'S disease. Symptoms are similar to Parkinson's disease but:
	  – Rapid progression
	  – Poor response to levodopa
	  – Bulbar symptoms (swallowing difficulty, gaze palsy, etc.)
	  – Early-onset postural instability
	  – Dysautonomia
	Parkinson plus includes:
	  – MSA: multisystem atrophy (Shy–Drager syndrome)
	  – CBD: corticobasal degeneration
	  – PSP: progressive supranuclear palsy
	  – DLB: dementia with Lewy body disease
		1. **Medications:**
		  • Dopaminergic agents
		  • Anticholinergics
		  • Amantadine
		2. **Surgery:**
		Indications:
		  • Acceptable operative risk
		  • Responsiveness to levodopa and frequent "off" periods with dyskinesia.
		Goal is to reduce "off" periods and subsequently reduce medication with less dyskinesias
		A. *Deep brain stimulation:*
		  • Reversible and adjustable
		  • Procedure causes no lesion.
		  • Contraindications:
		    – Dementia
		    – Parkinson's plus syndrome
		  • Complications of DBS procedures:
		    – Most common: device complications (lead fracture, disconnection, etc.)
		    – Infection (>5%)
		    – Clinically significant hemorrhage in 1%/per lead (identified on CT in 2% per lead)
		Targets:
		  I. Globus pallidus interna (GPi):
		    • Treats all Parkinson's symptoms especially severe dyskinesias
		    • Coordinates:
		      – 20 mm lateral to midline
		      – 3 mm anterior to mid-AC/PC
		      – 5 mm inferior to mid-AC/PC (see ▶ Fig. 7.1)

Presentation	Diagnostics/demographics	Treatment

		• Tract (firing pattern):
		  i. Globus pallidus externa (regular firing with irregular interruption of silence) →
		  ii. Border cells (low frequency and regular rhythm) →
		  iii. GPi (significant increase in firing rate, dense irregular activity, and firing modulated by passive and active movement of the extremities)
		  iv. Neuronal activity decreases upon exit from GPi
		• Increase stimulation to 10 V to ensure the correct placement by absence of side effects
		• If a new tract is needed, make sure a 2-mm distance from previous one exists
		• There may be delay (hours to days) in therapeutic response
		
		REMEMBER: If deep brain stimulation (DBS) lead is:
		  a. Too medial to GPi → increased arm tone and contraction of face (internal capsule)
		  b. Too deep from GPi → flashing lights (optic tract)
		  c. Too lateral: → no effect
		
		Effectiveness:
		• 40% improvement in motor scores
		• 65% improvement in dyskinesias
		II. Subthalamic nucleus (STN):
		• Treats all Parkinson's symptoms
		• Medication reduction after DBS surgery
		• Coordinates:
		  – 11 mm lateral to midline
		  – 3 mm posterior to mid-AC/PC
		  – 5 mm inferior to mid-AC/PC (see ▶Fig. 7.1)
		• Typical tract (firing pattern):
		  – Thalamus (bursting units and irregular tonic firing) →
		  – Zona incerta (quiet) →
		  – Subthalamic nucleus (significant increase in firing)

Presentation	Diagnostics/demographics	Treatment

		REMEMBER: If DBS lead is:
		  a. Too medial to STN: → eye deviation (nucleus of CN III)
		  b. Too deep from STN: → depression, crying (substantia nigra)
		  c. Too posterior to STN: → dysesthesia (medial lemniscus)
		  d. Too lateral to STN: → contralateral muscle contractions (internal capsule)
		Effectiveness: 50–60% improvement in use of medication and symptom
		B. Pallidotomy
		  • Consider for patients with limited medical access or when cost of DBS surgery is prohibitive
		  • Target: same as for GPi DBS
		  • Uni- or bilateral
		  • Staged or both sides at the same time
		  • RF lesion with 1.1-mm probe with 3-mm exposed tip; first lesion at target, second lesion with probe 3 mm withdrawn superficially
		  • Complications:
		    – Cerebral hemorrhage
		    – Contralateral weakness
		    – Visual field defects

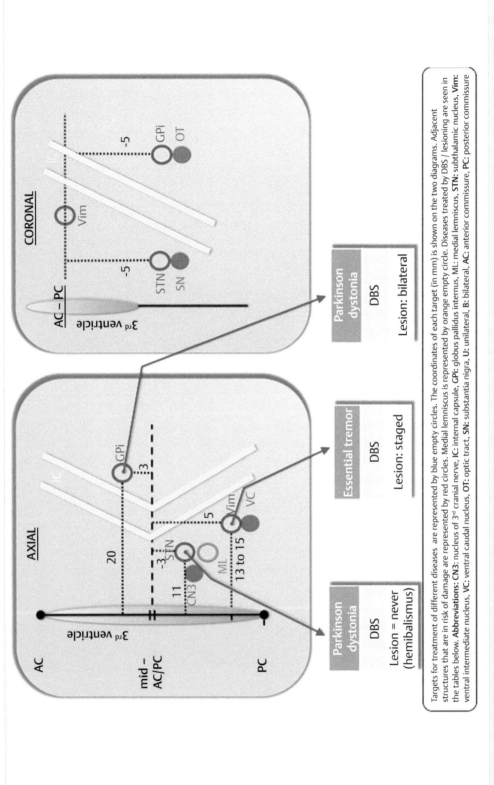

Fig. 7.1 Location of STN, GPi, and ventral intermediate nucleus on axial and coronal images

Targets for treatment of different diseases are represented by blue empty circles. The coordinates of each target (in mm) is shown on the two diagrams. Adjacent structures that are in risk of damage are represented by red circles. Medial lemniscus is represented by orange empty circle. Diseases treated by DBS / lesioning are seen in the tables below. **Abbreviations: CN3:** nucleus of 3rd cranial nerve, **IC:** internal capsule, **GPi:** globus pallidus internus, **ML:** medial lemniscus, **STN:** subthalamic nucleus, **Vim:** ventral intermediate nucleus, **VC:** ventral caudal nucleus, **OT:** optic tract, **SN:** substantia nigra, **U:** unilateral, **B:** bilateral, **AC:** anterior commissure, **PC:** posterior commissure

7.2.2 Hemifacial Spasm (Table 7.2b)

Presentation	Diagnostics	Other	Treatment

• **Muscle contractions:**
  – Unilateral
  – Intermittent
  – Painless
  – Starting with orbicularis oculi with caudal progression
  – May involve platysma
  – Possibly lacrimation
  – Also present while sleeping
• **Frequently associated with:**
  – CN VIII dysfunction
  – Trigeminal neuralgia
  – Geniculate neuralgia
  – Tic convulsive
• **Differential diagnosis:**
  – Blepharospasm
  – (it is bilateral)
  – Facial myokymia (muscle quivering)
  – Postparalytic Bell's palsy
  – Rule out seizures
• **Atypical hemifacial spasm:**
  – Begins in buccal muscles
  – More resistant to treatment
	1. **MRI brain** (rule out tumor)
	2. **MRA brain** (vascular compression)
		Offenders (in order of frequency):
		a. Anteroinferior cerebellar artery (AICA)
		b. PICA
		c. Vertebral artery
		d. Vein
		Compression may be caused by more than one vessels
			1. **Medications:**
			  • Botox injection every 4 mo (>90% effectiveness)
			  • Antiepileptics (carbamazepine, phenytoin): usually not helpful
			2. **Surgery: Microvascular decompression:**
			  • Intraoperative EMG of facial nerve and brainstem auditory evoked potentials (BAEP)
			  • The crucial point of vascular compression is at the DREZ near the brainstem
			  • Retract the inferolateral angle of cerebellum to superomedial direction
			  • Place a small retractor at 60-degree angle to cerebellar folia and retract superiorly
			  • Identify CN IX and dissect on superior aspect to find CN VII. DO NOT retract laterally as you can avulse CN VIII
			  • Any change in recordings of CN VII or CN VIII: relax the retractors
			  • Avoid overmanipulation of vessels: risk of vasospasm (in that case use papaverine)
			  • Preserve branches and place pledget or sling
			Main complication: Ipsilateral complete (2%) or partial (10%) hearing loss and facial weakness
			Prognosis:
			  • 95% find some relief and 70% have complete resolution at 1 mo
			  • Sometimes improvement takes time (even 3 mo)
			  • Younger patients with short history of spasm do better
			Recurrence:
			  • 10% within 2 y
			  • Do not re-explore (75% complication rate)
			  • Use botulinum toxin

341

7.2.3 Spasticity (Table 7.2c)

Presentation	Other	Treatment

• **VELOCITY-DEPENDENT** increased muscle tone and unidirectional resistance to passive movement
 • Increased deep tendon reflexes
 • Spontaneous or elicited clonus
 • Typically upper limb flexor and lower limb extensor muscles
 • Possibly also spastic bladder
 • Orthopaedic deformities may follow (as equinovarus deformity)
 REMEMBER: Rigidity is:
 • Velocity INDEPENDENT
 • Bidirectional
 • Normal reflexes
 • No clonus
	• Loss of inhibition on alpha and gamma motor neurons
	 • **Modified Ashworth's scale** (evaluation of muscle tone): 0: normal tone
	 1: catch with flexion or extension at the end of movement
	 2: catch with flexion or extension throughout movement
	 3: passive movements are easy
	 4: passive movements are hard
	 5: unable to flex or extend at joint
		Remember that the patient may rely on spasticity to:
		 • Improve functional activities (standing, walking, etc.)
		 • Maintain muscle size and bone strength
		 • Prevent deep venous thrombosis
		 • Help the patient identify a urinary tract infection
		 1. **Physical therapy**
		 2. **Oral medication:**
		   a. *Diazepam*
		     • GABA-A agonist
		     • Increases presynaptic inhibition of α motor neurons
		     • Begin with 2 mg TID and increase gradually up to 20 mg TID
		     • Do not discontinue abruptly (risk of seizures, depression, withdrawal syndrome)
		   b. *Baclofen*
		     • GABA-B agonist
		     • Begin with 5 mg TID and increase gradually up to 20 mg QID
		     • Do not discontinue abruptly (risk of seizures)
		   c. *Dantrolene*
		     • Reduces influx of Ca^{++} into skeletal muscle after depolarization
		     • Begin with 25 mg every day and gradually increase to twice, thrice, and four times a day—max dose 100 mg four times a day.
		     • Risk of severe hepatitis and muscle weakness
		 3. **Surgery:**
		   Indications:
		   • No response to oral medication
		   • Side effects to oral medications
		 A. *Nonablative:*
		   I. *Intrathecal baclofen:*
		     • Before pump placement perform test injection via:
		       a. consecutive bolus injections of 50–75–100 μg
		       b. intrathecal catheter trial

Presentation	Other	Treatment
		• Reduction of 2 points on Ashworth's scale for more than 4 h along with no significant side effects is a good prognostic sign for response to Tx
		• May be contraindicated in patients with other implanted programmable device (as a pacemaker), history of hepatic, gastrointestinal, renal disease, pregnancy
		• Pump implantation and management: see Table 7.4c
		• Baclofen overdose and withdrawal: see Table 11.3d
		II. *Botulinum toxin:*
		• Injection in spastic muscles for focal spasticity causes inhibition of acetylcholine release with blocking of neuromuscular transmission
		• Very good results for small muscle groups (hands, feet, etc.)
		• Must be repeated every 3–6 mo
		B. *Ablative: Selective dorsal rhizotomies*
		• Disruption of afferent signal in reflex arc
		• EMG-guided cutting of <50% of sensory rootlets
		• Best results in young patients with maintained ambulation
		• Possible recurrence
		C. *Rarely performed procedures* (typically for nonambulatory patients and as last resort):
		a. Selective neurectomy (for scissoring, sciatic / pudendal)
		b. Percutaneous RF lesion (foraminal rhizotomy) from S1 to T12 (affects sensory > motor)
		c. Myelotomy:
		• Midline incision in spinal cord
		• May relieve spasticity and pain
		d. Phenol nerve block
		e. Intrathecal phenol ablation of T12 to S1
		f. Anterior rhizotomies
		g. Cordectomy:
		• Only when everything else fails
		• Patient becomes totally flaccid
		4. Orthopaedic surgeries: tenotomy transposition

7.2.4 Torticollis (Table 7.2d)

Presentation	Diagnostics	Other	Treatment

Head turned and tilted with:
• Limited movement
• Pain
• Muscle stiffness
	1. **MRI brain/neck** in selected or persistent cases
	2. **EMG** may help define accurately the muscles and nerves involved (when operation is planned)
	3. **ENT** evaluation may also be needed
		May be due to:
		• Congenital (congenital dysplasia of hip may coexist)
		• Associated with bulbar palsy and extrapyramidal abnormalities
		• Infection (remember retropharyngeal abscess)
		• Atlantoaxial rotatory subluxation
		• Compression of CN XI
		• Hematoma of sternocleidomastoid muscle
		• Syringomyelia
		• Psychiatric comorbidity
		• Pediatric cerebellar tumor
		• Diplopia
			1. **Medication:**
			• Muscle relaxants
			• Benzodiazepines
			• Injections of botulinum toxin (not effective for anterocollis)
			2. **Physiotherapy and transcutaneous electrical nerve stimulation (TENS)**
			3. **Surgery:** consider it in case of no response to conservative treatment
			  a. *CN XI sectioning:*
			    • Dissect posterior border of sternocleidomastoid muscle (avoid injury to greater auricular and lesser occipital nerves) until you identify CN XI (to trapezius muscle)
			    • Cut sternocleidomastoid muscle 3 cm below mastoid and reflect down to find the branches of CN XI to sternocleidomastoid and trapezius muscles
			    • Possible cuts depend on torticollis, but always cut the recurrent branch that connects the branches of CN XI to sternocleidomastoid and trapezius
			    • Use nerve stimulation and EMG to identify and confirm you have cut all branches needed
			  b. *Microvascular decompression of CN XI* (responsible artery is usually vertebral or rarely PICA)
			  c. *Deep brain stimulation* (globus pallidus for contralateral symptoms)
			  d. *Dorsal column stimulation*
			  e. *Sternocleidomastoid muscle release*

7.3 Epilepsy

7.3.1 Epilepsy (Table 7.3)

Treatment	Indications	Other	Surgical technique

Vagus nerve stimulator (VNS)	• Patients older than 12 y with partial-onset seizures resistant to pharmacotherapy (Food and Drug Administration [FDA] approved)
	• Patients of any age, both partial and generalized seizures (off label)
	• Good results may be observed both with idiopathic and secondary to structural lesion epilepsy
		• Also FDA approved for treatment of chronic pharmacoresistant depression in adults
		• Risk of:
		  – Vocal cord paralysis (even permanent-recurrent laryngeal nerve is in tracheoesophageal groove)
		  – Swallowing difficulty
		  – Bradycardia
		• The device stimulates at regular intervals. Using a magnet, the patient can self-initiate a stimulation (useful in patients with aura)
		• Battery life of 5–10 y
		• MRI is not recommended (but there are reports of MRI performed on patients with VNS in literature)
		• Do not use diathermy
		• The first FDA-approved neuromodulatory therapy for the treatment of epilepsy
			1. **Location:** LEFT SIDE ONLY
			  • Right vagus innervates sinoatrial node
			  • Left vagus innervates atrioventricular node
			2. **Skin incision:**
			  a. *For electrode:* At C5–C6 level like anterior cervical discectomy and fusion (ACDF)
			  b. *For battery:* Subclavicular or in axilla along anterior fold
			3. **Vagus nerve:**
			  • Dissect a 3-cm segment between carotid and internal jugular vein
			  • Avoid pulling on the nerve (risk of recurrent laryngeal stretching)
			4. **Intraoperative test stimulation:**
			  • Notify anesthesiologist before stimulating → CAUTION: bradycardia or asystole can occur
			  • Assure that superior and inferior cervical cardiac branches are NOT inside electrode (connect below their separation from vagus
			5. **Battery placement:** DO NOT turn on device for 2 wk after surgery (allow swelling to decrease and electrode to fix to nerve).
			Complications (usually improve with time):
			  • Hoarseness
			  • Paresthesias
			  • Cough
			Outcome:
			  • Improvement is often delayed (>1 y)
			  • 50% of patients
			  • 50% reduction in seizures
			Surgery to remove electrode:
			  • Cut the electrode or
			  • Dissect off vagus cephalad
			  • Electrode removal has high risk of complications (recurrent laryngeal palsy)

Treatment	Indications	Other	Surgical technique

Multiple subpial transection	• Focal area of epileptogenic cortex that resides in eloquent area
	• Epileptogenic brain that extends into eloquent area (resection + multiple subpial transection)
	• Pediatric patients with Landau–Kleffner syndrome (acquired epileptic aphasia)
		• **PET** is done preoperatively (in addition to MRI) to determine the target area
		• **Video EEG** may also be helpful
		• Technique is considered a subpial disconnection of nerve fibers
			Awake craniotomy with intraoperative EEG
			• Outline the area for transection and always keep hook perpendicular to pial surface
			• Transections are performed perpendicular to long axis of gyrus:
			  – Depth of 5 mm
			  – Every 5 mm
			• After each cut, move to another distant cut so as bleeding has time to stop
			• Start in dependent part of gyrus so that you can deal with pooling of expected subarachnoid hemorrhage (SAH)
			• If you feel resistance on hook, stop (possibly a vessel has been encountered) and move around it
			• Each transection: pull hook across gyrus, push back and stop
			• A transient postoperative deficit may be present but resolves within 6 mo

Treatment	Indications	Other	Surgical technique

Callosotomy	• Drop attacks
	• Secondarily generalized seizures
	• Rasmussen's syndrome (encephalitis)
	• Lennox–Gastaut syndrome (patient may suffer from 50 drop attacks per day!)
	• Exclude patients with focally resectable abnormality
		• WADA test Identify handedness, speech, and memory dominance before surgery
		• Callosotomy better than VNS in reducing the frequency of drop attacks and atonic seizures
			A. One stage: Complete callosotomy
			B. Two stages:
			  i. anterior two-thirds first
			  ii. Posterior one-third later if the first operation is not sufficient
			  iii. REMEMBER: Two-stage callosotomy reduces risk of disconnection syndrome
			IV. *Anterior two-thirds callosotomy:*
			  • Use frameless stereotaxis to determine the extent of callosotomy
			  • Skin incision:
			    – U-incision (not for two-stage procedure)
			    – Bicoronal OR
			    – Straight midline
			  • Craniotomy two-thirds anterior and one-third posterior to coronal suture
			  • Approach via the nondominant hemisphere
			  • Identify cingulate gyrus (callosomarginal arteries)
			  • Callosotomy
			    – Between pericallosals OR
			    – Lateral to pericallosals
			  • Do not violate the ependymal
			V. *Posterior one-third callosotomy:*
			  • Craniotomy centered 2–3 cm anterior to lambdoid suture
			
			Complications:
			a. *Retraction on supplementary motor cortex:*
			  • Decreased spontaneity of speech
			  • Paresis of contralateral extremities
			b. *Disconnection syndrome:*
			  • Tactile anomia
			  • Dyspraxia
			  • Smell anomia
			  • Speech difficulty
			  • Usually temporary for several months

Treatment	Indications	Other	Surgical technique
Temporal lobectomy	Ideal candidate: drug-resistant temporal lobe epilepsy associated with mesial temporal sclerosis	• **Surgical options:** – Extensive temporal lobectomy – Anterior temporal lobectomy – Selective amygdalohippocampectomy • **Presurgical evaluation:** 1. Detailed history 2. Clinical assessment 3. *MRI* (investigate on hippocampal sclerosis, cortical dysplasias, gliomas, structural lesions) 4. Consider functional MRI 5. *Long-term video EEG* with several recorded seizures 6. Neuropsychological testing 7. *WADA test* (selective carotid sodium amytal injection) to localize speech and memory dominance (may not be necessary for right-sided epilepsy in right-handed individuals) 8. *Interictal PET:* – localizes epileptic areas as hypometabolic – During seizures, the same areas present as hypermetabolic – Very useful when epileptic foci are difficult to localize • Dominant temporal lobe resections are associated with risk of memory and speech deficits	**Four steps** **1. Neocortical resection** • Resection below superior temporal gyrus (that remains intact) • *From temporal tip:* – 4 cm dominant lobe – 6 cm in nondominant lobe • Find the ventricle (3 cm deep to middle temporal gyrus) • *Temporal horn borders:* – Superior: white matter and tail of caudate – Inferior: hippocampus – Medial: arachnoid of choroidal fissure – Anterior: amygdala • Resect tissues from temporal tip posteriorly to entry point into temporal horn **2. Dissect through fusiform gyrus** (posteriorly to the level of calcar avis): Connection between temporal horn and the floor of middle fossa **3. Resect amygdala + mesial temporal structures in front of hippocampus** • From anterior temporal horn to front of middle fossa) • NEVER above superior temporal sulcus (damage to basal ganglia, anterior perforated substance) • Subpial dissection • After resection, identify: – Free tentorium – CN III – PCA **4. Remove hippocampus until it starts to curve medially behind quadrigeminal plate and also remove parahippocampal gyrus:** • NEVER advance into choroidal fissure (medial border of temporal horn)—risk of anterior choroidal artery injury • Remain subpial at all times • Advancing superior will cause lesion to internal capsule, thalamus • Tail of hippocampus is bordered superiorly by internal capsule and pulvinar

Treatment	Indications	Other	Surgical technique
			Complications: a. *Contralateral superior homonymous quadrantanopia* ("pie in the sky"): Lesion of Meyer loop when resection exceeds 6–7 cm from temporal tip b. *Speech disturbance:* When resection exceeds 4–5 cm from temporal tip in dominant lobe c. *Injury to anterior choroidal artery:* Infarct of internal capsule, thalamus **Prognosis:** • Best results in epileptic patients who present with *hippocampal sclerosis* in MRI (atrophy + increased T2 signal) • *Quality of life* improves in more than 80% of patients • *Better neuropsychological performance* are observed in more selective resections (temporal lobectomy vs. amygdalohippocampectomy)

Hemispherectomy	Infantile seizures without response to nonsurgical treatment	a. Functional hemispherectomy:
		  • Preservation of basal ganglia
		  • Associated with lower surgical risk
		b. Anatomic hemispherectomy
			• **Goal:** disconnect all white matter tracts from cortex in the affected hemisphere
			• **Four steps:**
			  1. Mesial temporal lobectomy and amygdalohippocampectomy
			  2. Sylvian dissection and longitudinal opening of the entire lateral ventricle length (i.e., disconnection of temporoparietal white matter)
			  3. Corpus callosotomy with cingulotomy
			  4. Disconnection of orbitofrontal cortex

Note: The workup for seizures may include placement of subdural grids for up to 3 weeks in selected cases of difficult localization. Intraoperative seizures (stimulation evoked for mapping) respond well to ice-cold Ringer's lactate.

7.4 Various

7.4.1 Deep Brain Stimulation (Table 7.4a)

Indications	Other	Surgical technique
Parkinson's disease	Parkinson's disease is a FDA approved indication for DBS (see Table 7.2a)	

Essential tremor	• Typical family history (AKA familial tremor)
	• Symmetrical intention tremor (increases with movement)
	• Decreases at rest and with alcohol
	• Frequency of 5–10 Hz
	• Movement is flexion-extension
	• Head and voice may be involved
	
	Treatment options:
	1. **Medication (first-line treatment):**
	  • beta-blockers
	  • primidone
	  • gabapentin
	  • topiramate
	2. **Surgery:**
	  a. *Deep brain stimulation (Vim):*
	    • Can be performed bilaterally
	    • *Indications:*
	     – Patients with contralateral thalamotomy
	     – Tremor with MS
	     – Poststroke tremor
	    • Up to 80% *success rate*
	    • *Most common side effect:* paresthesias
	    • *Complications* identical to other DBS procedures (STN, GPi)
		Essential tremor is an FDA-approved indication for DBS:
		• **Target** for DBS, thalamotomy, and radiosurgical thalamotomy: Vim of thalamus
		• *Coordinates:*
		  – 3 mm anterior to PC
		  – 15 mm from midline (for normal ventricles and 11–12 mm lateral to lateral wall of enlarge 3rd ventricle)
		  – at the AC–PC (see ▶Fig. 7.1)
		• Distance from medial to lateral depends on the target of treatment (12–14 mm for face, 14–16 mm for upper extremity, 16–18mm for lower extremity)
		• Patient should be off medication for 24 h and no sedation or narcotics are used (tremor suppression)
		• *Results:*
		  – Better for distal tremors (hand) than proximal (arm)
		  – Poor results for head and voice tremors

Indications	Other	Surgical technique
	b. *Unilateral ventral intermediate nucleus (Vim) RF thalamotomy:* • Procedure steps identical to GPi pallidotomy • Can cause transient contralateral weakness, numbness, dysarthria • Success rate: 80% **c. *Stereotactic radiosurgical VIM thalamotomy:*** • consider for patients with high surgical risk • patients on anticoagulation • short-term results are similar to DBS and open thalamotomy	
Dystonia	**Indications:** a. Early-age dystonia usually associated with DYT1 gene b. Adult-onset dystonia **Not recommended for: dystonia due to** • Injury • Hypoxic • Toxic cause • Metabolic	**Dystonia is an FDA-approved indication for DBS:** • *Target:* globus pallidus internus or STN (▶ Fig. 7.1) • Neurophysiology of GPi and STN not very different from Parkinson's disease • Benefits from stimulation may present with delay • Electrode placement depends very much on microelectrode recording and less on verifying intraoperative effectiveness with stimulation (because often there is no immediate visible effect)

Cluster headaches	First-line therapies (see cluster headache in Table 12.14):
	• Oxygen
	• Triptans
	• Dihydroergotamine
	• Verapamil
	• Topiramate
	• Steroids
	• Lithium
	• Lidocaine nasal swab
	• Occipital nerve blocks
		Cluster headache is *not* an FDA-approved indication for DBS
		• Consider only if first-line therapies have failed
		• *Target:* posterior hypothalamus
		• *Coordinates:*
		  – 2 mm lateral to midline
		  – 3 mm posterior and 5 mm inferior to midcommissural point
		• *Stimulation parameters:* 185 Hz, 60- to 90-μs pulse width and 1 to 3 V amplitude
		• *Complications (side effects):*
		  a. transient reversible diplopia
		  b. intracranial hemorrhage
		• *Prognosis:* effectiveness of 70% at 2 y

351

Indications	Other	Surgical technique

Chronic pain syndromes	Consider DBS when all other pain therapies (medication, spinal cord stimulation therapy, intrathecal medication therapy) have been tried and have failed	Chronic pain is *not an FDA-approved indication for DBS*
		
		 1. *DBS of somatosensory nucleus of thalamus* (AKA ventralis caudalis [Vc] or ventralis posterior [Vp])
		 • For neuropathic pain (burning paresthesias) and denervation pain in broad distribution
		 • Coordinates:
		   – 4 mm anterior to PC
		   – 12 mm from midline
		   – At the AC–PC plane
		
		 2. *DBS for periventricular and periaqueductal gray matter:*
		 • For nociceptive pain
		 • Low-voltage stimulation (1–3 V)
		 • Coordinates:
		   – 0 to 3 mm anterior to PC
		   – 3 mm from midline
		   – 3 mm in below AC–PC plane
		 • Complications and side effects:
		   – Diplopia
		   – Oscillopsia
		   – Anxiety and fear
		 • Stimulation of periventricular gray matter is well tolerated
		 • Prognosis:
		   – Effectiveness of 50% in 50% of patients
		   – Loss of effectiveness in time does not always respond to change of stimulation parameters
		
		 3. *Other targets* have also been described (internal capsule, centromedian thalamic nucleus, etc.)

7.4.2 Spinal Cord and Stimulation (Table 7.4b) G

Indications	Other	Surgical technique
Spinal cordstimulation (SCS) AKA Dorsal column stimulation **Most common indications:** • Failed back syndrome (AKA postlaminectomy syndrome) • Complex regional pain syndrome • Peripheral neuropathy • Postherpetic neuralgia • Ischemic limb pain • Chronic intractable angina pectoris *Effectiveness:* neuropathic pain > nociceptive pain	**Pain syndromes:** *a. Nociceptive pain:* Pain from tissue damage (i.e., low back pain) *b. Neuropathic pain:* Related to nerve damage (i.e., radiculopathy) *c. Mixed pain:* Features of nociceptive and neuropathic pain **Proposed mechanism of action:** **Gate control theory** • Gate (in the spinal cord) to transmit pain information gets closed by nonpainful stimuli (i.e., paresthesia) • In other words: spinal cord can only transmit paresthesia information OR pain information but not both at the same time	**1. Patient selection:** • Failed nonsurgical pain management (medications, interventional procedures, etc.) • Chronic pain is limited to anatomical structure (i.e., not whole-body pain) • No secondary gain issues • Psychogenic causes have been excluded (i.e., neuropsychology testing) • No contraindications to surgery • Patient is able to cooperate • Patient is educated and understands how to operate the SCS patient controls **2. SCS trial:** • Trial is MANDATORY • Performed in MAC (patient has to be awake during intraoperative test stimulation) • SCS leads are implanted temporarily into epidural space • Position of leads corresponds to area of pain (i.e., cervical spinal cord for arm pain, lower thoracic spinal cord for leg pain, etc.) • Intraoperative stimulation and lead repositioning as needed • **Goal:** all painful areas are covered with paresthesia from SCS • Paresthesias extending beyond painful area are usually well tolerated and not always preventable • *Trial period:* typically 3–7 d • *Before end of trial period and removal of trial electrodes:* take X-ray showing exact lead position • Trial is successful if pain relief is >50% (higher numbers have better prognosis for long-term relief)

Indications | Other

Surgical technique

3. **Permanent implantation:**
   - Typically 2–4 wk after trial
   - Mark the area where patient wants implantable pulse generator (IPG) implanted (i.e., buttock, flank, etc.)
   - MAC or general anesthesia
   - Lead implantation in exactly the same position as for trial as documented by X-ray
   - Leads need to be secured to paravertebral fascia; otherwise, lead migration will occur
   - Pocket for IPG must be in superficial subcutaneous fat (not more than 1.5 cm deep from skin surface)
   - Leads + connecting wires if needed tunneled to IPG pocket

Complications:
   - Loss of effective pain control (>25%)
   - Lead migration or malfunction (10%)
   - Pain at IPG implantation site (10%)
   - Infection (5%)
   - CSF leak (rare)

7.4.3 Intrathecal Pain Pump Therapy (Table 7.4c) G

Indications	Other	Surgical technique

Intrathecal pump AKA pain pump AKA morphine or baclofen pump
Indications:
• Cancer-related pain
• Chronic non-cancer-related pain of nociceptive or neuropathic origin that fails to respond medication or other nonintrathecal interventions
• Spasticity
 	
Most common indications:
• Failed back syndrome
• Spinal cord injury
• Complex regional pain syndrome
• MS spasticity
 	
Not recommended for patients with:
• Psychiatric disorders (depression, bipolar, etc.)
• Personality disorders
• Drug addiction
• Suicidality
	a. **FDA approved for intrathecal pump and FIRST-LINE CHOICE:**
	  – Morphine
	  – Ziconotide
	  – Baclofen
	b. **Not FDA approved but commonly used (with scientific support):**
	  – Bupivacaine
	  – Clonidine
	  – Hydromorphone
	  – Fentanyl
	REMEMBER:
	• Medication mixtures are common
	• Intrathecal pumps currently used only have one medication chamber
	• Medications can only be titrated *independently* by changing their CONCENTRATIONS at the time of refill
	• **Maximum recommended intrathecal concentration of medications:**
	  – Morphine: 20 mg/mL
	  – Ziconotide: 100 µg/mL
	  – Baclofen: 2,000 mcg/mL
	• **Maximum daily recommended intrathecal dose:**
	  – Morphine: 15 mg/24 h
	  – Ziconotide: 19.2 µg/24 h
	  – Baclofen: no known limit but doses above 1,000 µg/24 h are rarely needed
	• *Medication titration:*
	  – 10–30% increase/24 h maximum
	  – Consider hospital admission with monitoring for faster titration
		1. **Intrathecal trials:**
		Recommended for noncancer pain / spasticity
		  a. *Single bolus injection trial:*
		    Single bolus medication doses:
		    – Morphine: 20–50 µg
		    – Ziconotide: 1–5 µg
		    – Baclofen: 50, 75, and 100 µg on consecutive days until effect is seen
		  b. *Long-term trial (3–7 d) with intrathecal catheter and continuous infusion:*
		    – Morphine: 25–50 µg/24 h
		    – Ziconotide: 0.5–2.5 µg/24 h
		    – Baclofen: 25–50 µg/24 h
		If trial is successful proceed to implantation of intrathecal pump system
		2. **Intrathecal pump implantation:**
		• Intrathecal catheter implantation: enter in lumbar intrathecal space
		• Catheter tip should be positioned several vertebral levels above entry level to minimize risk of catheter pullout →
		  Catheter tip typically advanced into low thoracic spine
		• Catheter tip can be advanced to cervical levels (may be desirable with some medications, i.e., baclofen for treatment of upper extremity spasticity)
		• Catheter must be secured with tie-down device to prevent catheter pullout
		• Pump implantation site between rib cage and pelvic ring in subcutaneous tissues

7.5 Cases

7.5.1 Trigeminal Neuralgia

Chief complaint/History of present illness	• A 77 y/o man presents to the ER with severe right facial pain.
	• He has had the pain for 6 weeks and was initially treated for dental problems resulting in two root canal procedures and extraction of two molars, all of which did not relieve his pain.
	• He describes his pain as occurring in attacks lasting seconds to minutes, lancinating, and electric- shooting. The location is in the right jaw and cheek.
	• His past medical history is remarkable for coronary artery disease.
Physical examination	• He is found to have normal cranial nerve function without facial weakness and normal facial sensation.
	• During examination, touching his right nose and right cheek triggers pain attacks.

1. **What is your diagnosis?**
   Patient suffers from trigeminal neuralgia. (See Table 7.1a: Trigeminal neuralgia, presentation).

2. **What is your plan?**
   MRI brain should be ordered to rule out tumor or multiple sclerosis (MS). Furthermore, an MRA brain could reveal microvascular compression of trigeminal nerve. Treatment depends on the cause of trigeminal neuralgia. (See Table 7.1a: Trigeminal neuralgia, diagnostics).

3. **After you start treatment, the patient's pain is greatly relieved and the patient is lost to follow-up. He returns 3 years later again to the ER with severe pain recurrence. He describes the same pain as on his first presentation but with more severe intensity and longer duration of the attacks. He is unable to eat and has lost 5 pounds in the past 2 weeks. Neurological examination is unchanged to his previous examination.**
   Updated medical history: Stenting of coronary artery branches 18 months ago. What is your plan?
   Conservative treatment options should be offered to this patient due to his advanced age (80 years) and his recent history of stenting of coronary artery branches. (See Table 7.1a: Trigeminal neuralgia, treatment, indications for percutaneous procedures).

4. **Discuss the treatment options for this patient.**
   We should administer IV phenytoin in the ER. Then we should prescribe any of the oral medications either alone or in combinations (carbamazepine, gabapentin, baclofen). If patient does not respond to the oral medications, he could undergo a percutaneous procedure (balloon compression, glycerol injection, or radiofrequency [RF] rhizotomy), which produces immediate pain relief. If oral medications produce adequate but not complete pain suppression, the patient could consider stereotactic radiosurgery of the root entry zone instead of the percutaneous procedures. (See Table 7.1a: Trigeminal neuralgia, treatment).

7.5.2 Baclofen Withdrawal

Chief complaint/History of present illness	• A 27 y/o woman is brought to the ER by her family because of confusion and agitation progressive over the past 36 hours. • Past medical history: Remarkable for motor vehicle accident (MVA) 2 years prior which left her paraplegic at the T8 level. Because of severe leg spasticity she underwent implantation of an intrathecal baclofen pump 1 year prior which resulted in great relief of the spasticity.
Physical examination	• She is oriented ×1 but able to speak, very agitated, and restless on the stretcher with severe spasticity (5/5 on modified Ashworth scale). • Severe and painful spasms spontaneously occurring in both legs. • During your examination the patient sudden loses consciousness, turns blue in her face, and suffers a tonic-clonic seizure.

1. **What is your plan?**
   Patient presents symptoms of baclofen withdrawal. Patient should be intubated and IV benzodiazepines or antiepileptics should be administered. The patient should be admitted to ICU. The pump should be interrogated and anteroposterior (AP) and lateral X-rays abdomen/lumbar spine or CT abdomen should be performed. (See Table 11.3d).

2. **Your evaluation reveals that pump is filled with medication; no error messages on pump interrogation; last pump refill 3 weeks ago with unchanged medication dose of 175 µg/24 h of intrathecal baclofen; dose has been stable for 8 months. X-ray of the pump reveals that the catheter is disconnected (see image, *arrow*). What is your plan?**

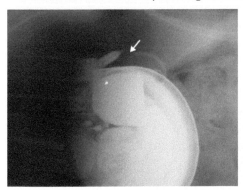

   Patient should be admitted to ICU and be treated for baclofen withdrawal. Then the disconnected catheter should be surgically repaired. (See Table 11.3e).

Suggested Readings

Bennett DS, Cameron TL. Spinal cord stimulation for complex regional pain syndromes. In: Simpson BA, ed. Electrical stimulation and the relief of pain: Pain research and clinical management. Amsterdam: Elsevier; 2003:111–129

Brown JA. Percutaneous balloon compression for trigeminal neuralgia. Clin Neurosurg. 2009; 56:73–78

Brown JA, Barbaro NM. Motor cortex stimulation for central and neuropathic pain: current status. Pain. 2003; 104(3):431–435

Coffey JR, Cahill D, Steers W, et al. Intrathecal baclofen for intractable spasticity of spinal origin: results of a long-term multicenter study. J Neurosurg. 1993; 78(2):226–232

Ebel H, Rust D, Tronnier V, Böker D, Kunze S. Chronic precentral stimulation in trigeminal neuropathic pain. Acta Neurochir (Wien). 1996; 138(11):1300–1306

Gorecki JP, Nashold BS. The Duke experience with the nucleus caudalis DREZ operation. Acta Neurochir Suppl (Wien). 1995; 64:128–131

Han Y, Zhang J, Chen N, He L, Zhou M, Zhu C. Corticosteroids for preventing postherpetic neuralgia. Cochrane Database Syst Rev. 2013; 28(3):CD005582

von Heideken J, Green DW, Burke SW, et al. The relationship between developmental dysplasia of the hip and congenital muscular torticollis. J Pediatr Orthop. 2006; 26(6):805–808

Kemler MA, de Vet HC, Barendse GA, van den Wildenberg FA, van Kleef M. Effect of spinal cord stimulation for chronic complex regional pain syndrome type I: five-year final follow-up of patients in a randomized controlled trial. J Neurosurg. 2008; 108(2):292–298

Linklater GT, Leng ME, Tiernan EJ, Lee MA, Chambers WA. Pain management services in palliative care: a national survey. Palliat Med. 2002; 16(5):435–439

Maesawa S, Salame C, Flickinger JC, Pirris S, Kondziolka D, Lunsford LD. Clinical outcomes after stereotactic radiosurgery for idiopathic trigeminal neuralgia. J Neurosurg. 2001; 94(1):14–20

Møller MB, Møller AR. Loss of auditory function in microvascular decompression for hemifacial spasm. Results in 143 consecutive cases. J Neurosurg. 1985; 63(1):17–20

Müller-Schwefe G, Penn RD. Physostigmine in the treatment of intrathecal baclofen overdose. Report of three cases. J Neurosurg. 1989; 71(2):273–275

Peyron R, Garcia-Larrea L, Deiber MP, et al. Electrical stimulation of precentral cortical area in the treatment of central pain: electrophysiological and PET study. Pain. 1995; 62(3):275–286

Ponce FA, Theodore N, Dickman CA. Thoracoscopic approaches to the spine. In: Winn HR. Youmans Neurological Surgery. 6th ed. Philadelphia, PA: Elsevier Saunders; 2011:3097–3108

Ramirez LF, Levin AB. Pain relief after hypophysectomy. Neurosurgery. 1984; 14(4):499–504

Rolston JD, Englot DJ, Wang DD, Garcia PA, Chang EF. Corpus callosotomy versus vagus nerve stimulation for atonic seizures and drop attacks: a systematic review. Epilepsy Behav. 2015; 51:13–17

Samii M, Bear-Henney S, Lüdemann W, Tatagiba M, Blömer U. Treatment of refractory pain after brachial plexus avulsion with dorsal root entry zone lesions. Neurosurgery. 2001; 48(6):1269–1275, discussion 1275–1277

Sartorius CJ, Berger MS. Rapid termination of intraoperative stimulation-evoked seizures with application of cold Ringer's lactate to the cortex. Technical note. J Neurosurg. 1998; 88(2):349–351

Shamim S, Wiggs E, Heiss J, et al. Temporal lobectomy: resection volume, neuropsychological effects, and seizure outcome. Epilepsy Behav. 2009; 16(2):311–314

Shils JL, Arle JE. Treatment applications of cortical stimulation. In: Winn HR. Youmans Neurological Surgery. 6th ed. Philadelphia, PA: Elsevier Saunders; 2011:1059–1064

Uthman BM, Reichl AM, Dean JC, et al. Effectiveness of vagus nerve stimulation in epilepsy patients: a 12-year observation. Neurology. 2004; 63(6):1124–1126

Viswanathan A, Burton AW, Rekito A, McCutcheon IE. Commissural myelotomy in the treatment of intractable visceral pain: technique and outcomes. Stereotact Funct Neurosurg. 2010; 88(6):374–382

Wendling AS, Hirsch E, Wisniewski I, et al. Selective amygdalohippocampectomy versus standard temporal lobectomy in patients with mesial temporal lobe epilepsy and unilateral hippocampal sclerosis. Epilepsy Res. 2013; 104(1–2):94–104

8 Other Diseases

8.1 Hydrocephalus (Table 8.1)

Definition/condition	Diagnosis and comments	Treatment
Imaging criteria for diagnosis of hydrocephalus 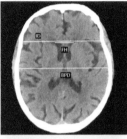 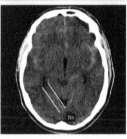 Obstructive Hydrocephalus (AKA Noncommunicating Hydrocephalus)	**Hydrocephalus suspected if:** a. Ballooning of lateral ventricles and 3rd ventricle b. Transependymal CSF (hypodense on CT, hyperintense on T2WI MRI) c. Frontal horn (FH)/internal diameter (ID) ratio > 0.5 d. FH/biparietal diameter (BPD; Evan's ratio) > 0.3 e. Temporal tip diameter > 2 mm **Obstruction of the normal CSF flow pathways at:** a. Foramen of Monro (colloid cyst, etc.) b. Cerebral aqueduct (aqueductal stenosis, tectal glioma, etc.) c. Foramen magnum (Chiari's malformation. Dandy–Walker malformation, etc.) d. Trapped ventricle (see below)	**1. Nonsurgical management of hydrocephalus:** • Useful for premature newborns with low birth weights • Temporizing measures a. Serial spinal or ventricular taps b. Acetazolamide + steroids **2. Surgical management of hydrocephalus** **A. Ventriculoperitoneal shunt:** • *Indications:* communicating / NPH AND noncommunicating hydrocephalus • *Ventricular catheter entry point:* see Table 8.2 • *Peritoneal catheter:* a. Midline—between rectus abdominis muscles b. Subcostal: 3 cm below ribcage in mammillary line • *Alternative locations for distal shunt catheter (if peritoneum is contraindicated):* a. Right atrium or superior vena cava b. Pleural cavity c. Gallbladder d. Ureter or bladder e. Sagittal sinus

(Continued) ▶

Definition/condition	Diagnosis and comments	Treatment
Communicating Hydrocephalus	A. Inadequate absorption of CSF because of "plugged" arachnoid granulations: • Posthemorrhage • Postinfection • Tumor • Arteriovenous malformation (AVM) • Postsurgery B. Overproduction of CSF: • Very rare • Typically related to choroid plexus papilloma	B. Endoscopic third ventriculostomy: • *Indications:* Recommended for obstructive hydrocephalus (especially aqueductal stenosis) • There are reports of successful treatment of communicating hydrocephalus although mechanism poorly understood • Requires very thin (transparent) floor of the 3rd ventricle • Approach with rigid endoscope through frontal horn into foramen of Monro into the 3rd ventricle • Direct endoscopic visualization of mammillary bodies and tip of basilar artery through the 3rd ventricular ependyma MANDATORY—if not visualized, abort the procedure
Normal-pressure hydrocephalus (NPH)	• A type of communicating hydrocephalus • **Cause:** unknown • **Presentation** with typical triad of symptoms: a. Gait disturbance (small steps, difficulty turning) b. Urinary incontinence c. Memory impairment • **Diagnosis:** a. Clinical presentation PLUS MRI brain consistent with hydrocephalus b. If diagnosis likely or probable, perform ancillary test: 1. **Lumbar puncture:** opening pressure >10 cm H_2O is a positive predictor of good outcome after shunt (opening pressure >24 cm H_2O is not consistent with NPH but indicative of obstructive hydrocephalus)	C. Lumboperitoneal shunt • *Indications:* communicating hydrocephalus / NPH ONLY • Placement of lumbar catheter with C-arm guidance • To reduce valve migration or difficulty tapping shunt → Place valve over iliac bone just below crest To reduce risk of overshunting → Place programmable shunt valve

Definition/condition	Diagnosis and comments	Treatment

	2. Large-volume CSF removal: spinal tap → remove 40–50 mL → then check for improvement in symptoms
	3. Continuous CSF drainage: place lumbar drainage → remove 10 mL/h for 3 - 5 d → then check for improvement in symptoms
	• **Improvement after treatment (best response first):**
	   1. Incontinence
	   2. Gait
	   3. Memory	

Arrested Hydrocephalus (AKA Compensated Hydrocephalus)	**Three criteria:**
	  a. Near-normal ventricular size
	  b. Normal head growth
	  c. Normal development
		• Spontaneous third ventriculostomy has been suggested
		• Close clinical follow-up for signs of high intracranial pressure (ICP)

Trapped ventricle	• Can occur in ventricles containing choroid plexus (ALL but frontal and occipital horns) • Outflow of ventricle is obstructed, but CSF production continues • For the 4th ventricle: inflow into the 4th ventricle AND outflow (foramina Luschka and Magendie) are obstructed • Typically seen postinfection (4th ventricle) or with tumors (all others)	• Remove cause of obstruction (i.e., tumor) • Implant separate shunt for trapped ventricle
External Hydrocephalus	• Large subarachnoid space (bifrontal) and wide interhemispheric fissure (frontally) in infants • Ventricles are mildly dilated or normal • Head perimeter crosses percentiles • Possibly frontal bossing • Look for "cortical vein sign" (veins extend from inner skull to cortical surface, which is not to be seen in subdural hematoma)	• Close follow-up • Self-resolving by 2–3 y of age
Siphoning	• Patient with shunt has orthostatic headache • Possibly slit ventricles • Possible subdural hematomas	• Anti-siphon device OR • Increase programmable valve pressure

(Continued) ▶

Definition/condition	Diagnosis and comments	Treatment

Slit Ventricle Syndrome	• Slit ventricles on imaging studies AND
	• Signs of intermittent or constant shunt malfunction
	• **Causes:**
	  a. Permanent scarred down ventricles
	  b. Intermittent ventricular collapse that temporarily occludes the catheter
		• Always rule out shunt malfunction first, because ventricles may just be scarred down slit
		• Steroids may help
		• Increase valve pressure setting

Shunt malfunction in pregnancy		• **In trimesters 1 and 2:** new ventriculoperitoneal shunt • **In trimester 3:** new ventriculoatrial or ventriculopleural shunt • **Prophylactic antibiotics** in labor and continue until 48 h after birth (Ampicillin 2 g IV every 4 h + Gentamicin 1.5 mg/kg IV every 8 h)

8.2 Ventricular Catheter Placement Tips (Table 8.2)   G

Entry point	Specifics
Kocher's point 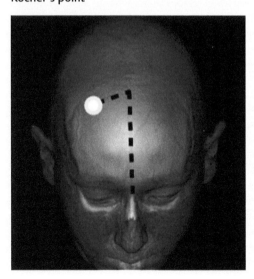	**Coordinates:** • 11 cm up from nasion (= 1 cm anterior from coronal suture) on midline • 3 cm lateral of midline (midpupillary line) **Trajectory:** • *Aim* toward ipsilateral medial canthus (ipsilateral eye) and external acoustic meatus • *Length:* NOT DEEPER than 6.5 cm from the skull It is the Preferred entry point for ventricular access

Entry point	Specifics

Frazier's point

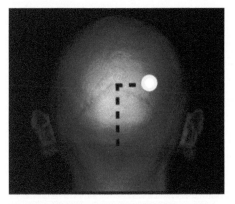

Coordinates:
- 7 cm up from inion on midline
- 3 cm lateral

Trajectory:
- *Aim* toward nasion
- *Length:* 10 cm

For emergency access, if needed during posterior fossa craniotomy

Keen's point

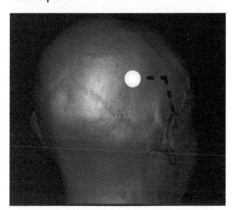

Coordinates:
- 3 cm above and
- 3 cm posterior to pinna

Trajectory:
- *Aim* toward nasion
- *Length:* 7–10 cm

Dandy's point

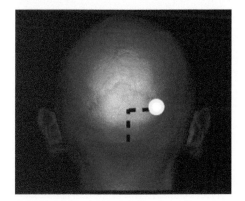

Coordinates:
- 3 cm up from inion on midline
- 2 cm lateral to inion
  Beware of transverse sinus

Trajectory:
- *Aim* toward nasion
- *Length:* 7 cm

Remember:

a. *Conversion from cm H_2O to mm Hg:*
- Multiply pressure in cm H_2O × 0.74
- 10 cm H_2O = 7.4 mm Hg

b. *Conversion from mm Hg to cm H_2O:*
- Multiply pressure in mm Hg × 1.36
- 10 mm Hg = 13.6 cm H_2O

8.3 Intracranial Hypotension and Hypertension (Table 8.3)

Clinical presentation	Diagnostic studies	Treatment
A. Spontaneous intracerebral hypotension		
• Spontaneous positional (orthostatic) headache • No history of trauma or iatrogenic cause **REMEMBER:** Spontaneous subdural hemorrhage (without trauma): search for spine CSF leak	1. **Spinal tap:** Low CSF pressure (<6 cm H$_2$O) (not always) 2. **MRI brain and spine with contrast:** • Pachymeningeal enhancement • Sagging brain • Pituitary hyperemia • Subdural collections • Engorged veins 3. **CT brain (coronal thin cuts) and spine with intrathecal contrast** with immediate (45 min) and delayed (4 h) images: • Skull base leaks • Spinal meningeal cysts Delayed diagnosis makes treatment more difficult	**A. Symptomatic treatment:** • Treat like postlumbar puncture headache: – Bed rest – Hydration – Caffeine • Epidural blood patch that can be repeated (inject 10–20 mL of autologous blood in epidural space and place the patient placed in Trendelenburg after the injection) **B. Surgical repair** (exact site of leak must be known)
B. Pseudotumor cerebri AKA benign (or idiopathic) intracranial hypertension		
• **Most common in (4 F's):** – Female – Fat – Fertile – Forty (usually 40 y old) • **Common symptoms:** – Headache – Papilledema – Enlarged blind spot – Constricted visual field (the best test for following vision) – Blindness may occur but rarely • **Uncommon symptoms:** – CMVI palsy – Tinnitus – Nausea – Neck stiffness	1. **MRV brain:** exclude venous sinus thrombosis or stenosis 2. **MRI brain** • Slit ventricles • Possible empty sella 3. **Lumbar puncture:** CSF pressure > 20 cm H$_2$O (remember the possible variations during day; so if there is strong suspicion, repeat the test)	**A. General treatment recommendations:** • Weight loss (recent gain can worsen vision) • Salt restriction • Diuretics (acetazolamide, furosemide) • Topiramate • Steroids (short term if no response to other medications) • Serial lumbar punctures (consider especially in pregnancy) **B. Surgery:** 1. **Headache ± visual disturbance:** • Ventricular peritoneal shunt • Lumbar peritoneal shunt • Always consider programmable shunt systems 2. **Visual disturbance without headache:** • Shunt • Optic fenestration **REMEMBER:** Spontaneous remission, but also relapse, is common. Close follow-up necessary.

8.4 Arachnoid Cyst (Table 8.4 ◀))) G

Epidemiology/classification	Histology/ Presentation/ diagnostics	Treatment
Arachnoid cyst AKA leptomeningeal cyst (CAUTION: not synonymous with posttraumatic leptomeningeal cyst; see Pediatric Head Injury in Chapter 6) **Location:** • Middle cranial fossa (the most common) • Cerebellopontine angle • Suprasellar area • Posterior fossa • Intraventricular • Optic nerve • Spine (most commonly thoracic spine) Male:female = 3:1 **Galassi classification of the middle cranial fossa arachnoid cysts:** a. **Type 1:** • Small, temporal tip • Free communication with cisterns b. **Type 2:** • Intermediate size • Rectangular shape • It originally communicated with subarachnoid space and later sealed off c. **Type 3:** • Large • No communication to subarachnoid space • Causing local mass effect	**Proposed mechanisms:** • Cyst formation and brain hypoplasia secondary to cyst development • Primary brain hypoplasia of brain (i.e., temporal lobe) with arachnoid cyst "filling the void" **Histology:** • Splitting of arachnoid membrane • Thickening of the collagen layer in cyst wall • No arachnoid trabeculations within the cyst • Hyperplastic arachnoid cells in cyst wall **Clinical presentation:** • Commonly an incidental finding • Macrocephaly • Asymmetric head growth with focal skull protrusion • Seizures (controversial) • Signs of increased ICP • Pituitary dysfunction (suprasellar cysts) • Hydrocephalus (suprasellar cysts) • Visual impairment (optic nerve cyst) **Diagnostic tests:** • CT and MRI • Follows CSF intensity on all MRI sequences (difference from dermoid cysts)	**A. Asymptomatic:** • Repeat MRI imaging at 6 mo • If no change in size or appearance, no further imaging studies are needed **B. Symptomatic:** • Craniotomy with cyst fenestration and opening cyst to subarachnoid space • Endoscopic cyst fenestration and cyst wall marsupialization • Cystoperitoneal shunt • CT-guided needle aspiration (spinal arachnoid cysts) • Cyst amputation at the stalk (spinal arachnoid cysts) **REMEMBER:** Cysts are a known *RISK FACTOR for development of subdural hematomas.* Patients need to be counseled regarding contact sports and head trauma

8.5 Central Nervous System Infections (Table 8.5)

Bacterial infections

General antibiotics suggestions:
- *Gram-positive (except Staphylococcus):* Ampicillin ± Gentamicin
- *Staphylococcus:* Nafcillin
- *MRSA:* Vancomycin
- *Gram-negative (except Pseudomonas):* Ceftriaxone
- *Pseudomonas:* Cefepime or Ceftazidime
- *Anaerobes:* Metronidazole
- *Penicillin or Cephalosporin allergy:* Meropenem
- *Cryptococcus, Aspergillus, Candida:* amphotericin B + flucytosine
- *Empiric therapy (no pathogen isolated):* Vancomycin + Cefepime ± metronidazole

Condition	Presentation/ causative agent	Diagnostic tests/ comments	Treatment
Posttraumatic meningitis	**Risk factor:** CSF leak **Pathogens:** • Gram-positive cocci (*Staphylococcus*, *Streptococcus*) • Gram-negative bacilli (*Escherichia coli*, *Klebsiella*, *Acinetobacter*)	• LP with CSF cell count with differential, glucose, protein and Gram stain / cultures • Diagnostic imaging to determine leak site	• Continue iv antibiotics for at least 1 wk after sterile CSF culture • Persistent or recurrent CSF leaks must be surgically explored and repaired
Brain abscess (including nocardiosis)	**Three possible ways of spreading:** • Hematogenous (the most common) • Posttraumatic (including postsurgical) • Contiguous spread (sinusitis, otitis, dental) **Risk factors:** • Pulmonary abnormality (lung abscess, bronchiectasis) • Congenital cyanotic heart disease • Immunocompromised state **Pathogens:** • Streptococcus (adults) • Anaerobes • Staphylococcus (posttraumatic) • Fungi (immune- compromised) • Gram negatives (infants)	**Send specimen for:** • Gram stain • Acid-fast stain (*Nocardia*, *Mycobacterium*) • Aerobic and anaerobic culture • Fungal culture • TB culture • Polymerase chain reaction (PCR) testing • Pathological examination (rule out tumor) **Rule of one-third:** • One-third single agent • One-third polymicrobial • One-third sterile (or organism cannot be isolated)	**A.** Surgery (resection or needle aspiration) in case of: • Mass effect • Signs of increased ICP • Possible rupture into ventricle • Fungal abscess • Failure of medical management **B.** Nonsurgical management: • Causative agent has been identified • Small (< 2 cm) abscess • Multiple abscesses • Brain stem abscess • Poor surgical candidates **C.** IV antibiotics for at least 6 wk + 6 wk oral **D.** Regular MRI follow-up

Condition	Presentation/ causative agent	Diagnostic tests/ comments	Treatment

		Diagnostic workup MRI (or CT) with contrast:
		1. **Acute stage:** Low T1, high T2
		2. **Consolidated stage:**
		  • **Center:** Low T1, high T2
		  • **Capsule:** High T1, low T2
		  • **Perifocal area:** Low T1, high T2
		CAUTION: lumbar puncture has no role in diagnostic workup of brain abscess
			Nocardiosis abscess:
			• Caused by the bacterium *N. asteroides* or *N. brasiliensis*
			• May form abscesses or present as diffuse infection
			• *Affects patients with chronic conditions like:*
			  – Cancer
			  – Long-term steroid use or Cushing's disease
			  – AIDS
			  – Transplant patients
			• **Treatment:**
			  – Surgery as for other brain abscesses
			  – Trimethoprim-sulfamethoxazole
			  – Imipenem alternatively

Subdural empyema	• Often direct extension of infection (sinusitis)
	• Rare complication of otitis
	• Patients presenting with:
	  – Fever
	  – Headache
	  – Meningismus
	  – Swelling or tenderness over affected sinus
	  – Focal neurological deficits
		• CT or MRI with contrast
		• Signs of mass effect are common
		• **Sometimes difficult to diagnose:**
		  – Imaging findings look too benign for severity of patient's sickness
		  – When in doubt, repeat CT or MRI
			1. Surgical drainage is treatment of choice
			2. Seizure prophylaxis
			3. Antibiotics similar to abscess
			CAUTION: lumbar puncture is potentially dangerous

Osteomyelitis of the skull	Contiguous spread (sinus, skull lesion) **Pathogen:** • *S. epidermidis* • *S. aureus*	**CT, MRI:** • Bone enhancement • Osteolytic lesion	1. Surgical debridement until normal bone is encountered 2. Cranioplasty (at the same time or delayed) 3. Antibiotic therapy for 3 mo

(Continued) ▶

Condition	Presentation/ causative agent	Diagnostic tests/ comments	Treatment
Viral infections			
Herpes encephalitis	**Pathogen:** herpes simplex virus 1 (HSV1) Hemorrhagic encephalitis **Typical location:** temporal lobes **Patient presentation:** Encephalitis with • Seizures • Confusion • Fever • Lethargy • Coma	**Diagnostic tests:** a. *CSF:* • RBC > 500 mm³ • HSV antibodies (after 2 wk) b. *MRI:* temporal edema across Sylvian fissure (transsylvian sign) c. *Open brain biopsy* of anterior temporal lobe for direct virus isolation (rarely needed)	• Early IV acyclovir • Supportive therapy
Fungal infections			
Cryptococcosis	Most frequent fungal disease affecting the CNS	**Diagnostic test:** a. *Lumbar puncture:* elevated opening pressure b. *Cryptococcal antigen titer:* high	**Antifungal therapy** (amphotericin B + fluconazole) **For increased ICP:** a. Daily lumbar puncture OR b. Lumbar drain OR c. CSF shunt
Candidiasis	See "Shunt Infection"		
Parasitic infections			
Toxoplasmosis	• **Pathogen:** Toxoplasma gondii • **Patient presentation:** Immunecompromised patients	a. **MRI findings:** • Multiple small lesions • Ring enhancement • Typically in basal ganglia • Perifocal edema b. **Toxoplasmosis titer:** positive and high	A. If toxoplasmosis titer high AND MRI findings typical (multiple lesions in basal ganglia): empiric therapy for 2–3 wk with Sulfadiazine + folic acid B. **Brain biopsy for:** • Negative toxoplasmosis titer • Lesions close to surface (atypical for toxoplasmosis) • Diagnosis questionable

Condition	Presentation/ causative agent	Diagnostic tests/ comments	Treatment

Neurocysticercosis	• **Pathogen:** Larva (*Cysticercus cellulosae*) of pork tapeworm (*Taenia solium*)
	• **Patient presentation:**
	  – Seizures
	  – Increased ICP
	• **Acquired from** ingestions of eggs that hatch in intestines and embryo burrows through intestinal wall into blood stream
		CT, MRI findings:
		• Ring-enhancing cyst
		• Cyst is hypodense with hyperdense area (= scolex; head of tapeworm)
		• Parenchymal calcifications
		• Hydrocephalus (common)
			1. **Medications**
			  • Steroids
			  • Albendazole or Praziquantel
			  • Antiepileptics
			2. **Brain biopsy** for diagnosis in questionable cases
			3. **Surgery for:**
			  • Large cysts > 5 cm (Cysticercus *racemosus*: contains no larva)
			  • Persistent increased ICP
			  • Spinal cysts
			  • Intraventricular andsubarachnoid cysts (more resistant to medical treatment)
			4. **CT or MRI** every 6 mo until cysts disappear or calcify

Echinococcosis **AKA hydatid cyst**	• **Pathogen:** Larva of dog tapeworm *Echinococcus granulosa*
	• **Endemic areas:**
	  – Australia
	  – New Zealand
	• **Life cycle:** Humans infected by eating contaminated food (larva eggs from infected dogs feces)
	• **Presentation:**
	  – Increased ICP
	  – Seizures
	  – Focal deficits
		CT, MRI:
		• Cysts isodense to CSF
		• No enhancement
		• Cysts enlarge slowly
			Goal of treatment: removal of cyst without rupture
			Dowling's surgical technique:
			1. Place patient in such a position that the cyst points to the ceiling
			2. Craniotomy
			3. Careful dura opening away from cyst
			4. Corticectomy
			5. Place soft irrigation catheter between cyst wall and white matter
			6. Irrigate through catheter, while lowering head end of table and "float" cyst out of the brain
			7. *If cyst ruptures:* immediate suction, remove capsule, and irrigate for 5 min, then change instruments and gloves

(Continued) ▶

Condition	Presentation/ causative agent	Diagnostic tests/ comments	Treatment
Protozoal infections			
Naegleria fowleri AKA Amoeba fowleri	• **Pathogen** lives in warm fresh water • **Acquired** during swimming through nasal mucosa • **Causes** meningoencephalitis with hemorrhagic necrosis of brain and spinal cord	CSF: • Often hemorrhagic • Increased leucocytes • High protein • Culture and gram stain: negative • Wet prep: motile trophozoites	• Amphotericin B + miconazole • Possible need for **ventriculostomy** • Possible brain abscess
Prion diseases			

Creutzfeldt–Jakob disease (CJD)	• **Incidence:** 1:1 million
	• **Typical age** > 50 y
	• 10% are **inherited** with autosomal dominant pattern (chromosome 20)
	• **Sporadic** occurrence
	• **Iatrogenic** transmission (including neurosurgeons)
	• **Presentation:**
	  – short duration: <12 mo
	  – mental impairment
	  – myoclonic jerks
		a. **Histology:** typical triad
		  • Neuronal loss
		  • Astrocyte proliferation
		  • Spongiform vacuoles in neurons and astrocytes
		b. **Imaging studies:** no specific findings
		c. **EEG:** 1- to 2-Hz periodic complexes
		d. **CSF:** 14–3–3 present (> 95% sensitivity)
		e. **Tonsillary biopsy** (for atypical CJD)
			Brain biopsy:
			• Necessity is questionable
			• Open biopsy with manual saw and personnel precautions
			Sterilization of instruments:
			• 1 h at 132°C OR
			• Immersion in 1 molar NaOH for 1 h at room temperature
			• Other methods ineffective
			Treatment:
			• None
			• Uniformly fatal typically within 1 y

Postsurgical and wound Infections			

Post-surgical meningitis	Pathogens:
	• Coagulase-negative staphylococci
	• *S. aureus*
	• *Pseudomonas*
	• Pneumococci (skull base, ENT surgery)
			1. Start empiric therapy after obtaining cultures, then
			2. Adjust antibiotic therapy according to sensitivity
			3. Consider intrathecal therapy for severe cases
			  • Vancomycin
			  • Gentamicin
			  • Amikacin
			  • Colistin

Condition	Presentation/ causative agent	Diagnostic tests/ comments	Treatment
Shunt infection	**Pathogens:** • Staphylococcus (coagulase negative and aureus) • Gram-negative rods • E. coli and Streptococcus (neonates) • Candida (infants)	**Diagnosis:** a. Suggestive history + b. General markers of infection • white blood cell (WBC) • C-reactive protein (CRP) • erythrocyte sedimentation rate (ESR) + c. CSF analysis + d. Cultures (blood or shunt tap CSF) **REMEMBER:** CSF gram stain or CSF culture ALONE have up to 50% false negatives	**Treatment:** 1. Surgical removal of shunt hardware 2. Send hardware for culture 3. EVD if necessary 4. Antibiotics as directed by Gram stain and culture (or empiric therapy if no cultures available) 5. Place new shunt system after CSF is clean (i.e., 3 clean serial CSF cultures) 6. Postoperative antibiotics for at least 2 wk **Candida shunt infection:** 1. After shunt removal (and placement of EVD if necessary), treat with antifungal therapy for 1 wk 2. Place new shunt 3. Continue antifungal therapy for 6–8 wk
Shunt contamination from peritonitis	**Peritonitis from:** • Ruptured appendix • Bowel perforation • Spontaneous bacterial peritonitis (e.g., from liver cirrhosis)	• Contamination of peritoneal catheter possible • Daily CSF cultures recommended	**Treatment options:** a. Cleaning and soaking of peritoneal catheter in antibiotic solution during abdominal surgery and immediate reimplantation b. Externalization of peritoneal catheter with re-implantation of new peritoneal catheter once CSF cultures are clean x 3 c. Externalization followed by implantation of new catheter at alternate distal site once CSF cultures are clean x 3

(Continued) ▶

EVD infection

Suggestive of EVD infection:
- Low CSF glucose
- CSF cell count > 1,000
- WBC > 15,000
- Positive Gram stain
- Positive cultures

Treatment:
1. Remove EVD and place new EVD at different site
2. Send EVD and CSF for culture
3. Start empiric antibiotics (see general suggestions above)

Prevention:
- Antibiotic-impregnated drain
- Tunneling of EVD catheter > 5 cm from burr hole
- Routine EVD rotation DOES NOT reduce infection rate
- Prophylactic prolonged antibiotics in patients with EVD DO NOT reduce the infection rate

8.6 Cases

8.6.1 Normal pressure hydrocephalus

Chief complaint/History of present illness

- A 75 y/o woman presents with 1-year history of progressive difficulties with walking, urinary incontinence, and memory problems.

Physical examination

- Not oriented to time and space.
- Walks with help due to severe unsteadiness, wide base stance.
- Upper and lower extremity strength is within normal limits, sensation within normal limits.
- Urinary incontinence.

1. Describe the CT and MRI of the patient.

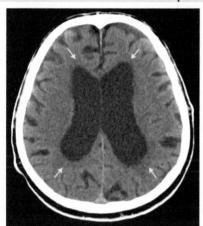

CT head (axial) shows enlarged lateral ventricles, atrophy and slight periventricular hypodensity (*arrows*), which can be attributed to transependymal CSF transudation in normal pressure hydrocephalus (NPH).

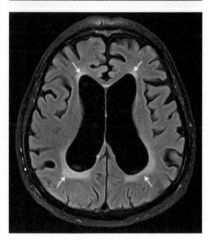

MRI head (fluid-attenuated inversion recovery [FLAIR], axial) shows enlarged lateral ventricles, atrophy, and periventricular high signal (*arrows*), which can be attributed to transependymal CSF transudation in NPH.

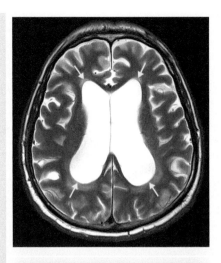

MRI head (T2, axial) shows enlarged lateral ventricles, atrophy and periventricular high signal (*arrows*), which can be attributed to transependymal CSF transudation in NPH.

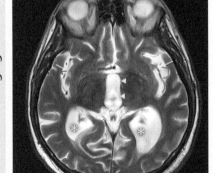

MRI head (T2, axial) shows atrophy with enlarged Sylvian fissures bilaterally (*arrows*), enlarged atrium bilaterally (*asterisks*), and enlarged third ventricle with round edges (*arrowheads*).

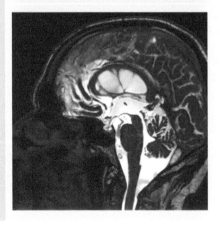

MRI head (T2, midsagittal section) shows an enlarged fourth ventricle (*arrow*) and no obstruction of the aqueduct (*arrowheads*).

Imaging

2. **What's the typical triad of symptoms in NPH?**
   (See Table 8.1: Normal pressure hydrocephalus, diagnosis and comments).

3. **How can the diagnosis of NPH be supported?**
   The diagnosis of NPH can be supported by typical triad of symptoms, MRI head, normal opening pressure, large volume CSF removal, or continuous CSF drainage (via lumbar drainage). (See Table 8.1: Normal pressure hydrocephalus, diagnosis and comments).

4. **What are some risk factors for NPH (secondary NPH)?**
   • History of previous: cranial surgery, head trauma, subarachnoid surgery, central nervous system (CNS) infection.
   • Aqueductal stenosis.

5. **The patient underwent a lumbar puncture. The opening pressure was 18 cm H_2O. Around 40 cc of CSF were removed. However, there was no improvement of her symptoms. The clinical suspicion of NPH is high. What is your plan?**
   Patient should undergo a continuous CSF drainage using a lumbar drainage. (See Table 8.1: Normal pressure hydrocephalus, diagnosis and comments).

6. **Patient improved after the continuous CSF drainage. What are the treatment options?**
   VP shunt OR lumboperitoneal shunt. Prefer programmable shunt valves. (See Table 8.1: Treatment).

7. **What are the different entry points for ventricular catheter placement? Describe the technique for ventricular catheter placement for each one of the different entry points.**
   Kocher's point, Keen's point, Frazier's point, Dandy's point.
   (See Table 8.2).

8. **What are the indications of endoscopic third ventriculostomy (ETV)?**
   ETV is mainly recommended for obstructive hydrocephalus. (See Table 8.1: Treatment).

9. **Which is the first symptom of the triad to improve after shunt placement?**
   Incontinence > gait > memory. (See Table 8.1: Normal pressure hydrocephalus, diagnosis and comments).

10. **The patient underwent a programmable lumboperitoneal shunt placement. Postoperatively the patient's gait progressively improved and she was oriented to place and time. However, 20 days after surgery she started having headaches, which were worse when she was upright and improved when she was lying flat. She also reported dizziness. What complication do you suspect and what study would you like to obtain? What is your treatment plan?**

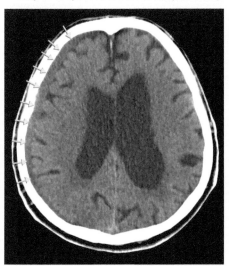

The most likely complication is subdural hematoma/hygroma due to overdrainage. The patient should undergo a head CT. The head CT (see CT on the left) showed a subdural hematoma (slightly hypodense to isodense, extra-axial collection, and crescentic shape) extending from right frontal lobe to parietal lobe without midline shift. Since the lumboperitoneal shunt is programmable, we should consider setting the valve to a higher resistance and repeat head CT after around 2 to 4 weeks, as long as the patient improves clinically.

8.6.2 Cerebral abscess

Chief complaint/History of present illness

- A 7 y/o girl presents with persistent headaches for 10 days. In addition, today the mother reports episodes of vomiting and mentions that her daughter is sleeping more than usual and it is difficult to awaken her.
- Previous medical history: Otitis media 1 month ago treated with antibiotics for 10 days.

Physical examination

- Temperature is 100.4°F (38°C).
- Patient is drowsy, but when awake she is oriented ×3.
- The rest of neurological examination is within normal limits without focal neurological deficits.

1. Describe the MRI of the patient.
   (See Table 8.5: Brain abscess, diagnostic tests/comments).

Imaging

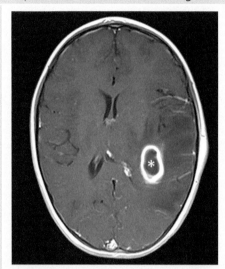

MRI head (enhanced T1WI, axial) shows a lesion (*asterisk*) with peripheral enhancement located in the left parietal lobe in close proximity to the left atrium. There is slight midline shift.

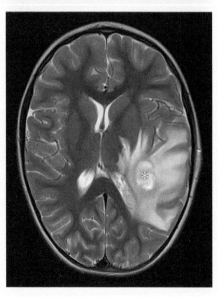

MRI head (T2WI, axial) shows a hyperintense lesion (*asterisk*) surrounded by a hypointense margin located in the left parietal lobe in close proximity to the left atrium. There is marked vasogenic perilesional edema (hyperintense signal) contributing to slight midline shift.

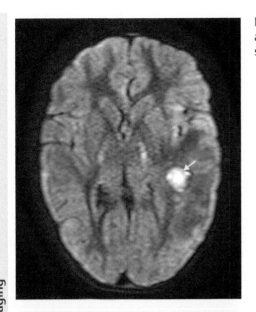

MRI head (diffusion-weighted image [DWI], axial) shows hyperintense lesion (*arrow*) representing restricted diffusion.

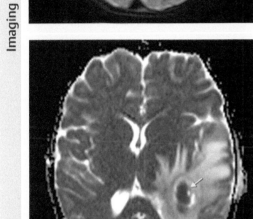

Diffusion coefficient map shows a lesion (*arrow*) with marked central diffusion restriction, resulting in low apparent diffusion coefficient (ADC) values seen as low signal. The lesion is surrounded by a large hyperintense area due to lack of diffusion restriction, representing vasogenic edema.

2. **What is the differential diagnosis of intra-axial brain lesions with ring enhancement? What is the most likely diagnosis?**
   The most likely diagnosis is abscess due to fever and the recent history of otitis media.
   (See Table 4.19).

3. **What are the MRI findings that can differentiate brain abscesses from a cystic or necrotic tumor? What are the magnetic spectroscopy findings of an abscess and a tumor?**
   • On DWI brain abscesses typically demonstrate restricted diffusion whereas cystic or necrotic brain tumors do not.
   • On MRS lactate peak can be increased in both tumors and abscesses, but amino acid, succinate, and acetate peaks are increased only in abscesses. (See Table 4.18).

4. **What are some risk factors for brain abscesses? What are the three possible ways of spread?**
(See Table 8.5: Brain abscess, presentation/causative agents).

5. **What are the four histologic stages of brain abscess formation? What are the MRI findings depending on the stage of the abscess?**
   - Early cerebritis (days: 1–3), late cerebritis (days: 4–9), early capsule (days: 10–13), late capsule (days >14).
   - MRI findings of acute stage and consolidated stage. (See Table 8.5: Brain abscess, diagnostic tests/comments).

6. **What is the diagnostic workup for brain abscesses?**
   - Workup to differentiate brain abscess from tumor:
     - MRI brain (DWI), MRS.
     - CT chest, abdomen, pelvis to rule out a metastatic origin.
   - Workup to support diagnosis of infection
     - Laboratory tests (CRP, ESR, CBC with differential).
   - Workup to find a source of infection
     - cultures (blood, urine).
     - CTs: Facial/temporal bone CT (rule out sinus/ear/dental infection), chest, abdomen, pelvis.
     - Serologic tests depending on Hx / clinical suspicion.
     - Transesophageal echocardiogram.

7. **Would you perform a lumbar puncture to confirm brain abscess diagnosis and to isolate a pathogen?**
Lumbar puncture should be avoided due to risk of herniation and low rates of positive CSF culture. (See Table 8.5: Brain abscess, diagnostic tests/comments).

8. **What are the indications for nonsurgical management and surgical management? What are the surgical options?**
(See Table 8.5: Brain abscess, treatment).

9. **How would you treat this patient and why?**

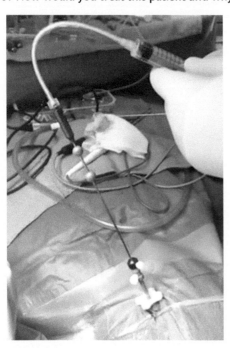

The patient should undergo surgery due to abscess size, close proximity to ventricle, midline shift in MRI, and signs of increased ICP (somnolence, headache, vomiting). Due to the deep location of the abscess, needle aspiration with use of neuronavigation was performed. (See intraoperative image on the left.)

10. What tests are you going to perform on the specimen? What are the most usual pathogens isolated in brain abscesses?

    (See Table 8.5: Brain abscess ,presentation/causative agent, diagnostic tests/comments).

11. What are the treatment steps after abscess aspiration?
    - Start broad-spectrum empirical antibiotics until cultures are obtained (continue empirical antibiotics if no pathogen is isolated).
    - After final culture results are obtained switch to antibiotics based on sensitivities of pathogen.
    - Administer IV antibiotics for at least 6 weeks followed by p.o. antibiotics for 6 weeks.
    - F/U with regular enhanced head MRI.
      (See Table 8.5: Brain abscess, treatment).

9 Anatomy

We selected the images to be included in this chapter not based on the need for fundamental anatomical information, but rather based on the utility for clinical tips and the ability to master complex neurosurgical anatomy through the study of the least amount of images. Anatomical structures are identified by numbers, while relevant clinical anatomic tips are identified by letters.

Sellar Region and Cavernous Sinus: Superior View (▶Fig. 9.1)

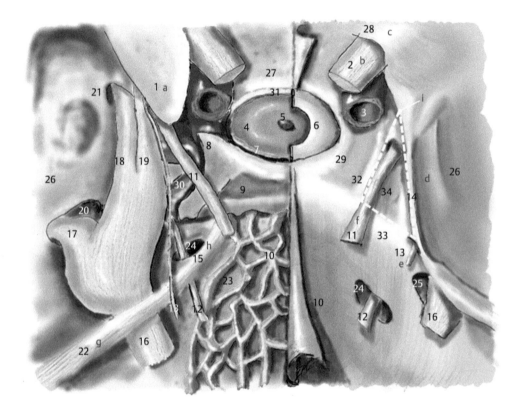

Anatomy: Superior view of the sellar region and the cavernous sinus. In the left half of the image, the dura has been removed from the floor of the middle fossa. Furthermore, in the left half of the picture, both layers of the dura of the lateral wall of the cavernous sinus have also been removed, exposing the nerves coursing along the cavernous sinus. (**1**) Anterior clinoid process (ACP); (**2**) optic nerve; (**3**) internal carotid artery (ICA; supraclinoid portion); (**4**) pituitary gland (hypophysis); (**5**) pituitary stalk; (**6**) diaphragm; (**7**) posterior intercavernous sinus; (**8**) posterior clinoid process; (**9**) dorsum sellae; (**10**) basilar sinus (in the right half of the image, it is located below the dura); (**11**) oculomotor nerve (cranial nerve [CN] III); (**12**) abducens nerve (CN VI); (**13**) trochlear nerve (CN IV); (**14**) anterior petroclinoid dural fold (part of tentorial edge); (**15**) petrosphenoid ligament (ligament of Gruber); (**16**) trigeminal nerve (CN V); (**17**) mandibular nerve (third branch of CN V, V3); (**18**) maxillary nerve (second branch of CN V, V2); (**19**) ophthalmic nerve (first branch of CN V, V1); (**20**) foramen ovale; (**21**) foramen rotundum; (**22**) edge of tentorium; (**23**) clivus; (**24**) Dorello's canal; (**25**) Meckel's cave; (**26**) middle cranial fossa; (**27**) tuberculum sellae; (**28**) falciform ligament; (**29**) cavernous sinus; (**30**) ICA (cavernous portion); (**31**) anterior intercavernous sinus; (**32**) interclinoid dural fold; (**33**) posterior petroclinoid dural fold; (**34**) oculomotor triangle.

Clinical information and surgical tips: (a) When **drilling ACP**, beware of CN III deep to the ACP. Furthermore, beware of pneumatized clinoid, which may communicate with sphenoid air sinus. **(b)** Use optic nerve to identify the ICA laterally. **(c)** In case of compressing masses, **cut falciform ligament** to decompress optic nerve. **(d)** There are **two layers of dura covering the cavernous sinus**. To achieve hemostasis, peel one layer and then inject Floseal into triangles to control venous bleeding. **(e)** When entering tentorial edge, beware of the trochlear nerve (CN IV). **CN IV** enters the tentorium approximately 10 mm posterior to the point where CN III touches the tentorium. **(f) CN III** enters the roof of the cavernous sinus through the oculomotor triangle (34). **(g)** Stop **bleeding from the superior petrosal sinus** by packing it with Gelfoam. The bleeding is usually caused by avulsion of the origin of Dandy's vein (superior petrosal vein). **(h) Dorello canal**, through which CN VI enters into the cavernous sinus, is not a bony canal. It is bounded by the petrous apex laterally and the superolateral clivus medially and its roof is formed by the petrosphenoid ligament (15). **(i) oculomotor triangle (Hakuba's triangle):** a triangular area of the dura formed by the anterior petroclinoid dural fold laterally (14), the posterior petroclinoid dural fold posteriorly (33), and the interclinoid dural fold medially (32). Through this triangle, CN III enters the roof of cavernous sinus.

Posterior View of Brainstem and Floor of Fourth Ventricle (▸Fig. 9.2)

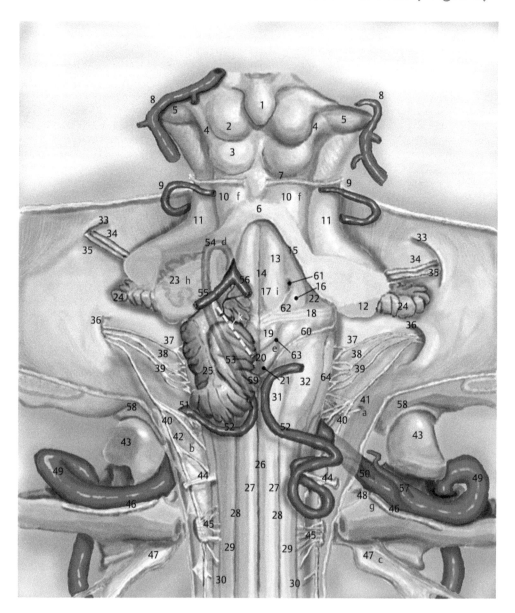

Anatomy: Posterior view of the brainstem and the floor of the fourth ventricle. Notice the different origin of the two posterior inferior cerebellar arteries (PICAs) from the vertebral arteries: on the left side, the origin is intradural (usual), whereas on the right side it is extradural (5–20%). On the left side, the dentate ligament is preserved. The left tonsil has also been preserved, so that its relationship with the PICA is better demonstrated.

(1) Pineal body (epiphysis), **(2)** superior colliculus, **(3)** inferior colliculus, **(4)** inferior brachium, **(5)** medial geniculate body, **(6)** superior medullary velum, **(7)** trochlear nerve (CN IV), **(8)** posterior cerebral artery (PCA), **(9)** superior cerebellar artery (SCA), **(10)** superior cerebellar peduncle, **(11)** medium cerebellar peduncle, **(12)** inferior cerebellar peduncle, **(13)** medial eminence, **(14)** dorsal median sulcus, **(15)** locus coeruleus, **(16)** vestibular area, **(17)** facial colliculus, **(18)** striae medullaris, **(19)** hypoglossal trigone, **(20)** vagal trigone, **(21)** area postrema, **(22)** lateral recess, **(23)** dentate nucleus, **(24)** flocculus, **(25)** tonsil, **(26)** posterior median sulcus, **(27)** gracile fasciculus, **(28)** posterior intermediate sulcus, **(29)** cuneate fasciculus, **(30)** posterolateral sulcus, **(31)** gracile tubercle, **(32)** cuneate tubercle, **(33)** internal acoustic meatus, **(34)** facial nerve (CN VII), **(35)** vestibulocochlear nerve (CN VIII), **(36)** jugular foramen, **(37)** glossopharyngeal nerve (CN IX), **(38)** vagus nerve (CN X), **(39)** cranial root of the accessory nerve (CN XI), **(40)** spinal root of the accessory nerve (CN XI), **(41)** hypoglossal nerve, **(42)** dentate ligament, **(43)** superior articulating facet of C1, **(44)** dorsal root of the C1 spinal nerve, **(45)** rootlets of the dorsal root of the C2 spinal nerve, **(46)** C1 spinal nerve, **(47)** dorsal root spinal ganglion of C2 spinal nerve, **(48)** groove for vertebral artery, **(49)** vertebral artery, **(50)** extradural origin of the PICA, **(51)** intradural origin of the PICA, **(52)** caudal loop of the PICA (belongs to the tonsillomedullary or posterior medullary segment of the PICA), **(53)** junction of tonsillomedullary with telovelonsillar segment of the PICA, **(54)** cranial loop or choroidal point (belongs to telovelonsillar segment of the PICA, **(55)** lateral trunk, **(56)** medial trunk, **(57)** posterior meningeal artery, **(58)** occipital condyles, **(59)** obex, **(60)** taenia, **(61)** superior fovea, **(62)** sulcus limitans, **(63)** inferior fovea, **(64)** trigeminal tubercle.

Clinical information and surgical tips: (a) In the far lateral approach, the **hypoglossal canal** obstructs access to the ventral brainstem. **(b) Dentate** ligament (42) separates rootlets of dorsal (sensory) root from rootlets of the ventral (motor) root. The intradural vertebral artery (49) courses anteriorly to the dentate ligament, whereas the spinal root of the accessory nerve (CN XI; 40) courses posteriorly to the dentate ligament. If the dentate ligament is divided, it can be used to rotate the spinal cord. **(c)** If there is significant venous bleeding, the **C2 root** (47) can be sacrificed for easier bleeding control. **(d)** The **choroidal point** (cranial loop) is defined as the superior-most point of the PICA. There are no perforators to brainstem distal to this. Occlusion of the PICA at or distal to the choroidal point does not usually result in a functionally significant neurological deficit. **(e)** Intraoperative irritation of **vagal trigone** (20) can cause bradycardia. **(f)** Bilateral damage to the **superior cerebellar peduncle** (10) is thought to be the anatomical basis of mutism in children after posterior cranial fossa tumor sugery.[1]**(g)** Palpate the **groove for the vertebral artery** (48) on the posterior arch of C1 with a Penfield no. 4 to estimate the location of the vertebral artery. May use Doppler. **(h)** Lesion to the **dentate nucleus** (23) can cause intention tremor of the ipsilateral extremities with voluntary movement. The dentate nucleus is located just superior to the rostral pole of the tonsil and is wrapped around the superolateral recess of the roof of the fourth ventricle forming a prominence (dentate tubercle, not depicted). The inferior medullary velum separates the rostral pole of the tonsil from the dentate tubercle. **(i)** Lesion to **facial colliculus** (17) can cause facial palsy. **(k) Telovelar approach to the fourth ventricle**[2]: In the telovelar approach to the fourth ventricle, the medullotonsillar and the uvulotonsillar space of the cerebellomedullary fissure are dissected and the tonsils are released from the uvula and the medulla oblongata and retracted superolaterally. In this step, care should be taken to avoid injury to the PICA. An oblique incision is made to the tela choroidea starting near the foramen of Magendie and extended superolaterally through the telovelar junction to the inferior medullary velum (*dashed green line*). The telar incision can also be extended laterally toward the foramen of Luschka. If needed, the approach can be bilateral for greater exposure. This approach was developed in order to replace the older transvermian approach (splitting of inferior vermis), which was associated with high incidence of postoperative cerebellar mutism.

Annulus of Zinn, Cavernous Sinus, and Middle Fossa: Lateral View (►Fig. 9.3)

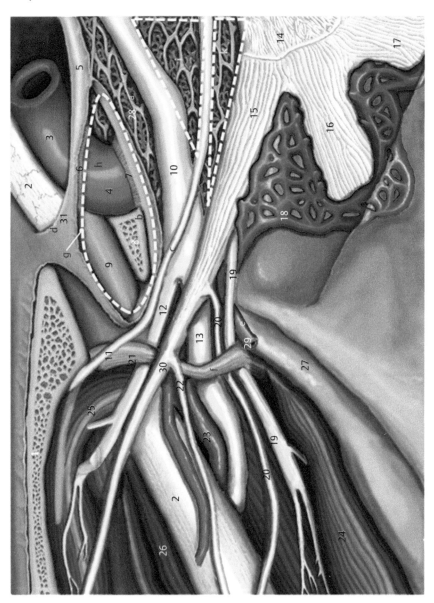

Anatomy: Lateral view of the left orbit, cavernous sinus, and middle fossa. The lesser sphenoid wing has been removed and the superior orbital fissure is open. The ACP has been removed. The annulus of Zinn can be seen. **(1)** orbital roof (drilled); **(2)** optic nerve; **(3)** supraclinoid portion of the ICA; **(4)** clinoid segment of the ICA; **(5)** tentorial edge; **(6)** upper or distal dural ring; **(7)** lower or proximal dural ring; **(8)** optic strut; **(9)** optic nerve covered by optic sheath; **(10)** oculomotor nerve (CN III); **(11)** trochlear nerve (CN IV); **(12)** superior division of CN III; **(13)** inferior division of CN III; **(14)** trigeminal ganglion (gasserian ganglion); **(15)** ophthalmic nerve (first branch of CN V, V1); **(16)** maxillary nerve (second branch of CN V, V2); **(17)** mandibular nerve (third branch of CN V, V3); **(18)** pericavernous venous plexus; **(19)** abducens nerve (CN VI); **(20)** nasociliary nerve (branch of V1); **(21)** annulus of Zinn (annular tendon); **(22)** lacrimal nerve (branch of V1); **(23)** ophthalmic artery; **(24)** lateral rectus muscle (pulled inferiorly); **(25)** superior rectus muscle (pulled superiorly); **(26)** medial rectus muscle; **(27)** residual greater sphenoid wing after drilling (lesser wing has been removed, thus unroofing the superior orbital fissure); **(28)** cavernous sinus; **(29)** superior ophthalmic vein (SOV); **(30)** frontal nerve (branch of V1); **(31)** falciform ligament.

Clinical information and surgical tips: (a) There are **two layers of the dura covering the cavernous sinus.** For hemostasis, peel one layer and inject Floseal into triangles to control venous bleeding. **(b)** The **optic strut** (8) is the posterior root of the lesser sphenoid wing and forms the floor of the optic canal. Thus, it separates the optic nerve from the superior orbital fissure. **(c) The trochlear nerve (CN IV**; 11) crosses over the oculomotor nerve (CN III; 10). Beware when dissecting on CN III not to injure CN IV. **(d)** When you manipulate optic nerve, first incise the **falciform ligament** (31). **(e) The SOV** (29) communicates directly to the cavernous sinus. That is the reason there is eye chemosis, pulsatile proptosis, and ocular bruit with carotid–cavernous fistula (CCF). The superior ophthalmic vein appears enlarged on MRI with CCF. **(f)** The **annulus of Zinn (annular tendon**; 21) is formed by fibrous tissue and serves as the origin of the four rectus muscles. The following structures pass through the annulus of Zinn: optic nerve, superior and inferior division of CN III, CN VI, nasociliary nerve (from V1), and ophthalmic artery. **(g) Clinoidal triangle:** this triangle is located between the optic nerve and oculomotor nerve and contains from anteriorly to posteriorly the optic strut (8), the clinoid segment of the ICA (4), and the cavernous sinus. Removal of the ACP is required for exposure of this triangle. **(h) Anterior clinoidectomy** is indicated in surgery for paraclinoid and ophthalmic aneurysms, as well as for resection of tumors involving the medial sphenoid ridge, the ACP, and the cavernous sinus (meningioma, craniopharyngioma, pituitary adenoma). The aim is to expose the ICA, the origin of the ophthalmic artery, and optic nerve, and to reduce the need for brain retraction. Furthermore, the ICA and the optic nerve are easier manipulated and mobilized after anterior clinoidectomy. Beware of possible pneumatization of ACP communicating with the sphenoid sinus, which could result in post-op cerebrospinal fluid (CSF) rhinorrhea after clinoidectomy. Beware not to injure CN III (deep to the ACP) and optic nerve (medial to ACP) during clinoidectomy. Also, CN IV can be injured. ICA maneuverability increases further if a dural incision around the distal dural ring (leaving a dural cuff) is made to release it from the surrounding dura. **(i) Supratrochlear triangle:** the triangular space formed between the lower margin of CN III (10) superiorly, the upper margin of CN IV (11) inferiorly, and an imaginary line connecting the dural entry points of these nerves (see ▶ **Fig. 9.4**). **(k) infratrochlear triangle (Parkinson's triangle):** the triangular space formed between the lower margin of CN IV (11) superiorly, the upper margin of V1 (15) superiorly, and an imaginary line connecting the dural entry point of CN IV and the entry point of CN V into Meckel's cave. This triangle usually contains the origin of the meningohypophyseal trunk from the cavernous portion of the ICA.

Cavernous Sinus and Middle Fossa: Lateral View (▸Fig. 9.4)

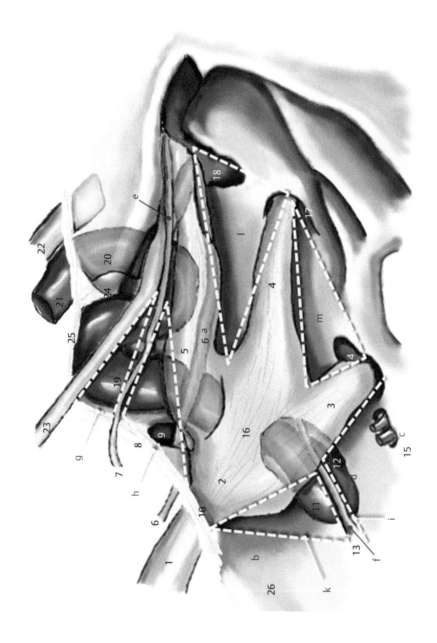

Anatomy: Lateral view of the right cavernous sinus area and the middle fossa. The middle fossa dura has been removed. Furthermore, the two layers of the dura of the lateral wall of the cavernous sinus have also been removed, exposing the nerves coursing along the cavernous sinus. **(1)** trigeminal nerve (posterior root); **(2)** trigeminal ganglion (gasserian ganglion); **(3)** mandibular nerve (third branch of CN V, V3); **(4)** maxillary nerve (second branch of CN V, V2); **(5)** ophthalmic nerve (first branch of CN V, V1); **(6)** abducens nerve (CN VI; medial to V1); **(7)** trochlear nerve (CN IV); **(8)** petrosphenoid ligament (ligament of Gruber); **(9)** Dorello's canal; **(10)** Meckel's cave; **(11)** petrous portion of the ICA (C2 portion); **(12)** carotid canal; **(13)** greater superficial petrosal nerve (GSPN) entering the middle cranial fossa through hiatus fallopii; **(14)** foramen ovale; **(15)** middle meningeal artery and vein in foramen spinosum; **(16)** petrolingual ligament (deep to trigeminal ganglion and over petrosal portion of the ICA); **(17)** foramen rotundum; **(18)** superior orbital fissure; **(19)** cavernous portion of the ICA (C3); **(20)** clinoid segment of the ICA (part of the cavernous portion between the upper and lower dural rings medial to the ACP); **(21)** supraclinoid portion of the ICA (C4); **(22)** optic nerve; **(23)** oculomotor nerve (CN III); **(24)** ACP; **(25)** tentorial edge; **(26)** petrous part of the temporal bone.

   Clinical information and surgical tips: (a) CN VI is located most medially of all cranial nerves in the cavernous sinus. **(b) peel the middle fossa dura** posterior to anterior. **(c)** Cauterize the **middle meningeal artery** above the foramen spinosum, and then cut high enough, so it does not retract and bleed. It may be required to drill around the foramen spinosum to expose the middle meningeal artery. If the middle meningeal artery retracts and bleed, first remove all soft tissue around the osseous foramen and then use bone wax. **(d)** Beware of **dehiscence of carotid canal roof** during middle fossa dissection. **(e) Trochlear nerve** (CN IV) crosses over the oculomotor nerve (CN III). Beware when dissecting on CN III not to injure CN IV. **(f)** Unilateral injury of the GSPN (13) causes reduction of tear production ipsilateral to the injury. **(g) Supratrochlear triangle:** the triangular space formed between the lower margin of CN III (23) superiorly, the upper margin of CN IV (7) inferiorly, and an imaginary line connecting the dural entry points of these nerves (see ▶ Fig. 9.3). **(h) infratrochlear triangle (Parkinson's triangle):** the triangular space formed between the lower margin of CN IV (7) superiorly, the upper margin of V1 (5) inferiorly, and an imaginary line connecting the dural entry point of CN IV and the entry point of CN V into Meckel's cave. This triangle usually contains the origin of the meningohypophyseal trunk from the cavernous portion of the ICA (see ▶ Fig. 9.3). **(i) The posterolateral middle fossa triangle (Glasscock's triangle):** this refers to an area of the middle fossa between the lateral margin of V3 (3) anteromedially (distal to its intersection with GSPN) and the anterior margin of GSPN (13; proximal to its intersection with GSPN) posterolaterally. It contains the middle meningeal artery and drilling of the middle fossa in this area leads to infratemporal fossa. **(k) The posteromedial middle fossa triangle (Kawase's triangle):** a triangular space defined by the lateral margin of CN V (proximal to its intersection with GSPN) medially, the GSPN (proximally to its intersection with CNV), and an imaginary line that connects the hiatus fallopii with the Meckel's cave (10) laterally. It contains the petrous portion of the ICA anteriorly and the cochlea laterally. Drilling of the petrous bone in the medial part of this triangle leads to posterior fossa. **(l) The anteromedial middle fossa triangle:** a triangular area defined by the lower margin of V1 medially (6), the upper margin of V2 laterally (4), and an imaginary line connecting the entry point of V1 into the superior orbital fissure (18) and the foramen rotundum (17) anteriorly. Drilling the middle fossa in this triangle leads to sphenoid sinus. **(m) The anterolateral middle fossa triangle:** a triangular area defined by the lower margin of V2 medially (4), the upper margin of V3 laterally (3), and an imaginary line connecting the foramen rotundum (17) with the foramen ovale anteriorly. Drilling the middle fossa in this triangle leads to the lateral wing of the sphenoid sinus.

Frontal Horn and Body of Lateral Ventricle and Third Ventricle: Sagittal Section (▶Fig. 9.5)

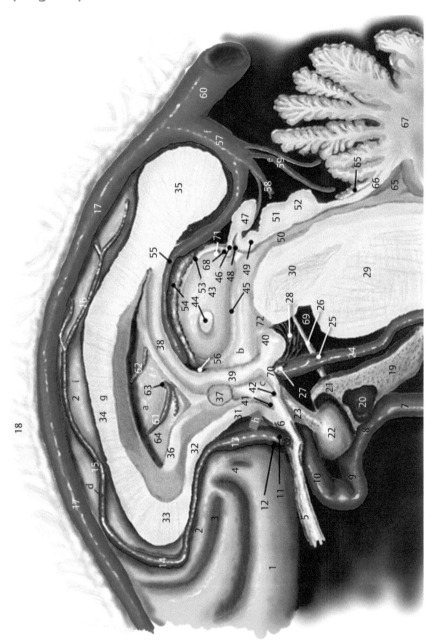

Anatomy: Parasagittal section, some millimeters lateral to midline to the left through corpus callosum (CC) and the body of the fornix. The septum pellucidum is removed, exposing the frontal horn and body of the right lateral ventricle. We also see the right lateral wall of the third ventricle. **(1)** Straight gyrus (gyrus rectus); **(2)** cingulate gyrus; **(3)** cingulate sulcus; **(4)** subcallosal area; **(5)** right optic nerve; **(6)** optic chiasm; **(7)** cervical portion of the right ICA (C1); **(8)** petrous portion of the right ICA (C2); **(9)** cavernous portion of the of right ICA (C3); **(10)** supraclinoid portion of the right ICA (C4); **(11)** anterior communicating artery (ACom); **(12)** A1 segment of the anterior cerebral artery (ACA; A1: from origin to ACom); **(13)** infracallosal segment of the ACA (A2, from ACom to junction of rostrum–genu of CC); **(14)** precallosal segment of the ACA (A3; anterior to genu of CC); **(15)** supracallosal segment of the ACA (A4, above the CC, from junction of genu–body of CC up to a point just posterior to the coronal suture); **(16)** postcallosal segment of the ACA (A5, above the CC, from a point just behind the coronal suture to the end); **(17)** inferior sagittal sinus; **(18)** falx; **(19)** clivus; **(20)** sphenoid sinus; **(21)** dorsum sellae; **(22)** pituitary gland (hypophysis); **(23)** pituitary stalk (infundibulum); **(24)** basilar artery; **(25)** SCA; **(26)** oculomotor nerve (CN III); **(27)** PCA; **(28)** thalamoperforating arteries from the P1 segment of the PCA terminating mostly to the interpeduncular fossa, posterior perforating substance, and the cerebral peduncles; **(29)** pons; **(30)** midbrain; **(31)** lamina terminalis; **(32)** rostrum of CC; **(33)** genu of CC; **(34)** body of CC; **(35)** splenium of CC; **(36)** septum pellucidum (removed); **(37)** anterior commissure; **(38)** body of fornix; **(39)** columns of fornix; **(40)** left mammillary body; **(41)** chiasmatic recess; **(42)** infundibular recess; **(43)** medial surface of the right thalamus; **(44)** massa intermedia; **(45)** hypothalamic sulcus; **(46)** habenular commissure; **(47)** pineal body (epiphysis); **(48)** pineal recess; **(49)** posterior commissure; **(50)** aqueduct; **(51)** superior colliculus; **(52)** inferior colliculus; **(53)** striae medullaris thalami; **(54)** choroid plexus of the third ventricle; **(55)** internal cerebral vein; **(56)** foramen of Monro; **(57)** great cerebral vein of Galen; **(58)** basal vein of Rosenthal (cut); **(59)** precentral cerebellar vein (aka vein of the cerebellomesencephalic fissure); **(60)** straight sinus; **(61)** anterior caudate vein; **(62)** posterior caudate vein; **(63)** confluence of the anterior caudate vein, anterior septal vein thalamostriate vein, and superior choroidal vein to form the internal cerebral vein passing through the foramen of Monro into the third ventricle; **(64)** caudate nucleus; **(65)** lingula; **(66)** superior medullary vellum; **(67)** cerebellum; **(68)** habenula; **(69)** pontomesencephalic sulcus; **(70)** tuber cinereum; **(71)** suprapineal recess; **(72)** posterior perforated substance.

Clinical information and surgical tips: (a) The **body of the lateral ventricle** extends from the foramen of Monro (56) anteriorly up to the point where the body of the fornix meets CC. It has a floor (thalamus), a roof (body of CC; 34), lateral wall (body of caudate nucleus; 64), and a medial wall (septum pellucidum and body of fornix; 38). **(b)** The **third ventricle** has (1) **a roof** (body of fornix anteriorly and the crura of fornix with the commissure of fornix posteriorly); (2) **a floor** (from anterior to posterior, chiasm, infundibulum, tuber cinereum, mammillary bodies, posterior perforated substance, midbrain up to aqueduct); (3) **an anterior wall** (from superior to inferior, columns of fornix, foramen of Monro, anterior commissure, lamina terminalis, chiasmatic recess, chiasm); (4) **a posterior wall** (from superior to inferior, suprapineal recess, the habenular commissure, the pineal body and pineal recess, the posterior commissure, and the aqueduct); and (5) **two lateral walls** (thalamus superiorly and hypothalamus inferiorly). The roof of the third ventricle apart from the fornix is also formed by two layers of tela choroidea below the fornix, a space between these membranes called velum interpositum, where the vessels course and the choroid plexus. **(c)** The floor of the third ventricle is fenestrated in the area between the mammillary bodies and the infundibular recess in the **endoscopic third ventriculostomy**. Beware of the basilar artery while fenestrating the floor. **(d)** The **pericallosal arteries** are defined as the portion of ACAs distal to ACom around and on the corpus callosum. For identification of midline during callosotomy, find both pericallosal arteries. The midline lies in between. **(e)** The **precentral cerebellar vein** (aka vein of the cerebellomesencephalic fissure; 59) can be sacrificed during the supracerebellar infratentorial approach. This vein drains directly (like in the illustration) or indirectly via the superior vermian vein into the great cerebral vein of Galen. **(f) Veins draining into the great cerebral vein of Galen (usually):** the two internal cerebral veins (55), the two basal veins of Rosenthal (58), superior vermian vein (which receives occasionally the precentral cerebellar vein), the tectal veins, the posterior pericallosal veins, the medial occipitotemporal veins, and the internal occipital veins. Additional veins draining usually in the internal cerebral veins have been described to drain into the great cerebral vein of Galen and vice versa. **(g)** When you are about to finish the **callosotomy**, just before entering the ventricle, look for a small midline groove. **(h)** Opening of the **lamina terminalis** via the subfrontal approach leads to the third ventricle. **(i)** Excessive bilateral **cingulate gyrus** retraction may cause postoperative transient akinetic mutism.[3] Furthermore, during the interhemispheric approach to the corpus callosum, have in mind that below the falx the two cingulate gyri may be adherent to each other and can be mistaken for corpus callosum. Identify corpus callosum by its bright white color and its relative hypovascularity.

389

Lateral Ventricles: Superior View (▸Fig. 9.6)

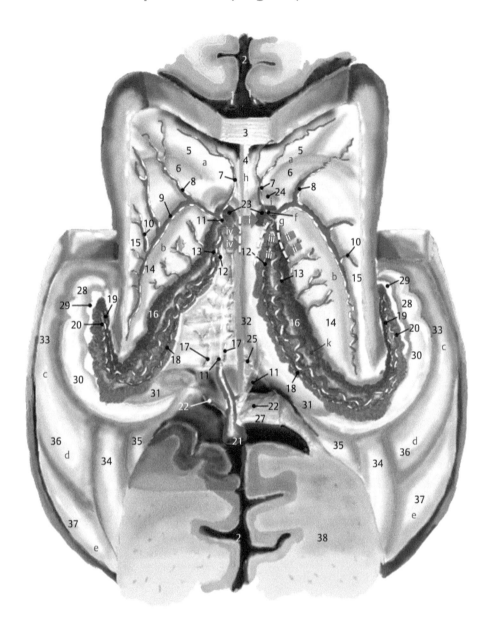

Anatomy: Superior view of the lateral ventricles. The upper part of the hemispheres and the corpus callosum have been removed and the floor of the lateral ventricles (frontal horn, temporal horn, occipital horn, atrium, and body) was exposed. On the left side, the body of the fornix has been removed, exposing the translucent superior membrane of tela choroidea, through which the vessels coursing in the velum interpositum can be seen. The two membranes of the tela choroidea with the intervening velum interpositum form three of the five layers of the roof of the third ventricle (body of fornix and the choroid plexus form the remaining two). **(1)** Pericallosal artery, **(2)** longitudinal cerebral fissure, **(3)** genu of corpus callosum (cut), **(4)** septum pellucidum, (5) rostrum of corpus callosum (part of the frontal horn floor), (6) head of the caudate nucleus, (7) anterior septal vein, (8) anterior caudate vein, (9) thalamostriate vein coursing along thalamostriate sulcus between the thalamus and the body of the caudate nucleus, (10) posterior caudate vein, (11) internal cerebral vein, (12) arterial blood supply of the choroid plexus of body of the lateral ventricle near the foramen of Monro from the medial posterior choroidal artery, (13) superior choroidal veins, (14) thalamus, (15) body of the caudate nucleus, (16) choroid plexus attached along the choroidal fissure between the thalamus and the fornix, (17) medial posterior choroidal arteries, (18) arterial blood supply of choroid plexus in the body of the lateral ventricle near the atrium, in the atrium, and in the posterior temporal horn from lateral posterior choroidal artery, (19) arterial blood supply of the choroid plexus in the anterior temporal horn and atrium from the lateral posterior choroidal arteries, (20) inferior choroidal veins, (21) great cerebral vein of Galen, (22) basal vein of Rosenthal, (23) foramen of Monro, (24) column of fornix, (25) commissure of fornix, (26) superior membrane of tela choroidea (velum interpositum can be seen with coursing vessels), (27) splenium of CC, (28) pes hippocampus (hippocampus head), (29) fimbria, (30) body of hippocampus, (31) crura of fornix, (32) body of fornix, (33) collateral eminence (overlies collateral sulcus), (34) calcar avis (overlies calcarine sulcus), (35) bulb of corpus callosum (overlies forceps major), (36) collateral trigone (overlies collateral sulcus), (37) occipital horn, (38) occipital cortex.

Clinical information and surgical tips: (a) The frontal horn is located in front of the foramen of Monro and has an anterior wall and a roof (genu of CC; 3), a floor (rostrum of CC; 5), a lateral wall (head of caudate nucleus; 6), and a medial wall (septum pellucidum; 4). **(b)** The body of the lateral ventricle is located between the foramen of Monro and the point where CC meets the fornix. It has a floor, a medial and lateral wall, and a roof (see ▶ **Fig. 9.5**). **(c)** The temporal horn extends from the atrium to the medial temporal lobe. It has a floor (formed by the hippocampus medially and the collateral eminence laterally; 33), a roof (formed by the thalamus and tail of the caudate nucleus medially and tapetum of CC laterally), a medial wall (choroidal fissure between thalamus and fimbria), a lateral wall (tapetum), and an anterior wall (overlies amygdaloid nucleus). **Caution:** when entering into temporal horn or in anterior temporal lobectomy, there is a risk of contralateral superior homonymous quadrantanopia due to injury to the Meyer loop (= fibers of optic radiation coursing over the roof of the temporal horn up to its tip, then looping back along the lateral wall). **(d)** The atrium communicates with the body of the lateral ventricle anteriorly, the temporal horn inferiorly, and the occipital horn posteriorly. It has a roof (formed by the body, splenium, and tapetum of CC), a medial wall (formed by the bulb of CC superiorly and the calcar avis inferiorly; 34), a lateral wall (formed by the caudate nucleus anteriorly and tapetum posteriorly), an anterior wall (formed by the crus of fornix medially and the pulvinar laterally), and a floor (collateral trigone; 36). **(e)** The occipital horn has a medial wall (bulb of CC and calcar avis), roof and lateral wall (both formed by tapetum), and a floor (collateral trigone). **(f)** The venous angle is defined as the "**U**"-shaped junction of the thalamostriate vein and internal cerebral vein at the posterior margin of the foramen of Monro (like in both hemispheres of the illustration). In the false venous angle variation, the "**U**"-shaped junction of the thalamostriate vein and internal cerebral vein is located posterior to the posterior margin of the foramen of Monro. **(g)** In the anterior transcallosal–transforaminal approach, study the pre-op MRV. If the junction of the anterior septal vein with the internal cerebral vein is located posterior to the posterior margin of the foramen of Monro (usual location of junction), then we recommend enlarging the foramen of Monro posteriorly by opening the choroidal fissure along the taenia choroidea (between choroid plexus and thalamus) up to the junction of the two veins. Do not sacrifice the thalamostriate vein.[4] **(h)** When you are about to complete the callosotomy, just before entering the ventricle, look for a small midline groove. **(i)** In the transcallosal–transforaminal approach, do not retract the columns of the fornix. There is risk of memory deficits. **(k)** In order to confirm entry into either the right or the left ventricle, identify the choroid plexus and the thalamostriate vein both coursing anteriorly toward the foramen of Monro. Choroid plexus is always medially to the thalamostriate vein. Also identifying and following choroid plexus anteriorly can help in finding the foramen of Monro. **(l)** The choroid plexus courses along the choroidal fissure. It is attached medially to the fornix by the taenia fornicis and laterally to the thalamus by the taenia choroidea. The approaches to the third ventricle are the following (see Latin numbers on arrows): **(i)** transforaminal (through the foramen of Monro), **(ii)** subchoroidal (incision in the taenia choroidea and upward reflection of choroid plexus), **(iii)** suprachoroidal (incision in the taenia fornicis and downward deflection of choroid plexus), **(iv)** interforniceal (between bodies of fornices by dividing the interforniceal raphe; see also the transcallosal approach in Chapter 10: Surgical Procedures).

Transsphenoidal Approach to the Sellar Region (▶Fig. 9.7)

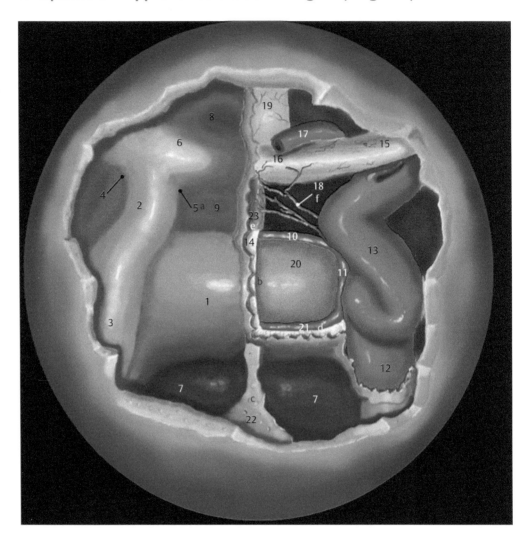

Anatomy: Transsphenoidal approach to the sellar region (endoscopic view). On the left side, the sellar floor and the bone of the anterior cranial fossa have been removed and the dura has been opened to expose the intradural anatomical structures. The left ICA has also been exposed. **(1)** sellar floor, **(2)** parasellar carotid protuberance, **(3)** paraclival carotid protuberance, **(4)** lateral opticocarotid recess (corresponds to the optic strut of the ACP intracranially), **(5)** medial opticocarotid recess (corresponds to the lateral portion of the tuberculum sellae), **(6)** optic protuberance, **(7)** clivus, **(8)** planum sphenoidale, **(9)** tuberculum sellae, **(10)** anterior intercavernous sinus, **(11)** cavernous sinus, **(12)** petrous portion of the ICA, **(13)** cavernous portion of the ICA, **(14)** dura mater (opened), **(15)** left optic nerve, **(16)** optic chiasm, **(17)** left ACA, **(18)** superior hypophyseal arteries, **(19)** lamina terminalis, **(20)** pituitary gland (hypophysis), **(21)** inferior cavernous sinus, **(22)** sphenoid septum, **(23)** pituitary stalk.

Clinical information and surgical tips: (a) Beware of the ICA in the **medial opticocarotid recess** (5). Also, beware of dehiscence of bone overlying the ICA. **(b)** Open the dura from midline to laterally. Avoid going too laterally (risk of ICA injury). **(c)** The **sphenoid septum** (22) may not be in midline. See where the septum is located relative to midline on pre-op CT or use navigation. Be very careful when removing septa located in the carotid protuberance. **(d)** Beware of the **inferior intercavernous sinus** (21) when opening the dura. **(e)** Identify **pituitary stalk** (23) by the vessels coursing on it. Try not to pull or manipulate the pituitary stalk during tumor removal to minimize the risk of postoperative diabetes insipidus. **(f)** The **superior hypophyseal arteries** (18) originate from the posteromedial or medial aspect of the ophthalmic segment of the ICA and supply blood to the anterior lobe of the pituitary gland, to the stalk, the chiasm, optic nerves, and the floor of the third ventricle.

Suprasellar Area: Anterior View (▶Fig. 9.8)

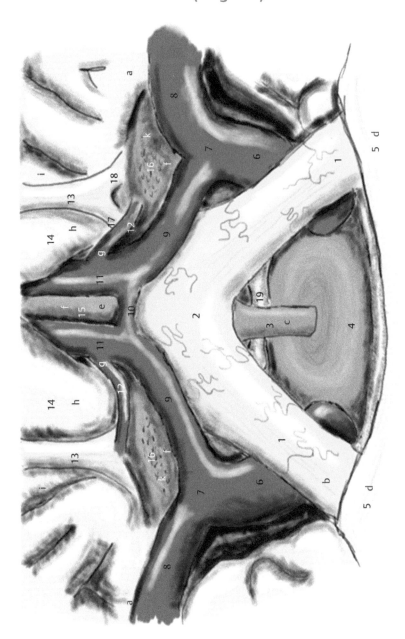

Anatomy: Anterior view of the suprasellar area. The frontal lobes are retracted superiorly. The olfactory nerves have been detached from the cribriform plate and retracted together with the orbital surface of the frontal lobes. (**1**) Optic nerve, (**2**) optic chiasm, (**3**) pituitary stalk, (**4**) pituitary gland (hypophysis), (**5**) falciform ligament, (**6**) supraclinoid portion of the ICA, (**7**) ICA bifurcation, (**8**) sphenoidal segment (M1) of the middle cerebral artery (from ICA bifurcation to MCA genu at the junction of sphenoidal-operculoinsular compartments of the sylvian fissure; in 90% of cases, the MCA bifurcation takes place proximal to genu), (**9**) A1 segment of the ACA (from ICA bifurcation to ACom), (**10**) ACom, (**11**) infracallosal (A2) segment of the ACA (from ACom to the junction of rostrum–genu of corpus callosum), (**12**) recurrent artery of Heubner, (**13**) olfactory tract of olfactory nerve in olfactory sulcus, (**14**) straight gyrus (gyrus rectus), (**15**) lamina terminalis, (**16**) anterior perforated substance, (**17**) medial olfactory stria, (**18**) lateral olfactory stria, (**19**) dorsum sellae.

Clinical information and surgical tips: (a) Open sylvian fissure further to allow more retraction of frontal lobe. (**b**) Use optic nerve (1) to identify the ICA laterally. (**c**) Identify the **pituitary stalk** (3) by the vessels coursing on it. (**d**) In case of masses compressing optic nerve/chiasm, **early cut of the falciform ligament** (5) can help in decompressing the nerve. (**e**) Opening of the **lamina terminalis** allows entry into the third ventricle (e.g., via the subfrontal approach). (**f**) Beware of **perforators** in these areas (not depicted). All the arteries of the area give rise to perforators: (**1**) **the ICA** (6) gives rise to perforators to pituitary stalk, to optic chiasm, and nerve, to the floor of the third ventricle, to the anterior perforated substance, to the optic tract, and to the uncus. These arise mainly from the posteromedial surface of the ICA. (2) The **A1, A2 segments of the ACA and the Acom** (10) give rise to perforators to the anterior perforated substance, to the dorsal surface of optic chiasm and optic nerve, to the optic tract, to the suprachiasmatic portion of hypothalamus, to the columns of fornix, to the anteroinferior striatum, to the sylvian fissure, and to the lower surface of frontal lobe. (3) **The M1 segment of the MCA** (8) gives rise to perforators (aka lenticulostriate branches) to the anterior perforated substance (16). They arise mostly from the posterior or superior aspect of M1 (but few also from proximal M2). They supply not only the basal ganglia (lateral globus pallidus, body and head of the caudate nucleus) but also the internal capsule. These perforators are end arteries. Thus, their damage can cause contralateral hemiparesis and hemihypesthesia and aphasia (in dominant hemisphere). (**g**) The **recurrent artery of Heubner** (12) arises from ACA at any point between distal A1 and proximal A2 (more often from A2). It follows a recurrent course anterior or anterosuperior to A1, then above the ICA bifurcation and the proximal MCA to enter the anterior perforated substance. The recurrent artery supplies the internal capsule (anterior limb), the uncinate fasciculus, the basal ganglia (anterior caudate, anterior one-third of the putamen, the anterior part of the external globus pallidus), and less frequently the anterior hypothalamus. Failure to identify the recurrent artery during vascular surgery in the area of A1–Acom complex can lead to its inadvertent occlusion with clipping of the aneurysm. Occlusion of the recurrent artery can cause hemiparesis (more prominent in face and upper extremity) and aphasia (in the dominant hemisphere). (**h**) During dissection for clipping of ACom aneurysms, the ipsilateral A2 has to be identified by lifting the ipsilateral **gyrus rectus** (14). In cases of brain edema or high location of ACom complex, resection of the gyrus rectus can be performed. (**i**) In surgery for anterior circulation aneurysm, place the tip of the brain retractor lateral to the **olfactory tract**[5] (13) to lift the frontal lobes before opening the chiasmatic cistern. Tracing the olfactory tract posteriorly leads to optic nerve. (**k**) **The anterior perforated substance** (16) has a rhomboid shape and is located in the roof of the sphenoidal compartment of the sylvian fissure. It is defined by the medial and lateral olfactory striae anteriorly, the optic tract posteromedially, and the stem of the temporal lobe and the limen insulae laterally. The surface of the anterior perforated substance is penetrated by numerous perforators from the ICA, the anterior choroidal artery, the lenticulostriate arteries (from the MCA), from the ACA (A1, A2), ACom, and recurrent artery of Heubner. Superiorly to the anterior perforated substance are located the frontal horn, the anterior limb of the internal capsule, the head of the caudate nucleus, and the anterior part of the lentiform nucleus.[6,7]

Atlas (C1): Superior View (▸Fig. 9.9)

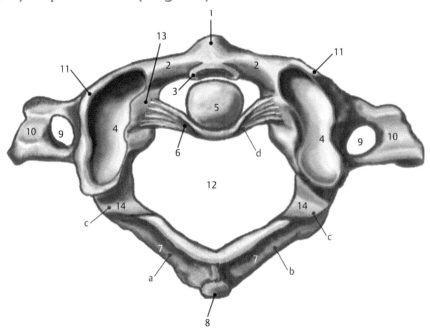

Anatomy: Superior view of the atlas (C1). The anterior arch articulates with the dens. The transverse ligament is one of the ligaments participating in the atlantoaxial joint. The other ligaments are not depicted. **(1)** Anterior tubercle, **(2)** anterior arch, **(3)** articular facet for the dens, **(4)** superior articulating facet of the lateral mass (articulates with the occipital condyle), **(5)** dens, **(6)** transverse ligament of the atlas, **(7)** posterior arch, **(8)** posterior tubercle, **(9)** transverse foramen, **(10)** transverse process, **(11)** lateral mass, **(12)** vertebral foramen, **(13)** tubercle for transverse ligament of the atlas, **(14)** groove for the vertebral artery.

    Clinical information and surgical tips: (a) The **posterior arch** (7) bone may not be contiguous (bifid posterior arch of the atlas). Be cautious when dissecting muscles off the posterior arch. **(b)** It is safe to resect bone up to 1 to 1.5 cm laterally from midline. Do not extend **laminectomy** more laterally to avoid vertebral artery injury. **(c)** On the lateral part of the upper surface of the posterior arch, there is a **groove for the vertebral artery** (14). The C1 spinal nerve also courses on this groove between the inferior aspect of vertebral artery and the bone. There may be a bridge of bone extending from the superior articulating facet of the lateral mass to the posterior arch forming a foramen (instead of a groove), through which the vertebral artery courses. We can estimate the location of the vertebral artery by palpating the groove with a no. 4 Penfield elevator. We could also use Doppler for the localization. The vertebral artery after exiting through the transverse foramen courses posteromedially around the lateral mass and atlanto-occipital joint and then on the groove of the posterior arch of C1, where it lies in a layer of dense fibrofatty tissue in the floor of the suboccipital triangle (formed by rectus capitis posterior major muscle superomedially, the inferior oblique muscle inferolaterally, and the superior oblique muscle superolaterally). Then, the vertebral artery enters the vertebral canal sequentially through the lateral part of the posterior atlanto-occipital membrane (which arches over the groove of the posterior arch) and through a funnel-shaped dural foramen, becoming intradural. We know we are approaching the vertebral artery during dissection in the area by the brisk venous bleeding from the venous plexus surrounding it. This bleeding can be controlled with thrombin-soaked morselized Gelfoam. For the far lateral approach, this venous plexus should be cauterized and divided and then dissected off the vertebral artery (see ▸ **Fig. 9.2** see far lateral approach in Chapter 10: Surgical Procedures). **(d)** The **transverse ligament of atlas** (6) is the horizontal component of the cruciform ligament. There is also a vertical component, which consists of a superior longitudinal band (attached to the clivus) and an inferior longitudinal band (attached to the body of axis). The transverse ligament is a thick, very strong band, which is attached bilaterally to a tubercle (on the medial side of the C1 lateral masses) and in the midline courses behind the dens trapping it against the anterior C1 arch. The transverse ligament plays an important role in determining management options for C1 and C2 fractures and for atlantoaxial rotatory deformities. Specifically, insufficiency/injury or disruption of transverse ligament assessed directly or indirectly warrants more aggressive treatment options (see Table 2.2a).

C4 Vertebra: Superior View (▸Fig. 9.10)

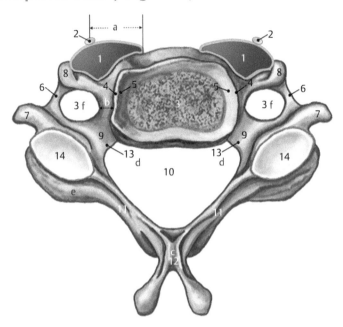

Anatomy: Superior view of the C4 vertebra. The longus colli muscles and the cervical sympathetic trunk can be seen bilaterally. (**1**) Longus coli muscle, (**2**) sympathetic trunk, (**3**) foramen transversarium, (**4**) uncinate process, (**5**) articular surface of uncinate process, (**6**) transverse process, (**7**) posterior tubercle, (**8**) anterior tubercle, (**9**) groove for spinal nerve, (**10**) vertebral foramen, (**11**) lamina, (**12**) spinous process, (**13**) pedicle, (**14**) superior articular process and facet.

    Clinical information and surgical tips: (**a**) From superior to inferior, the **sympathetic trunks** (1) converge medially to midline, whereas the **longus colli muscles** (1) diverge laterally. This implies that the sympathetic trunk is more vulnerable to injury during anterior procedures in the lower cervical spine and the surgeon should avoid excessive detachment of longus colli muscles in this area. There are studies that measure the distance between the medial border of the longus colli muscle and the sympathetic trunk in the cervical spine. At the level of C7 vertebra, the medial border of the longus colli is closer to the sympathetic trunk than any other level (≈13 mm). Injury to the sympathetic trunk causes Horner's syndrome (ipsilateral ptosis, miosis, anhidrosis, enophthalmos).[8-10](**b**) The mean distance between the medial border of the **uncinate process** (4) and **foramen transversarium** (3) is approximately 5 mm.[11] Beware of this in order to avoid vertebral artery injury during cervical decompression surgery. Furthermore, the distance of the vertebral artery from midline of the vertebral body increases from superior to inferior (at C3 level, the mean distance is measured around 15 mm and at C6 level around 17 mm).[12] The uncovertebral joints is a marker that we are approaching the vertebral artery. Brisk venous bleeding may occur prior to vertebral artery injury. (**c**) There may be a bone defect in the **lamina** (11; bifid lamina). Be cautious when dissecting muscles off the posterior arch. (**d**) If unsure about the anatomy of the **pedicles**, perform a small laminotomy to palpate the pedicles for pedicle screw placement. (**e**) If lateral mass screws are directed too medially, they may injure the vertebral artery. (**f**) The **transverse foramen** (3) transmits the vertebral artery. The vertebral artery enters the foramen of C6 (87–89%), but it can also enter the foramen at C7 (≈4%) or at C5 (6%) and even above C5 (<1.5%).[13] The vertebral artery ascends through the transverse foramina anterior to the cervical spinal nerves.

Cervical Spine: Posterior View (▸Fig. 9.11)

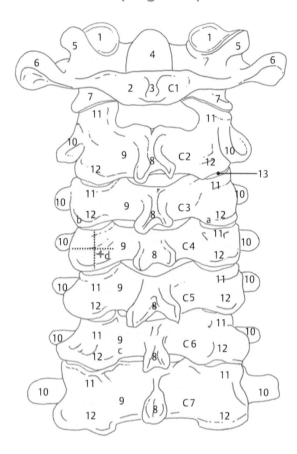

Anatomy: Posterior view of the cervical spine. **(1)** Superior articulating facet of the lateral mass of the atlas (articulates with occipital condyle), **(2)** posterior arch, **(3)** posterior tubercle, **(4)** dens, **(5)** lateral mass of the atlas, **(6)** transverse process of the atlas, **(7)** inferior articulating facet of the lateral mass of the atlas, **(8)** spinous process, **(9)** lamina, **(10)** transverse process, **(11)** superior articular process, **(12)** inferior articular process, **(13)** zygapophyseal joint (facet joint).

    Clinical information and surgical tips: (a) You can drill the facet joint and place a no. 4 Penfield elevator into the facet, in order to (1) obtain orientation for screw trajectory and (2) to decorticate for fusion. **(b)** You can drill to expose the lateral edge of the facet (especially in severe degenerative spine disease) to identify anatomic entry point for screws. **(c)** The medial edge of the facet joint is located at the point where the lamina meets the lateral mass. The vertebral artery and the exiting nerve root is located anteriorly to this point. **(d)** The **entry point for subaxial lateral mass screws** is located 1 mm inferiorly and 1 mm medially to the midpoint of the lateral mass (*red cross*). Lateral mass must be very well exposed and all its four borders (medial, lateral, superior, and inferior) must be identified (see also Chapter 2: Spine and Spinal Cord).

Thoracic Spine and Costovertebral Joints: Posterior View (▸Fig. 9.12)

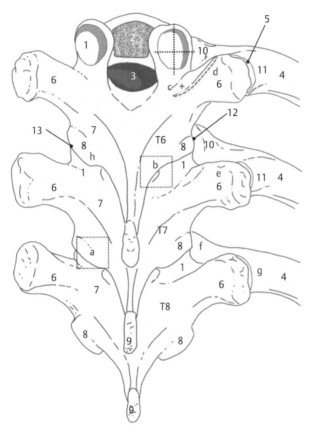

Anatomy: Posterior view of the thoracic spine and costovertebral joints. **(1)** Superior articular process and facet, **(2)** vertebral body, **(3)** spinal canal, **(4)** rib, **(5)** costotransverse joint, **(6)** transverse process, **(7)** lamina, **(8)** inferior articular process, **(9)** spinous process, **(10)** head of the rib, **(11)** tubercle of the rib, **(12)** costocentral joint (articulation of head of the rib with vertebra), **(13)** zygapophyseal joint.

   Clinical information and surgical tips: (a) Remove the inferior articular process (*dashed square*) to identify the underlying superior articular process and understand the anatomy for the pedicle screw entry point. **(b)** A small laminotomy (*dashed square*) can be performed in this area to palpate the pedicle, in order to determine its anatomy and direction for pedicle screw placement. **(c)** The entry point for the pedicle screw placement in the thoracic spine is the intersection between a point just lateral to the midpoint of the superior articular process and the top one-third of the transverse process (*red cross*). **(d)** A small ridge (*red dashed line*) is often present on the transverse process, which can be used as useful landmark for pedicle screw entry point in the thoracic spine. **(e)** Screws can be placed through the costotransverse joint as well. **(f) Head of the rib** (10) is tucked deep. Place a Cobb elevator in the costotransverse joint space to disarticulate the head of the rib for costotransverse exposure. **(g)** Insert a Penfield elevator in the **costotransverse joint** (5) to help rib head disarticulation. **(h)** In thoracic spine, the inferior articulating facet (inferior articular process; 8) is located posteriorly in the joint and faces anteriorly, whereas the superior articulating facet (superior articular process; 1) is located anteriorly in joint and faces posteriorly.

Thoracic Spine: Left Lateral View (▸Fig. 9.13)

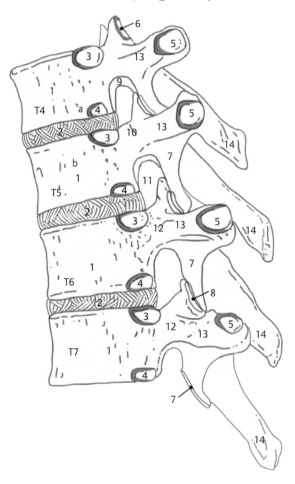

Anatomy: Left lateral view of the thoracic spine: (**1**) Vertebral body, (**2**) intervertebral disk, (**3**) superior costal facet, (**4**) inferior costal facet, (**5**) transverse costal facet, (**6**) superior articular process and facet, (**7**) inferior articular process and facet, (**8**) zygapophyseal joint, (**9**) inferior vertebral notch, (**10**) superior vertebral notch, (**11**) intervertebral foramen, (**12**) pedicle, (**13**) transverse process, (**14**) spinous process.

    Clinical information and surgical tips: (**a**) The rib number is based on the inferior articulating vertebral body. Each rib has two articulating surfaces with inferior vertebra (i.e., the inferior costal facet and the transverse costal facet; 5) and one articulating surface with the superior vertebra (superior costal facet; 4) and one articulating surface with the intervertebral disk between the superior and the inferior vertebra as well. The head of the rib articulates with the costal facets and the intervertebral disk (costocentral joint) and the tubercle of the rib articulates with the transverse costal facet (costotransverse joint; see ▸**Fig. 9.12**). (**b**) Beware not to avulse the segmental spinal artery, which originates directly from the aorta and courses posteriorly on the lateral surface of the vertebral body to enter through the intervertebral foramen into the spinal canal. Beware of the artery of Adamkiewicz (aka arteria radicularis anterior magna, which mainly supplies spinal cord from T8 to the conus). It is located in the left side in 80% cases. It usually enters the spinal canal between T9 and L2 (85%) and rarely between T5 and T8 (15%).

Lumbar Spine: Right Oblique View (▸Fig. 9.14)

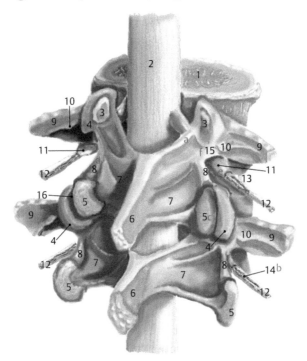

Anatomy: Right oblique view of the lumbar spine: **(1)** Vertebral body, **(2)** dural sac (contains the cauda equina), **(3)** superior articular process, **(4)** mammillary process, **(5)** inferior articular process, **(6)** spinous process, **(7)** lamina, **(8)** pars interarticularis, **(9)** transverse process, **(10)** accessory process, **(11)** spinal nerve covered by dural sleeve, **(12)** spinal nerve, **(13)** intervertebral disk, **(14)** segmental spinal artery, **(15)** pedicle, **(16)** zygapophyseal joint (facet joint).

   Clinical information and surgical tips: (a) If unsure about the orientation of the pedicles, perform a small laminotomy to palpate the pedicles for pedicle screw placement. **(b)** In thoracic spine scoliosis surgery, a thoracic spinal nerve (intercostal nerve) may be sacrificed, if needed for VCR (vertebral column resection) or PSO (pedicle subtraction osteotomy). However, first you should clamp the spinal nerve (12) for 6 minutes and watch somatosensory evoked potential (SSEP)/motor evoked potential (MEP) for changes, to ensure that spine cord blood supply is not compromised. Beware of the artery of Adamkiewicz (aka arteria radicularis anterior magna, which mainly supplies the spinal cord from T8 to the conus). It is located in the left side in 80% cases. It usually enters the spinal canal between T9 and L2 (85%) and rarely between T5 and T8 (15%). **(c)** In lumbar spine, the inferior articulating facet (**inferior articular process**; 5) is located medially in the joint and faces laterally, whereas the superior articulating facet (**superior articular process**; 3) is located laterally in joint and faces medially. **(d)** Be careful to always save the **pars interarticularis** (8) during lumbar decompressive surgery, in order to avoid iatrogenic instability. In spondylolysis, there is a defect in pars interarticularis areas causing instability back pain with or without spondylolisthesis. **(e)** The dura forms a **dural sleeve** around the ventral and dorsal root and the dorsal root ganglion. The two roots merge just distally to the ganglion and form a spinal nerve at the exit from the intervertebral foramen. At this point, the dural sleeve becomes adherent to the epineurium of the spinal nerve. After resection of dumbbell schwannomas (intradural tumors with extradural extension through the intervertebral foramen), the dural sleeve has to be repaired; otherwise, CSF leak will occur.[14] **(f)** In thoracic and lumbar spine, each spinal nerve exits below the pedicle of the vertebra with the same number. For example, the L4 spinal nerve exits under the pedicle of the L4 vertebra through the intervertebral foramen L4/L5. In the cervical spine, however, spinal nerves exit over the pedicle of the vertebra with the same number. For example, the C4 spinal nerve exits over the pedicle of C4, through the C3/C4 intervertebral foramen. The C8 spinal nerve exits through the intervertebral foramen C7/T1.

Lumbar Spine: Posterior View (▶Fig. 9.15)

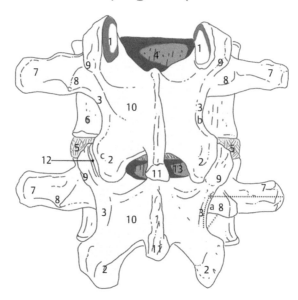

Anatomy: Posterior view of the lumbar spine. **(1)** Superior articular process and facet, **(2)** inferior articular process, **(3)** pars interarticularis, **(4)** vertebral foramen, **(5)** intervertebral disk, **(6)** vertebral body, **(7)** transverse process, **(8)** accessory process, **(9)** mammillary process, **(10)** lamina, **(11)** spinous process, **(12)** zygapophyseal joints (facet joints), **(13)** spinal canal.

    Clinical information and surgical tips: (a) There are different options for pedicle screw entry points based on landmarks: (1) the accessory process (8) and (2) the junction of a line along the midtransverse process with pars interarticularis (*red cross*). Sometimes the pars has a lateral wing toward the transverse process (*red dashed line*). Use the medial ridge instead of this wing to determine the entry point. **(b)** Be careful to always save the pars interarticularis (3) during lumbar decompressive surgery, in order to avoid iatrogenic instability. **(c)** In lumbar spine, the inferior articulating facet (inferior articular process; 2) is located medially in the joint and faces laterally, whereas the superior articulating facet (superior articular process; 1) is located laterally in the joint and faces medially.

Sacrum: Posterior View (▶Fig. 9.16)

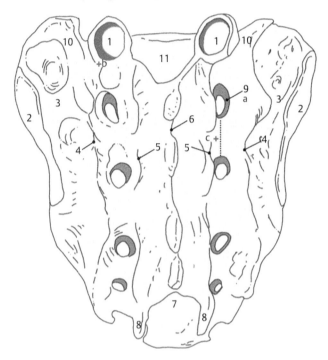

Anatomy: Posterior view of the sacrum. **(1)** Superior articular processes and facets, **(2)** auricular surface, **(3)** sacral tuberosity, **(4)** lateral sacral crest, **(5)** intermediate sacral crest, **(6)** median sacral crest, **(7)** sacral hiatus, **(8)** sacral cornu (horn), **(9)** posterior sacral foramen, **(10)** sacral ala, **(11)** sacral canal.

    Clinical information and surgical tips: (a) The posterior rami of the sacral spinal nerves exit from the **posterior sacral foramina** (9) and form the middle cluneal nerves, which contribute to the cutaneous innervation of the gluteal region (together with the superior cluneal nerve).[15] Posterior foramina are a usual site of significant bleeding. Use Gelfoam and pressure. **(b)** The **entry point for S1 pedicle screws** is just inferior and lateral to S1 facet joint (*red cross*). **(c)** The **entry point for S2 alar screws** is just medial to the midpoint of a line connecting the S1 and S2 foramina (*blue cross*; see also Chapter 2: Spine and Spinal cord).

Lumbosacral Spine: Left Lateral View (▸Fig. 9.17)

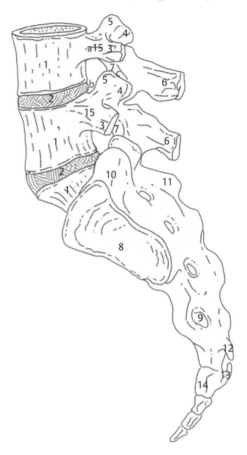

Anatomy: Lateral view of the lumbosacral spine. **(1)** vertebral body, **(2)** intervertebral disk, **(3)** transverse process, **(4)** mammillary process, **(5)** superior articular process, **(6)** spinous process, **(7)** pars interarticularis, **(8)** auricular surfaces (articulation with ilium), **(9)** posterior sacral foramina, **(10)** sacral ala, **(11)** median sacral crest, **(12)** sacral cornu **(13)** coccygeal cornu, **(14)** coccyx, **(15)** pedicle.

Clinical information and surgical tips: (a) always use a **pedicle** (15) for pre-op planning and intraoperative localization of correct vertebral level with fluoroscopy. Do not localize intraoperatively based on spinous processes. **(b)** in the lumbar spine, the spinal root exits just below the pedicle of the like-numbered vertebral. The pedicle is located well above the intervertebral disk. That explains why a lumbar disk herniation usually does not involve the spinal root exiting at the same level of the intervertebral foramen with the disk, but compresses the spinal root, which exits through the foramen one level below. **(c)** Be careful to always save the **pars interarticularis** (7) during lumbar decompressive surgery, in order to avoid iatrogenic instability. In spondylolysis, there is a defect in bilateral pars interarticularis areas causing instability back pain with or without spondylolisthesis.

References

[1] Ojemann JG, Partridge SC, Poliakov AV, et al. Diffusion tensor imaging of the superior cerebellar peduncle identifies patients with posterior fossa syndrome. Childs Nerv Syst. 2013; 29(11):2071–2077

[2] Mussi AC, Rhoton AL, Jr. Telovelar approach to the fourth ventricle: microsurgical anatomy. J Neurosurg. 2000; 92(5):812–823

[3] Apuzzo ML. Surgery of masses affecting the third ventricular chamber: techniques and strategies. Clin Neurosurg. 1988; 34:499–522

[4] Türe U, Yaşargil MG, Al-Mefty O. The transcallosal-transforaminal approach to the third ventricle with regard to the venous variations in this region. J Neurosurg. 1997; 87(5):706–715

[5] Fossett DT, Caputy AJ. Operative Neurosurgical Anatomy. New York, NY: Thieme; 2002

[6] Rhoton AL. Cranial Anatomy and Surgical Approaches. Philadelphia, PA: Lippincott Williams & Wilkins; 2003

[7] Lawton MT. Seven Aneurysms: Tenets and Techniques for Clipping. New York, NY: Thieme; 2011

[8] Ebraheim NA, Lu J, Yang H, Heck BE, Yeasting RA. Vulnerability of the sympathetic trunk during the anterior approach to the lower cervical spine. Spine. 2000; 25(13):1603–1606

[9] Civelek E, Karasu A, Cansever T, et al. Surgical anatomy of the cervical sympathetic trunk during anterolateral approach to cervical spine. Eur Spine J. 2008; 17(8):991–995

[10] Yin Z, Yin J, Cai J, Sui T, Cao X. Neuroanatomy and clinical analysis of the cervical sympathetic trunk and longus colli. J Biomed Res. 2015; 29(6):501–507

[11] Sangari SK, Dossous P-M, Heineman T, Mtui EP. Dimensions and anatomical variants of the foramen transversarium of typical cervical vertebrae. Anat Res Int. 2015; 2015:391823

[12] Güvençer M, Men S, Naderi S, Kiray A, Tetik S. The V2 segment of the vertebral artery in anterior and anterolateral cervical spinal surgery: a cadaver angiographic study. Clin Neurol Neurosurg. 2006; 108(5):440–445

[13] Schroeder GD, Hsu WK. Vertebral artery injuries in cervical spine surgery. Surg Neurol Int. 2013; 4(5, Suppl 5):S362–S367

[14] Wiltse LL. Anatomy of the extradural compartments of the lumbar spinal canal. Peridural membrane and circumneural sheath. Radiol Clin North Am. 2000; 38(6):1177–1206

[15] Tubbs RS, Levin MR, Loukas M, Potts EA, Cohen-Gadol AA. Anatomy and landmarks for the superior and middle cluneal nerves: application to posterior iliac crest harvest and entrapment syndromes. J Neurosurg Spine. 2010; 13(3):356–359

10 Surgical Procedures

10.1 Pterional (Frontotemporal Craniotomy)

10.1.1 Basic Information (Table 10.1a)

Indications	• Aneurysms (anterior circulation + basilar tip and superior cerebellar artery)
	• **Tumors:**
	  – Extra-axial: in sphenoid, parasellar, cavernous sinus, anterior + middle fossa
	  – Intra-axial: insula, lateral frontal/parietal/temporal areas
	• **Perisylvian AVMs**
	• Hematoma evacuation in lateral frontal/parietal/temporal areas
	• "Workhorse exposure" for most procedures

Contraindications	• **Sellar/parasellar tumors:**
	  – In midline (prefer transsphenoidal approach)
	  – With superoanterior extension (prefer bifrontal craniotomy)
	• **Aneurysms:**
	  – Distal aneurysms of anterior cerebral artery
	  – High-riding basilar aneurysms

Positioning	• **Patient position:**
	  – Supine
	  – Ipsilateral shoulder up
	• **Mayfield clamp:**
	  – Posterior paired pins → ipsilateral retromastoid region (equator)
	  – Anterior single pin → contralateral frontal bone (midpupillary line)
	• **Head** (aim: malar eminence at highest point)
	  – **Elevation:** above heart level
	  – **Rotation:** contralateral 30–60 degrees
	  – **Neck extension:** vertex down 10–30 degrees (allows gravity to retract frontal lobe away from anterior fossa floor)
	!! **Caution:** make sure neck is free, no venous compression

Incision	• **Curvilinear**
	  – **Starts:** 1 cm anterior to tragus at zygomatic root (some prefer incision more posterior for cosmesis)
	  – **Course:** up to linea temporalis → then anteriorly–superiorly
	  – **Ends:** midline behind hairline (if widow's peak present may get lower OR extend further contralaterally to midpupillary line)

Abbreviation: AVMs, arteriovenous malformations.

10.1.2 Key Procedural Steps (Table 10.1b)

1. Skin elevation

- **From midline – linea temporalis:** cut down to the bone—elevate scalp
- **From linea temporalis – zygoma root:** dissect scalp from temporal fascia and elevate scalp separating from temporalis muscle up to the superficial fat pad (frontal branch of superficial temporal artery (STA) may serve as a landmark)

2. Preservation of frontalis branch of CN VII

- **Subfascial technique:** incision of temporal fascia posterior to the superficial fat pad (stay 1 fingerbreadth behind fat pad) → in order to avoid injury to frontalis branch of CN VII, dissect temporalis fascia by staying in the plane right above the muscle→ reflect fat pad with scalp anteriorly[1,2]
- Use blunt dissection with bipolar coagulation for hemostasis, not monopolar cautery.

!! In the main author's opinion, although this is the bloodiest plane of dissection it is also the safest in order to avoid injury to the frontalis branch of the facial nerve.

3. Temporalis muscle elevation

- **Muscle incision:** from root of zygoma along the skin incision up to superior temporal line→ anteriorly along the superior temporal line (leave muscle cuff by incising muscle 1 cm below superior temporal line)
- **Subperiosteal muscle dissection:** blunt dissection from inferior to superior to avoid injury to neurovascular supply of temporalis and atrophy
- Muscle reflection anteriorly–inferiorly

4. Burr holes

- McCarty keyhole*(= just above frontosphenoidal suture and behind frontozygomatic suture)[3,4]
- Above zygoma root*
- Inferior to superior temporal line in line to zygoma root
- Anterior to coronal suture
- Above orbit (!! avoid frontal sinus, study pre-op CT → if frontal sinus is large, harvest pericranial flap before scalp elevation)

!! Variable placement of burr holes depending on surgeon's preference and location of lesion. Burr holes with asterisk repre sent the essential ones.

(*Continued*) ▶

5. Craniotomy	• Drill trough between key hole – root of zygoma burr hole • Connect rest of burr holes with craniotome • Bone flap elevation

6. Further bone removal	• Inferior part of temporal bone → remove bone down to middle fossa floor (!! beware of bone air cells)
	• Connection of anterior–middle fossa (anterior cranial fossa floor should be flush with middle cranial fossa floor)
	  – Flatten orbital roof
	  – Remove lesser wing of sphenoid bone (as flat as possible) upto lateral edge of superi-or orbital fissure (meaning orbital artery)

7. Dural opening	• Dural tacking sutures • Semicircular flap (start incision from frontal dura) → reflect anteriorly (base at sphenoid bone)
8. Anterior clinoidectomy (intradural or extradural) (as needed)	**Intradural clinoidectomy:** semilunar incision of dura covering anterior clinoid process (ACP) with the base over optic nerve → strip dural flap away from ACP → drilling of ACP within the confines of cortical bone→ fracture gently and remove ACP → resect optic strut → open falciform ligament to mobilize optic nerve (see also ► Fig. 9.3)
9. Sylvian fissure dissection	• "Divide plane deep to superficial" like peeling an orange • Dissect Sylvian fissure along the frontal side of superficial Sylvian veins → mobilize these veins to the temporal side of the Sylvian fissure • May use cotton balls or retractors to help maintain fissure opening • Veins crossing the Sylvian fissure can be sacrificed
10. Closure	• Watertight dura closure + central tack-up suture • Bone flap fixation (cover any bone defects with mesh or cement, if needed) • Temporalis muscle suturing • Galea sutures • Skin sutures

10.1.3 Pearls for Each Procedural Step (Table 10.1c)

Positioning	Head elevation + slight extension	Allows gravity to retract frontal lobe away from anterior fossa floor
Incision	Superficial temporal artery preservation (STA)	• **Technique:** blunt dissection of scalp from superficial temporal fascia in the inferior part of the incision • **Significance:** – Sufficient blood supply of the skin flap (crucial in case of adjuvant radiotherapy, ensures good cosmetic outcome) – Could be used for bypass – Lower risk of post-op epidural hematoma due to STA bleeding
	Do not extend incision below zygoma	Extending the incision below the zygoma increases the risk of facial nerve and superficial temporal artery injury
Craniotomy + extra bone removal	Combination with other extensions (e.g., orbitozygomatic, anterior clinoidectomy)	• ↑ exposure • ↑ angle • Minimal brain retraction • Makes deep tumors superficial
	Large lesions	• Remove more bone to avoid brain retraction • First devascularize tumor and then debulk
	Inadvertend periorbital fat exposure	If periorbital fat gets exposed, cover with Gelfoam or use bipolar to shrink
	Additional bony removal before dura opening	• Extradurally flatten frontal fossa bony ridges • Drill off the sphenoid ridge down to the level of the lateral superior orbital fissure • If bleeding from middle meningeal artery, first completly expose and then cauterize vessel
	Meningorbital artery cauterization	Meningorbital artery can be cauterized w/ bipolar and divided to obtain slightly more exposure
	Beware of air cells in posterior portion of middle fossa	After craniotomy push wax into air cells rather than swipe wax across air cells

(Continued) ▶

409

Dural opening	Dural flap	• Initially cut away from Sylvian fissure (frontal dura) • Dissect bridging veins before dura elevation • Place wet patties over dura to avoid dehydration and shrinkage
	Dural tack-up sutures	Place dural tack-up sutures as deep as possible to tent dura flush with skull base
Closure	Check for inadvertent frontal sinus opening	Strip mucosa → plug nasofrontal duct → cover with vascularized pericranium (see also technique in Table 10.4c)

10.1.4 Complications: Avoidance + Mx (Table 10.1d)

Complications	Symptoms/consequences	Mx
Entry into frontal sinus	• CSF rhinorrhea • Infection • Pneumocephalus	strip mucosa → plug nasofrontal duct → cover with vascularized pericranium (see also technique in Table 10.4c)
Entry into orbit	Intraorbital bleeding	• Hemostasis • If periorbital fat gets exposed, cover with Gelfoam or use bipolar to shrink
Injury of frontalis branch of CN VII	Inability to raise ipsilateral eyebrow	Avoid by incising temporal fascia posterior to superficial fat pad during scalp elevation (see step 2 in Table 10.1b)
Retraction injuries to frontal or temporal lobe		• Head elevation + slight extension (allows gravity to retract frontal lobe away from anterior fossa floor) • Use cotton balls for retraction

Other general craniotomy complications: post-op hematoma, neurovascular injury, infection, cerebral infarction, and seizures

10.2 Pterional with Orbitozygomatic Osteotomy

10.2.1 Basic Information (Table 10.2a)

Indications	<ul><li>**Tumors in the following areas:**<ul><li>Anterior cranial fossa</li><li>Orbit</li><li>Medial sphenoid wing</li><li>Sellar region (suprasellar, parasellar)</li><li>Anterior cavernous sinus</li><li>Middle cranial fossa</li></ul></li><li>**Aneurysms:**<ul><li>Acom</li><li>Paraclinoid ICA, opthalmic artery</li><li>Basilar apex aneurysms</li><li>Complex anterior circulation aneurysms</li></ul></li></ul>!! combination w/ posterior clinoidectomy and/or anterior petrosectomy allows access to upper clivus
Contraindications	Sellar/parasellar tumors with superoanterior extension (prefer bifrontal craniotomy)
Positioning	<ul><li>**Patient position:**<ul><li>Supine</li><li>Ipsilateral shoulder up</li></ul></li><li>**Mayfield clamp:**<ul><li>Posterior paired pins → ipsilateral retromastoid area (equator)</li><li>Anterior single pin → contralateral frontal bone in midpupillary line (equator)</li></ul></li><li>**Head** (aim: malar eminence at highest point)<ul><li>**Elevation:** above heart</li><li>**Rotation:** contralaterally up to 30 degree</li><li>**Neck extension:** vertex down 10–30 degree (allows gravity to retract frontal lobe away from anterior fossa floor)</li></ul></li></ul>
Incision	Variable, C-shaped (usually)<ul><li>**Starts:** 1 cm anterior to tragus at zygomatic root</li><li>**Course:** up to linea temporalis → then anteriorly – superioriorly</li><li>**Ends:** contralateral midpupillary line behind widow's peak</li></ul>

10.2.2 Key Procedural Steps (Table 10.2b)

1. Skin elevation

- **From midline – linea temporalis** → cut down to the bone – elevate scalp
- **From linea temporalis – zygoma root:** dissect scalp from temporal fascia and elevate scalp separating from temporalis muscle up to the superficial fat pad (frontal branch of STA may serve as a landmark)

!! preserve STA if possible

2. Preservation of frontalis branch of CN VII

- Incision of temporal fascia posterior to the superficial fat pad (stay 1 fingerbreadth behind fat pad) → in order to avoid injury to frontalis branch of CN VII, dissect temporalis fascia by staying in the plane right above the muscle (use blunt dissection with bipolar coagulation for hemostasis, not monopolar cautery)
- At the junction of the fascia with the zygomatic arch, perform subperiosteal dissection releasing fascia from the top of the zygomatic arch
- Subperiosteal exposure of frontozygomatic process
- Reflect fat pad with scalp anteriorly

!! In the main author's opinion, although this is the bloodiest plane of dissection it is also the safest in order to avoid injury to the frontalis branch of the facial nerve.

3. Cuts to zygomatic arch and temporalis muscle reflection

- Perform osteotomy using reciprocating saw at the root of the zygoma and at junction of zygomatic arch with maxilla
- **Muscle incision:** from root of zygoma along the skin incision up to superior temporal line → anteriorly along the superior temporal line (leave muscle cuff by incising muscle 1 cm below superior temporal line)
- **Subperiosteal muscle dissection:** blunt dissection from inferior to superior to avoid injury to neurovascular supply of temporalis and atrophy
- Reflect temporalis muscle inferiorly with zygomatic bar attached to the muscle

4. Frontotemporal craniotomy

see steps 4, 5 in Table 10.1b

5. Bone exposure for osteotomies

Dissect off bone:
- **Periorbita:** from right above medial canthus through orbital roof → to right above lateral canthus
- **Frontal fossa intracranial dura:** from the level of the falx (avoid injury to olfactory nerve) → all the way to the sphenoid ridge at the level of the lateral border of the superior orbital fissure, over the entire superior orbital roof
- **Temporal fossa intracranial dura:** from the sphenoid ridge at the level of the lateral border of the superior orbital fissure posteriorly to the posterior margin of the frontotemporal craniotomy

6. Orbitozygomatic osteotomy (see ► Fig. 10.1)	• **Dissection of supraorbital neurovascular bundle**: depending on whether frontal osteotomy will be medial or lateral to supraorbital notch dissect neurovascular bundle free from notch

	• **Cut #1: vertical cut along orbital rim in the sagittal plane**: with brain ribbons protecting the frontal dura and the periorbita, use reciprocating saw to make vertical cut along orbital rim lateral to supraorbital notch in the sagittal plane, which extends:
	  – From intracranial space
	  – Through orbital roof
	  – Into orbital space

	• **Cut #2: curved cut along orbital roof in the coronal plane**: with brain ribbons protecting frontal dura, temporal dura, and periorbita, use reciprocating saw to perform perpendicular osteotomy in the coronal plane, that extends:
	  – From the level of the previous frontal cut
	  – Along orbital roof
	  – 1 cm deep into sphenoid bone
	  – Out into temporal fossa

	• **Cut #3: horizontal cut along sphenoid bone – lateral orbital wall in the axial plane**: with brain ribbons protecting temporal dura and lateral periorbita, use reciprocating saw to perform osteotomy that extends:
	  – From temporal fossa
	  – Into sphenoid bone at the level of the previous osteotomy
	  – Into the orbit

	• **Elevation of osteotomy flap**: orbital rim should now be free and mobile. Use handheld osteotome to free it completely and elevate
8. Additional craniectomy	Use high-speed drill and rongeurs to remove additional bone as desired: • Squamous temporal bone (down to middle fossa floor) • Lesser sphenoid wing (unroofing of superior orbital fissure, no bone between globe – ACP) • Anterior clinoidectomy (see step 8 in Table 10.1b) • Unroofing of optic canal
9. Dural opening	• C-shaped across Sylvian fissure (exposing half of frontal and temporal lobes) • Dural flap reflected anteriorly (also depressing gently periorbita – eye)
10. Closure	• Watertight dura closure + central tack-up suture • Fixation of orbitozygomatic osteotomy • Bone flap fixation (cover any bone defects with mesh or cement) • Temporalis muscle suturing • Galea sutures • Skin sutures

10.2.3 Orbitozygomatic Osteotomy Cuts (▶Fig. 10.1)

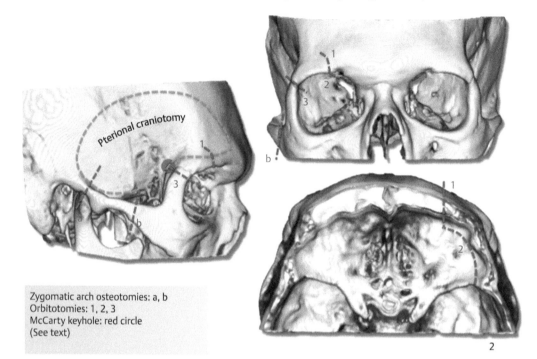

Zygomatic arch osteotomies: a, b
Orbitotomies: 1, 2, 3
McCarty keyhole: red circle
(See text)

10.2.4 Pearls for Each Procedural Step (Table 10.2c)

Pre-op preparation	Assess size of frontal sinus in pre-op CT	If frontal sinus is large, the risk to be opened during craniotomy is higher → harvest pericranial flap before scalp elevation
	Check for pneumatized ACP in pre-op CT	ACP may be pneumatized. In case of anterior clinoidectomy, this can be a route for CSF rhinorrhea. Try to not violate the mucosa during its removal. If there is a small violation, you may stitch, otherwise pack sphenoid with fat/muscle graft and place lumbar drain (LD)
Closure	Avoid extraocular muscle entrapment when replacing orbital osteotomy flap	While replacing the orbital flap there is a risk of extraocular muscles getting entrapped in bone gaps

Note: See also following pearls in frontotemporal craniotomy (also important for orbitozygomatic craniotomy):
• Head elevation + slight extension
• STA preservation
• Inadvertent periorbital fat exposure
• Beware of air cells in posterior portion of middle fossa
• Check for inadvertent frontal sinus opening

10.2.5 Complications: Avoidance + Mx (Table 10.2d)

Complications	Risks	Avoidance/Mx
Injury of frontalis branch of CN VII	Inability to raise ipsilateral eyebrow	• Avoid by incising temporal fascia posterior to superficial fat pad during scalp elevation (see Step 2 in Table 10.2b) • Avoid by placing incision at the root of the zygoma (not inferior)
Violation of periorbita	• Injury of intraorbital contents • No visualization of reciprocating saw during orbitozygomatic (OZ) osteotomy	• Avoid by carefully elevating periorbita off the orbital walls and protecting it at all time with brain ribbon during osteotomies • Hemostasis • If periorbital fat gets exposed, cover with Gelfoam or use bipolar to shrink
Injury of trochlear attachment of superior oblique muscle	Diplopia	Avoid periorbita dissection medial to supraorbital notch
Extraocular muscle entrapment when replacing orbital osteotomy flap	Diplopia	While replacing the orbital flap, check for extraocular muscles getting entrapped in bone gaps
Post-op pulsatile enopthalmos		• Avoid by preserving lateral orbital wall • Usually resolves in 3–6 months
Eye injury	Vision disturbances	Avoid by keeping periorbita intact and protecting it at all time with brain ribbon during osteotomies
Entry into frontal sinus	• CSF rhinorrhea • Infection • Pneumocephalus	Strip mucosa → plug nasofrontal duct → cover with vascularized pericranium (see also technique in Table 10.4c)
Retraction injuries to frontal or temporal lobe		• Head elevation + slight extension (allows gravity to retract frontal lobe away from anterior fossa floor) • Use cotton balls for retraction • Remove more bone

Other general craniotomy complications: post-op hematoma, neurovascular injury, infection, cerebral infarction, and seizures

10.3 Transcallosal Approach   G

10.3.1 Basic Information (Table 10.3a)

Indications	Exposure	• In body of lateral ventricle • Anterior two-third of third ventricle
	Tumors	• Colloid cysts • AVM • Thalamic gliomas • Craniopharyngioma etc.

Contraindications		• Lesion location in anterior frontal horn, posterior atrium, or temporal horn (prefer transcortical route)
		• **Crossed dominance[5]:**
		  – **Definition:** different hemispheres control dominant hand and speech/language
		  – Post-op writing/speech deficit in case of transcallosal approach

Positioning		• **Position:**
		  – Supine
		  – Thorax elevation
		• **Mayfield head holder**
		• **Head**
		  – **Elevation:** above heart level
		  – **Neutral position** (helps surgeon stay oriented to midline)
		  – **Extension:** 10 degree
		• Choose right-sided approach (preferrably)

Incision		**Modified bicoronal incision** • Shorter, centered to midline • 2–3 cm anterior to coronal suture • Anteroposterior skin flap retraction (exposure around 4 cm anterior and 2 cm posterior to coronal suture)

10.3.2 Key Procedural Steps (Table 10.3b)

| 1. Anterior parasagittal craniotomy | • Rectangular (size: AP)
• Nondominant hemisphere (usually)
• Extents:
  – **Mediolateral extent:** extending up to or encompassing midline (total width ≈ 4 cm)
  – **Anteroposterior extent relative to coronal suture** (two-third anterior + one-third posterior to coronal suture) (total length ≈ 5–6 cm)
!! **Criterion:** study pre-op magnetic resonance venography (MRV) for variations in draining veins
• **Craniotomy:**
  – **Drill a trough along sinus:** using an M8 bit w/ the non-cutting tip pointing toward the sinus. Unroof the edge of the superior sagittal sinus (SSS) along its entire length where it abuts the planned craniotomy
  – Two burr holes at the lateral two corners of the planned craniotomy (optional)
Using a craniotome, complete the parasagittal craniotomy, always cutting away from sinus |

2. Dural opening	• "U"-shaped dural flap based on SSS → reflect over midline • Preserve draining veins while retracting dural flap

3. Interhemispheric dissection	• **Aims:**
	  – Minimal retraction (≤ 2 cm)
	  – Avoid venous infarction (avoid too much retraction on sinus causing thrombus or occlusion)
	• **Technique:** combination of alternating sharp dissection + retractor blade advancement
	• **Anatomical structures to identify before corpus callosum (CC) (from superficial to deep):**
	  – Inferior falx
	  – Inferior sagittal sinus
	  – Cingulate gyri
	  – Callosomarginal arteries
	  – Pericallosal arteries
	• **CC features:** pearly white, relatively avascular (see Chapter 9, ▶Fig. 9.5)

4. Callosotomy	• **Technique:** split CC down the midline w/ bipolar cautery and suction (check pre-op imaging for midline asymmetry!) → widen opening (length < 2–3 cm) → advance retractor → side identification • **Identification of side:** choroid plexus (CP) courses medially to the thalamostriate vein (both structures if followed, guide surgeon to foramen of Monro [Fmo] (see Chapter 9, ▶Fig. 9.5) ! **Always** → fenestrate/excise septum pellucidum !! **Suspect entry into cavum septum pellucidum,** if after opening CC no veins or CP is identified !!! Make sure the trajectory of callosotomy is perpendicular to CC (ensures shorter route in CC)
5. Entry into body of lateral ventricle	Orientation: • Identify CP and trace it anteriorly up to the Fmo • CP is located medially to the thalamostriate vein

6. Approaches to third ventricle (if needed) (see Table 10.3c)	• Selection criteria:
	  – Lesion (size, location, and characteristics)
	  – Avoidance of post-op deficits
	• Options:
	
	  – Transforaminal
	  – Transchoroidal (sub-/suprachoroidal)
	  – Interforniceal

7. Closure	• Irrigation of ventricular system to wash out clots • Inspect ventricular system for obstruction • Layer-by-layer hemostasis (esp. callosotomy, cortex) • Leave external ventricular drain (EVD) (hydrocephalus prevention) • Watertight dura closure • Bone flap fixation • Galea closure • Skin closure

10.3.3 Approaches into Third Ventricle (Table 10.3c)

Approach		Definition	Indications	Caution	Pros	Cons
Transforaminal		Through FMo	• **Tumor location**: anterior third ventricle • **Tumor characteristics**: cystic/soft • Tumor dilates FMo	Avoid further dilation of FMo (risk for memory deficit)	Uses a natural opening (no need for creating a new one) → least traumatic	• May require unilateral thalamostriate vein sacrifice (neuro deficits) • May require sacrifice of venous tributaries from thalamus – basal ganglia
Transchoroidal	Subchoroidal	Incision in taenia choroidea → CP retracted upward	Extra access to the middle and posterior third ventricle	Beware of venous tributaries to superior choroidal veins	Less risk for forniceal injury	Risk of unilateral forniceal injury
	Suprachoroidal	Incision in taenia fornicis → CP deflected downward			Safer (preferred) → less manipulation of superficial caudate, thalamic veins	
Interforniceal		Between bodies of fornices by dividing the interforniceal raphe	↑ morbidity → reserved only for tumors distending upward 3rd ventricle roof located in the posterior two-third of third ventricle (rarely used)	Hippocampal commissure (avoid extending incision to the posterior component of fornices)		Risk of bilateral forniceal damage → memory impairment

Note: See ▶ Fig. 9.6

10.3.4 Pearls for Each Procedural Step (Table 10.3d)

Pre-op preparation	Pt selection	• Check for crossed dominance • Pre-op neuropsychological assessment in pts with cognitive impairment (esp. memory deficits) • Pre-op vascular anatomy study
	Pre-op imaging study	• **MRV:** find optimal surgical corridor between bridging veins • CC midline distortion • Beware of existence of cavum septum pellucidum
	Transcortical approach (alternative)	• Main author prefers transcortical approach in pts w/ hydrocephalus • There is higher risk of epilepsy but less cortical structures en route
Interhemispheric stage	Avoid venous infarction	• Vein preservation • Do not retract the medial hemisphere surface > 2 cm • Maintain pt well hydrated during surgery
	Interhemispheric dissection	• Wait 2–3 min between every advancement of the retractor blade (allows for ventricular pressures to equilibrate) • Brain relaxation measures (mannitol, hyperventilation)
	Do not mistake cingulate gyrus for CC	Below the falx and superior to CC, the two cingulate gyri may be adherent to each other and can be mistaken for CC. Identify CC by its bright white color and its relative hypovascularity (vs cingulate gyri, which are yellow white). Furthermore, pericallosal arteries lie on CC (see ▶ Fig. 9.5)
Intraventricular stage	Preservation of anatomical structures	• Draining cortical veins • Thalamostriate vein • Fornices
	Control of tumor blood supply	• **CP tumors (papilloma, meningioma)** → blood supply from choroidal arteries (ligate early) • **Ependymal tumors (gliomas, neurocytomas etc)** → blood supply from small ependymal vessels (require meticulous dissection)
	Tumor dissection	Always maintain plane between tumor – ependyma
Closure	Hydrocephalus prevention	Place cottonoid into FMo to prevent blood from pooling into third ventricle
	EVD	Always leave ventriculostomy post-op

10.3.5 Complications: Avoidance +Mx (Table 10.3e)

Complications	Consequences	Avoidance/Mx

• Venous injury/obstruction
• SSS injury/thrombosis
	• Venous infarcts
	• Hemiparesis
	• Brisk venous hemorrhage
	• Air embolism
		• **Avoid by:**
		  – Preserving draining cortical veins (no sacrifice, less manipulation)
		  – Minimizing midline retraction (≤ 2 cm)
		  – Preserving thalamostriate vein
		  – Keeping veins wet
		  – Placing two-third of craniotomy anterior to coronal suture (minimal risk for cortical veins draining motor or supplementary motor cortex to cross the surgical field – usually drain into SSS 2–3 cm behind to coronal suture
		  – Brain relaxation measures (mannitol, hyperventilation, CSF drainage after callosotomy)
		  – Adequate hydration
		• Mx: see Table 11.1d

Transient akinetic mutism (range: slow speech initiation → mutism)	**Other potential syndrome symptoms:** • Paraparesis • Incontinence • Seizures • Emotional disturbances	Avoid by: • Limiting CC incision (1–2 cm) • Minimizing retraction to anterior cingulate gyrus, fornix (take brain relaxation measures, avoid using retractors, prefer cotton balls or rolled cottonoids for retraction of cingulate gyri • Preserving vessels of supplementary motor area, basal ganglia, thalamus
Disorders of interhemispheric information transfer	• Disorder of visuospatial info transfer • Disorder of tactile info transfer • Bimanual learning difficulty • Alexia	Avoidance: • Limit CC incision (2–3 cm) • Avoid posterior callosotomy (splenium)
Unilateral thalamostriate vein injury/sacrifice	• Hemiplegia • Drowsiness • Mutism	Avoidance: • Preserving vein • Preferring suprachoroidal over subchoroidal approach
Fornix injury	Amnesia (usually transient amnesia of recent events)	Avoidance: • Do not distend FMo in transforaminal approach • Preserve fornix • Avoid interforniceal approach

Complications	Consequences	Avoidance/Mx
Obstructive hydrocephalus	Neurological deterioration Coma	**Avoidance:** • Irrigate ventricles at closure • Hemostasis • Leave EVD • Placement of cottonoid patties into ventricles to prevent debris and blood clot dispersal – remove them at closure • Open septum pellucidum (prevents occurrence of trapped ventricle)
Injury of pericallosal artery injury of callo-somarginal artery	• Contralateral hemiparesis with lower limb predominance • Sensory deficits of contralateral limbs, urinary incontince • Akinetic mutism (infarction of left supplementary motor area) • Ideomotor apraxia (pericallosal) • Decreased verbal fluency • Abulia	**Avoidance:** • Meticulous dissection • Good knowledge of regional anatomy and the anatomical structures encountered • Do not mistake cingulate gyri for CC and callosomarginal arteries for pericallosal arteries, thus entering into cingulate gyri and injuring the pericallosal arteries
CSF leak	• CSF leak from wound • Subgaleal CSF collection	• Avoid with watertight dura closure • Mx with running-locking sutures oversewing leak (see Chapter 11: Complications, CSF leak)

Other general craniotomy complications: post-op hematoma, infection, cerebral infarction

10.3.6 Approaches to Ventricles[6] (Table 10.3f)

Target		Approach
Lateral ventricles	Frontal horn (anteroinferior wall)	• Anterior frontal via rostrum of CC
	Body	• Anterior transcallosal • Anterior transcortical via middle frontal gyrus

	Atrium	• Transcortical approaches
		  – Posterior transcortical via superior parietal lobule
		  – Transcortical via posterior middle/inferior temporal gyrus
		  – Via isthmus of cingulate gyrus (occipital approach)
		• Posterior transcallosal (via posterior splenium)

	Temporal horn	Transcortical via inferior part of middle temporal gyrus or superior part of inferior temporal gyrus (via temporal or posterior frontotemporal approach)
	Occipital horn	Transcortical via isthmus of cingulate (gyrus occipital approach)

(Continued) ►

Target		Approach	

Third ventricle	Anterior	Midline approaches	• Anterior transcallosal approach
			  – Transforaminal approach
			  – Transchoroidal (sub/suprachoroidal) approach
			  – Interforniceal approach
			• Subfrontal approach:
			  – Opticocarotid approach (through opticocarotid triangle)
			  – Subchiasmatic approach (below optic chiasm between the optic nerves)
			  – The lamina terminalis approach (through lamina terminalis)
			  – Transfrontal – transsphenoidal (through planum sphenoidale – throughsphenoid sinus)
			• transsphenoidal approach

		Lateral approaches	• Posterior frontotemporal • Subtemporal
	Posterior		• Median/paramedian supracerebellar infratentorial • Posterior transcallosal • Occipital transtentorial • Posterior transcortical via superior parietal lobule
Fourth ventricle			• Midline suboccipital approachTranscortical via vermis • Telovelar approach

10.4 Bifrontal Craniotomy With Supraorbital Bar Removal ⬚G

10.4.1 Basic Information (Table 10.4a)

Craniotomy	Indications
Bifrontal	**Access to:** • Entire anterior cranial fossa • Anterior midline parasellar area (tuberculum, ACom, ICA, chiasm, optic nerve)
Plus supraorbital bar removal	• Smaller and more posterior lesions • Significant superior extension of lesions **! pros:** ↓ retraction and ↑ visualization
Contraindications	• Middle cranial fossa lesions • Sub-/retrochiasmatic lesions (prefer pterional or orbitozygomatic approach) • Paranasal sinus infection

Positioning	• **Patient position:**
	  – Supine
	  – Thorax elevation
	• **Mayfield clamp:**
	  – **Paired pins:** above mastoid in the coronal plane (push skin forward before fixating head to decrease tension on incision during closure
	  – **Single pin:** above the contralateral pinna
	• **Head** (aim: ipsilateral orbital rim at highest point)
	  – **Elevation**
	  – **Neutral position**
	  – **Neck:** slightly extended 10–15 degrees (allows gravity retraction)

Incision	**Bicoronal skin incision** • **Starts:** 1 cm anterior to tragus of one ear • **Ends:** 1 cm anterior to contralateral tragus * In midline the incision forms an anteriorly directed peak

10.4.2 Key Procedural Steps (Table 10.4b)

1. Soft-tissue elevation	• Scalp elevated anteriorly over orbital rim • Subfascial reflection of fat pad containing frontalis branch of CN VII posterior to frontal process of zygomatic bone (see step 2 in Table 10.2b) • Rectangular piece of vascularized forehead pericranium reflected separately anteriorly as far as nasofrontal suture (keep wet)

2. Bifrontal craniotomy	• Burr holes:
	  – McCarty keyholes bilaterally
	  – Drilling of bone over SSS near frontal fossa (anteriorly) and in front of coronal suture (posteriorly) → expose SSS and dura on each side of sinus
	• Bifrontal craniotomy (as close to the anterior cranial fossa as possible)

3. Further bony exposure for biorbitonasal osteotomy	• Free supraorbital nerve from supraorbital notch/foramen (after opening it with osteotome/drill) • Elevate scalp upto nasofrontal suture • **Frontal dura dissection:** dissect frontal dura off frontal fossa and orbital roofs preserving attachments at the crista galli • **Periorbita dissection:** dissect periorbita bilaterally from medial to supraorbital notch to just above medial canthus

(Continued) ▶

4. Biorbitonasal osteotomy (see ▸ Fig. 10.2)	Cut #1: horizontal osteotomy above nasofrontal suture	With brain ribbons bilaterally protecting medial periorbita and frontal dura → perform horizontal osteotomy using reciprocating saw just above nasofrontal suture: • **Starting** in one orbit • **Extending** 1 cm deep into nasal bone (not deeper, in order to avoid crista) • **Out** into the other orbit
	Cuts #2 and 3: vertical cuts along orbital rim in the sagittal plane	With brain ribbons bilaterally protecting the frontal lobe and the periorbita, → use reciprocating saw to make vertical cuts in the sagittal plane just medial to the supraorbital notches along orbital rim which extend: • From intracranial space • Through orbital roof • Into orbit
	Cut#4: coronal cut along orbital roofs – nasal bone	With brain ribbons bilaterally protecting medial periorbita and frontal dura, perform perpendicular cut using reciprocating saw in the coronal plane that: • **Starts** from the level of the previous sagittal frontal cut (cut #2) • **Along** one orbital roof • **Then** 1 cm deep into nasal bone down to the level of the previous horizontal nasal osteotomy (cut #1), anterior to crista • **Out** into the contralateral orbit, along the orbital roof • **To the level** of the previous contralateral sagittal frontal cut (cut #3)
	Elevation of osteotomy flap	Orbital rim should now be free and mobile. Use handheld osteotom to free it completely and elevate
5. Dura opening – division of SSS	b/l horizontal dural openings ligations (as close to anterior cranial fossa as possible) → b/l gentle retraction of frontal lobes away of falx → 2 SSS ligations (as close to anterior cranial fossa as possible) → division of SSS together with falx between the ligations	
6. Intradural dissection	Depending on pathology	

7. Closure	• **Frontal sinus closure** (see also Table 10.4c: technique for preventing CSF rhinorrhea from frontal sinus)
	• Repair of anterior cranial fossa with vascularized pericranial flap
	  – Cover frontal sinus (below orbital osteotomy piece)
	  – Cover defects on anterior cranial fossa (below frontal lobes)
	• **Dural closure:** circumferentially sew dura to pericranial flap, which has replaced basal dura
	• Craniotomy – osteotomy bone flap fixation + possible cranioplasty
	• Galea closure
	• Skin closure	

10.4.3 Biorbitonasal Osteotomy Cuts (▶Fig. 10.2)

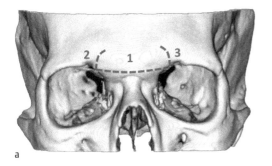
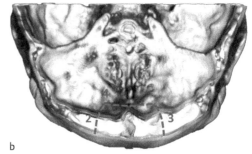

a   b

10.4.4 Pearls for Each Procedural Step (Table 10.4c)

Soft tissue elevation	Vascularized pericranium flap	• Always harvest a vascularized pericranium flap → utilities:
		  – Frontal sinus exclusion
		  – Repair of anterior cranial fossa defects
		  – Prevention of CSF rhinorrhea
		! Caution: when replacing biorbital rim/frontal craniotomy over vascularized pericranial graft, beware not to strangulate the graft → this may lead to graft venous congestion and associated mass effect.

Dura dissection	Ethmoidal artery cauterization	Early anterior ethmoidal artery cauterization to devascularize anterior midline skull base tumors
	Frontal fossa drilling	**Before opening dura extradurally, use diamond drill:** • To flatten frontal fossa bony ridges • To devascularize potential intradural lesion (such as olfactory groove meningioma) from ethmoidal feeders
Craniotomy	Drilling over SSS	**Pros vs burr holes straddling SSS:** • Better dura detachment for craniotomy → protection of bridging veins during craniotomy • Better SSS dissection → SSS protection during craniotomy – bone flap elevation * Main author always drills bone over sinuses instead of burr holes for craniotomies involving sinuses

(Continued) ▶

Osteotomy	Biorbitonasal osteotomy	Pros:
		• ↓ brain retraction
		• Low and flat trajectory for lesions located more posterior in anterior cranial fossa
		• Removes obstructions around lesser sphenoid wing
		! Main author is very liberal with use of biorbitonasal osteotomies in order to decrease frontal lobe retraction, particularly for large bilateral lesions
Closure	Technique for preventing CSF rhinorrhea from frontal sinus	• Strip mucosa (study frontal sinus drainage, beware of duplicate orbital roof)
		• Drill thin layer of bone from entire sinus wall (in order to ensure that all mucous secreting cells have been removed)
		• Plug nasofrontal duct with Gelfoam soaked with bacitracin ointment followed by muscle plug
		• Apply vascularized pericranium graft

10.4.5 Complications: Avoidance + Mx (Table 10.4d)

Complications	Consequences	Avoidance/Mx
Injury of frontalis branch of CN VII	Inability to raise ipsilateral eyebrow	Avoid by subfascial elevation of fat pad
Supraorbital nerve injury	Frontal numbness/pain	Avoid by freeing nerve from supraorbital notch/foramen during scalp elevation
Unilateral trochlear pulley injury	Diplopia	Avoid with careful dissection of periorbita from medial orbital roof
CSF rhinorrhea due to entry into frontal sinus	• Infection • Pneumocephalus	• Avoid by covering frontal sinus with pericranial flap (see Table 10.4c for technique) • Use lumbar drainage when indicated (for Mx, see Table 11.1f)
SSS injury	• Brisk venous bleeding • Air embolism	Avoid by drilling trough parallel to sinus edge instead of burr holes across sinus → better SSS dissection (for Mx, see Table 11.1d)

Complications	Consequences	Avoidance/Mx
Frontal lobe injury	• Brain contusions • Edema • Neurological deterioration	**Avoidance:** • Minimal frontal lobe retraction • Slight head extension (allows gravity to retract frontal lobe away from anterior fossa floor) • Supraorbital bar removal minimizes need for retraction • Brain relaxation measures (mannitol, hyperventilation)
Post-op pulsatile enopthalmos		• Usually resolves in 3–6 months
Eye injury	Vision disturbances	Avoid by keeping periorbita intact and protecting it at all time with brain ribbon during osteotomies
Olfactory nerve injury	Impaired olfaction	• Avoid by preserving dural attachments at the crista galli during elevation of dura from frontal fossa and orbital roofs • Avoid with minimal retraction of frontal lobes

Other general craniotomy complications: post-op hematoma, neurovascular injury, infection, cerebral infarction, and seizures

10.5 Subtemporal Approach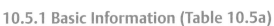

10.5.1 Basic Information (Table 10.5a)

Indications	Location of lesions	• **Middle fossa:** – Cavernous sinus – Medial temporal lobe – Petrous apex – Tentorial edge – incisura • **Posterior fossa:** – Extra-axial (upper petroclival region; may be reached by drilling petrous apex) – Intra-axial (anteromedial region of superior cerebellar hemispheres)
	Lesions	• Meningiomas • Gliomas • Aneurysms (located at basilar apex, posterior cerebral arteries, superior cerebellar arteries)

(Continued) ▶

Contraindications	• Lesion in left side (relative)
	• Vein of Labbé obstructing planned surgical trajectory
	• Lesions arising from cerebellopontine angle (CPA)
Surgical adjuncts	• Division of tentorium
	• Anterior petrosectomy
	• Zygomatic osteotomy
Positioning	• **Patient position:**
	– Supine
	– Ipsilateral shoulder roll
	• **Mayfield clamp**
	• **Head** (**aim:** zygoma at highest point)
	– **Rotation:** 90 degree from vertical plane contralaterally (make sure space between chin – contralateral clavicle is adequate)
	– **Neck extension:** 15 degree (vertex is lowered)
	– **Head elevation:** 20 degree
	!! **Positioning allows:**
	– Temporal lobe to fall with gravity
	– Direct visualization of the tentorium
Incision	**Horseshoe**
	• **Starts:** at zygomatic root (close to tragus)
	• **Course:** superiorly up to superior temporal line → turns posteriorly over the pinna
	• **Ends:** at asterion

10.5.2 Key Procedural Steps (Table 10.5b)

1. Musculocutaneous flap elevation	Subperiosteal elevation of musculocutaneous flap → flap reflected inferiorly
	!! **Caution:** cartilagenous portion of external auditory meatus
2. Craniotomy	• **Burr holes:**
	– Zygomatic root
	– Asterion
	– Superior temporal line (superior to zygoma root)
	• **Craniotomy**
	– Approximately two-third anterior to external acoustic meatus (EAM), one-third posterior to EAM
	– Drill temporal bone flush with the middle fossa floor
	! **Caution:** wax open mastoid air cells
3. Extradural dissection along middle fossa floor	• **Middle fossa landmarks:**
	– Tegmen tympani
	– Arcuate eminence (superior semicircular canal)
	– Greater superficial petrosal nerve (GSPN)
	– CN V3
	– Beware of dehiscence of carotid artery roof (see ▶ Fig. 9.1 and ▶ Fig. 9.4)
	• Dura is elevated (from lateral to medial and from posterior to anterior) up to petrous ridge → drilling of the petrous ridge can take place, if required

4. Dura opening	**Shape:** inferiorly based U-shaped
5. Subtemporal dissection	• Identify, trace, and preserve Labbé vein • Subtemporal dissection • Infratemporal veins may prevent subtemporal dissection (small bridging veins only can be divided) • Elevate temporal lobe. Be careful on dominant hemisphere • Proceed with subtemporal dissection until brainstem vessels are visualized
6. Division of tentorial edge (if required)	• **Pros:** access to p-fossa • **Technique:** trace CN IV → bipolar cautery of tentorium before incision → lateral-to-medial tentorial edge incision together with hemostasis → retract flaps !! Beware of location of 4th nerve
7. Closure	• Watertight dural closure • Bone flap fixation + possible cranioplasty for the extra bone defect near middle fossa floor • Closure in layers (temporalis fascia – galea – skin)

10.5.3 Pearls for Each Procedural Step (Table 10.5c)

Pre-op preparation	Alternative approaches when Labbè vein poses risks	Solutions for difficulties due to vein of Labbé (short vein in our surgical trajectory) in nondominant hemispheres: • Transcortical approach through inferior temporal gyrus for medial temporal lesions • Consider partially resecting inferior temporal gyrus rather than pulling upon temporal lobe for improved medial structure visualization
	Pre-op MRV study	Pre-op MRV study of the Labbé vein drainage
Craniotomy	Mastoid air cells	Push wax in to air cells rather than swipe wax across air cells
	Additional bone drilling	Drill temporal bone down to the middle fossa floor

(Continued) ▶

Extradural dissection	Middle meningeal artery ligation	For an extradural approach, the ligation of meningeal artery at foramen spinosum can facilitate dura elevation
	Bone dehiscence of carotid artery roof	Beware of bone dehiscence of petrous ICA roof → if not taken into consideration, ICA can be injured during the middle fossa dura dissection
	Avoid traction to greater superficial petrosal nerve	• Traction to GSPN can be transmitted to facial nerve causing facial palsy • Separate GSPN carefully from dura to prevent traction
Subtemporal dissection	Brain relaxation measures	Brain relaxation measures to facilitate temporal lobe elevation: • Diuretics (mannitol) • Hyperventilation • Pre-op LD placement

10.5.4 Complications: Avoidance + Mx (Table 10.5d)

Complications	Consequences	Avoidance/Mx
Vein of Labbé injury Injury of temporobasal veins	• Temporal lobe venous infarct/edema • Neurological deterioration	• Avoid by pre-op MRV study of Labbé vein • Avoid with use of brain relaxation rather than aggressive retraction
temporal lobe injury	• Seizures • Edema/contusions • Neurological deterioration • Hemiparesis	• Avoid with better positioning • Avoid excessive temporal lobe retraction with brain relaxation measures
CN IV injury (during tentorial edge incision) (also CN III can be injured)	Diplopia	Avoid by identifying and tracing CN IV before incision
CSF leak	• CSF otorrhea or rhinorrhea • CSF leak from wound • Subcutaneous CSF collection • Infection, meningitis	**Avoid by:** • Waxing mastoid air cells • Watertight dura closure • Meticulous layered closure (for Mx, see Table 11.1f)
Facial nerve injury		• To avoid, separate GSPN carefully from dura to prevent traction during middle fossa dura elevation • For Mx of CN VII palsy, see Chapter 11: Complications, CN VII palsy

Other general craniotomy complications: post-op hematoma, infection, cerebral or brainstem infarction, and seizures

10.6 Midline Suboccipital Craniotomy G

10.6.1 Basic Information (Table 10.6a)

Indications	Exposure	• Cerebellar hemispheres • Vermis • Fourth ventricle • Brain stem • Foramen magnum
	Lesions	• Tumors (meningiomas, ependymomas, gliomas, and metastases • Vascular lesions (aneurysms, AVMs, cavernous malformations) • Infections • Hematomas • Developmental anomalies (Chiari)
Contraindications		• Supratentorial extension of lesion → use combined supracerebellar–supratentorial approach • Lesions located on ventral cerebellum and brain stem • Extension of lesion to mid-fossa → use combined p-fossa + mid-fossa approach • Cervical spine pathology, which would oppose neck flexion

Positioning/ preparation		• **Patient position:**
		  – Prone Concorde position
		  – Chest rolls
		  – Arms tucked at sides
		  – Thorax elevation
		  – Flexed knees
		• **Mayfield clamp**
		• **Head:**
		  – Posterior translation of neck
		  – Neck flexion → opens C1 foramen magnum interval
		!!**Caution:** leave 2–3 fingerbreadths between chin and sternum
		Intra-op neuromonitoring: MEPs, SSEPs, brainstem auditory evoked potentials, cranial nerves (depending on tumor location)

Incision		Linear midline incision • Superior extent: 2–3 cm above inion • Inferior extent: C2 spinous process

10.6.2 Key Procedural Steps (Table 10.6b)

1. Soft tissue elevation	• Open fascia using "T"-shaped incision to have increased soft-tissue closure for a watertight seal (to prevent CSF leak) (see also Table 10.6c) • Subperiosteal muscle elevation from suboccipital bone • Subperiosteal elevation of paraspinal muscles along midline and lateral dissection of muscles off posterior C1 arch !! caution: during dissection of C1 arch beware of: • Vertebral artery (VA): 1–1.5 cm from midline, use low cautery microinstruments • Bone defect in posterior arch of C1 and C2 lamina (see ▶ Fig. 9.2 and ▶ Fig. 9.9)

(Continued) ▶

2. Craniotomy	• **Superior craniotomy edge**: drill trough along transverse sinus
	• **Craniotomy** (see also Table 10.6c):
	  – From one side of superior craniotomy edge to ipsilateral foramen magnum
	  – From other side of superior craniotomy edge to ipsilateral foramen magnum
	  – Further removal of foramen magnum rim laterally up to the occipital condyles (! caution: circular sinus)
	! landmarks for rough localization of sinuses: transverse sinus esimated along line from zygoma to inion; sigmoid/transverse junction often 1 cm inferolateral from mastoid emissary vein
	!! craniotomy extents: adjust rostral extent based on need; the more rostral the exposure, the less galea available to close
	!!! always drill away from sinuses with router

3. C1 laminectomy	**Indications:** • Existing tonsilar herniation • Chiari malformation • Foramen magnum lesions • Tumor extension to upper C-spine • Fourth-ventricle tumors (allows upward instrument angulation)
4. Dura opening	• Y-shaped incision (vertical limb extends up to foramen magnum or below, if tumor extends in upper C-spine) • Upward reflection of superior triangular dura flap over transverse sinus **!! Beware of circular sinus around foramen magnum**
5. Opening of cisterna magna	**Benefits:** • CSF drainage → brain relaxation • Full visualization of tonsils → if needed, mobilize tonsils by dividing arachnoid bands between them gaining access to foramen of Magendie
6. Closure	• Watertight dura closure (may require dural graft) • Bone flap fixation • Closure in layers (muscle fascia – galea – skin) **!! Consider a running suture for skin closure as extra reinforcement for watertight closure**

10.6.3 Pearls for Each Procedural Step (Table 10.6c)

Pre-op preparation	Suboccipital craniotomy in children	• Pre-op MRI: occipital bone in children may be full of venous lakes → always study pre-op MRI carefully • Mx: if venous lakes are present, consider pre-op embolization

Pre-op preparation	Pre-op EVD/Dandy-burr hole	• For all p-fossa approaches, main author places EVD pre-op OR leaves burr hole-ready pre-op
		• **Indications (when EVD is not placed routinely pre-op):**
		  – Tumor blocking access to cisterna magna
		  – Pre-op hydrocephalus
		• **Usefulness:**
		  – Brain relaxation
		  – Prevents acute obstructive HCP

Positioning	Head flexion	• Opens C1–foramen magnum interval → facilitates craniotomy • Facilitates trajectory into 4th ventricle

Soft tissue elevation	Create two fascial layers for watertight closure	• During opening, split fascia into two separate layers:
		  – Leave superficial layer attached to skin
		  – Leave deep layer attached to underlying muscles
		• Each artificially created layer will be closed separately → this allows a second watertight layer closure

	Identification of intermuscular septum	• Make fascial incision parallel to superior nuchal line • This allows immediate identification of intermuscular septum–muscle bundles along each side • Then open fascia in "T" fashion (vertical limb along intermuscular septum)

Craniotomy	Craniotomy procedure to reduce blood loss	• **Aim:** to reduce blood loss due to venous lakes usually located within midline suboccipital bony ridge (corresponds to internal–external occipital crest)
		• **Steps:**
		  – Perform all other craniotomy cuts leaving midline bony ridge (bone flap still attached to this bony bridge)
		  – Expose dura on either side of midline bony ridge
		  – Drill off midline ridge last (this tends to be the region with the most bony bleeding)

(Continued) ▶

Dura opening	Control of significant venous bleeding during dural opening around foramen magnum	• **Source of bleeding:** circular sinus and venous plexus
		• **Ways to control bleeding:**
		  – Bipolar cautery of both edges together (make sure you have both edges captured)
		  – Suture along both edges
		  – Use Weck clips

	Brain relaxation measures	• Diuretics • Hyperventilation • CSF removal (EVD, cisterna magna opening)

10.6.4 Complications: Avoidance + Mx (Table 10.6d)

Complications	Consequences	Avoidance/Mx
VA injury PICA injury	• Bleeding • Infarction • Neurological deterioration	• Avoid with pre-op CTA study of VA course • Avoid by use of bipolar cautery and careful dissection (less traumatic) with microinstruments in the foramen magnum area
Circular sinus injury or other sinus injury	• Brisk venous bleeding • Air embolism	• Mx bleeding with bipolar cautery and Gelfoam
Post-op hydrocephalus intra-op tight cerebellum	Post-op neurological deterioration, coma	• Avoid with pre-op EVD placement • Mx with EVD placement via Dandy burr hole
Cerebellar injury	• Edema • Neurological deterioration	• Avoid with brain relaxation measures (EVD, cisterna magna opening, etc.) • Avoid repositioning brain retractor too many times • Avoid static retractors
CSF leak	• CSF otorrhea or rhinorrhea • CSF leak from wound • Subcutaneous CSF collection • Infection, meningitis	**Avoid by:** • Watertight dura closure • Meticulous layered closure (for Mx, see Table 11.1f)

Others: hematoma, infection, post-craniectomy headache, cerebellar or brainstem infarct

10.7 Retrosigmoid Craniotomy

10.7.1 Basic Information (Table 10.7a)

Indications	Exposure	• CPA • In cephalocaudal axis from tentorium, CN V to jugular bulb and CN IX–XI

	Lesions	• Tumors:
		  – Extra-axial CPA and petroclival tumors (schwannomas, meningiomas, epidermoids, etc.)
		  – Intra-axial (petrosal cerebellum surface, cerebellar peduncles, brainstem)
		• Cascular lesions (aneurysms of vertebrobasilar system, brainstem cavernous malformations, AVMs)
		• Neurovascular compression syndromes → microvascular decompression for:
		  – Trigeminal neuralgia
		  – Geniculate neuralgia
		  – Glossopharyngeal neuralgia

Contraindications		Non-patent contralateral transverse – sigmoid sinus (relative) → ipsilateral sinus cannot be sacrificed in case of injury
Extended variation		Mastoidectomy → allows more anterior access to CPA and prepontine cistern

Positioning/ Preparation		• **Patient position:**
		• Park bench
		• Ipsilateral to lesion shoulder elevated
		• Consider taping ipsilateral shoulder down to increase working space between occiput and neck
		
		(!! Beware of excessive force – risk of brachial plexus palsy)
		• **Mayfield clamp:**
		  – Posterior paired pins → contralateral occipital bone (equator)
		  – Anterior single pin → ipsilateral frontal bone superior to orbit (equator)
		• **Head** (aim: petrous ridge perpendicular to floor)
		  – **Elevation:** above heart
		  – **Rotation:** to contralateral side of lesion
		  – **Neck flexion** (chin 2 fingerbreadths from sternum)
		  – **Lateral neck flexion:** vertex down
		• **Precordial Doppler + central venous line** (for prompt Dx and Tx of air embolism during skeletonization of sinuses)
		• **Intra-op neuromonitoring:** SSEPs, MEPs, brainstem auditory evoked potentials, facial EMG (esp. for lesions involving CN VII, CN VIII)

Incision		C-shaped (1 fingerbreadth behind pinna) • **Superior extent:** 2 cm superior to pinna • **Inferior extent:** 2 fingerbreadths below mastoid tip

10.7.2 Key Procedural Steps (Table 10.7b)

1. Soft tissue elevation	Subperiosteal muscle elevation in suboccipital area → bone exposure: • **Cephalocaudal axis:** from superior to asterion → foramen magnum (as low as needed by lesion) • **Anteroposterior axis:** from digastric groove of mastoid process → 4 cm posterior to sigmoid sinus

2. Retrosigmoid craniotomy	• Bony skeletonization of transverse – sigmoid sinus with high-speed M8 drill (= superior and lateral sides of square craniotomy)
	• **Craniotomy:**
	  – Use craniotome for the other two sides (medial and inferior) of the square craniotomy
	  – **Size of square craniotomy:** 3.5 cm posterior to sigmoid sinus
	! During craniotomy, always cut away from venous sinuses
	!! Main author prefers drilling a trough over transverse and sigmoid sinus and their junction and then unroofing them with Kerisson rongeurs rather than placing burr holes over sinuses

3. Limited posterior mastoidectomy (optional)	Aim: exposure of sigmoid sinus–jugular bulb junction ! Caution: • Wax mastoid air cells • Mastoid emissary vein injury (cauterize)(see Table 10.7c)
4. Dura opening	**C-shaped opening:** follows course of transverse–sigmoid sinus. Dural flap laid on cerebelum for protection
5. Opening of cisterna magna	• Place spatula on inferolateral cerebellar hemisphere • Retract cerebellum gently medially – superiorly • Gain access to lateral cerebellomedullary cistern and to cisterna magna • Open arachnoid of cisterns • Allow CSF drainage
6. Intradural dissection (depending on pathology)	Placement of retractor on the lateral cerebellar surface depending on location of pathology in the cephalocaudal axis
7. Closure	• Primary dura watertight closure • Bone flap fixation • Closure in layers (muscle fascia – galea – skin)

10.7.3 Pearls for Each Procedural Step (Table 10.7c)

Pre-op preparation	Pre-op MRV study	Pre-op evaluation of patency of contralateral transverse–sigmoid sinus → in case of occlusion of contralateral sinuses, we cannot risk injury of the ipsilateral to the approach sinuses – consider to avoid skeletonization of sinuses
	Pre-op high-resolution CT of petrous bone	Assess petrous bone pneumatization, position of vestibule and cochlea
	Surgical navigation	Information about location of venous sinuses for improved craniotomy placement (not used by main author)
	Anatomical landmarks for localization of sinuses	• Identify approximate location of transverse sinus along an imaginary line between zygoma – external acoustic canal – inion • Transverse–sigmoid sinus junction is located approximately superolaterally to the asterion (point where lambdoid, occipito-mastoid, and parieto-mastoid sutures meet) • Sigmoid sinus is located below mastoid groove
	Pre-op EVD/Dandy burr hole	For all p-fossa approaches, main author places EVD pre-op OR leaves burr-hole ready pre-op (see also Table 10.6c)
Soft-tissue elevation	Mastoid emissary vein	• During bony exposure (soft-tissue elevation), beware of mastoid emissary vein that usually tracks straight to sigmoid–transverse junction joint • **Hemostasis:** remove all soft tissue around bone before waxing; ideally isolate emissary vein and then cauterize and cut, but be prepared to encounter during craniotomy bone work
Craniotomy	Bony skeletonization of transverse–sigmoid sinus	**Pros:** ↑ working angle → view parallel to petrosal cerebellar surface + ventral brain stem
	Beware of mastoid air cells	After craniotomy, push wax into air cells rather than swiping wax across air cells
	Opening of foramen magnum depending on location of lesion	Foramen needs to be opened in case of large tumors extending inferiorly[7]

(Continued) ▶

Intradural work	Brain relaxation	• Diuretics • Hyperventilation • CSF removal (EVD, cisterna magna, and lateral cerebellomedullary cistern opening)
	Cisterna magna opening	It should be the first maneuver after dura opening to allow for CSF drainage and thus brain relaxation
	Beware of superior petrosal vein (Dandy's vein)	If superior petrosal sinus is torn off, the only way to stop sinus orifice bleeding is by packing if full of Gelfoam
	Drilling of internal acoustic canal (IAC)	• **Rationale:** should be done early for lesions involving the CN VII/VIII nerves to identify the parts of the nerves distal to the lesion and to untether them, in order to minimize risk of injury from manipulation • **Technique:** inverted U-shaped incision and elevation of dura overlying the superior part of IAC → drilling of bone superior and inferior to IAC (180 degree) up to the dura of the canal → open dura of IAC → identify intracanicular portions of CN VII, CN VIII

10.7.4 Complications: Avoidance + Mx (Table 10.7d)

Complications	Consequences	Avoidance/Mx

Venous sinus injury	• Brisk venous bleeding
	• Venous infarction/ neurological deterioration
		• Avoid with use of neuronavigation for burr hole placement
		• Avoid by preferring to unroof sinuses with drill than craniotome
		• Mx:
		  – Small defect: apply surgicel and gentle pressure
		  – Large defect: primary suture repair or with muscle graft. If unsuccessful and contra sinus patent (in pre-op MRV) sacrifice otherwise repair
		  (see also Table 11.1d)

Cerebellar injury or brainstem injury	• Ataxia • Cerebellar edema • Neurological deterioration	• Avoid with brain relaxation measures (EVD, cisterna magna opening, etc.) • Avoid repositioning brain retractor too many times • Avoid with extensive bone removal increasing exposure • Avoid by careful dissection of tumor from brain stem
CSF leak	• CSF otorrhea or rhinorrhea • CSF leak from wound • Subcutaneous CSF collection	**Avoid by:** • Waxing mastoid air cells • Watertight dura closure • Meticulous layered closure (for Mx, see Table 11.1f)

Complications	Consequences	Avoidance/Mx
Air embolism		• Precordial Doppler for quick Dx • Mx with pre-op placement of central vein catheter for air aspiration • Mx with lowering head, covering sinus defect, and irrigation
Hydrocephalus	• Neurological deterioration • Coma	• Avoid with pre-op EVD placement • Mx with EVD placement via Dandy burr hole
Cranial nerve injuries (CN V–XI)	depending on involved cranial nerve	• In case of CN V injury, beware of corneal ulceration due to impairment of corneal reflex (V1 branch) → eye patch at night, protective glasses, Lacri-Lube • For Mx of CVII palsy, see Chapter 11: Complications, CN VII palsy

Others: hematoma, aseptic meningitis, bacterial meningitis, other infections, post-craniectomy headache, cerebellar or brainstem infarct

10.8 Transnasal Transsphenoidal Approach G

10.8.1 Basic Information (Table 10.8a)

Variations	• Direct transnasal • Via submucosal tunnel • Sublabial		
Pros	• No visible scars • Minimal traumatic for brain (no retraction) vs. excellent pituitary visualization • ↓ morbidity vs. transcranial approaches		
Visualization	• Microscope (magnification, illumination, 3D view) • Endoscope • Combination		
Indications	**Tumor location**	• Sella • Suprasellar space • Sphenoid sinus • Clival or retroclival lesions (transclival approach)	
	Pathology	• Pituitary adenomas • Symptomatic apoplexis • Craniopharyngiomas • Rathke pouch cyst • Clival chordomas • Meningiomas • Metastases	

(Continued) ▶

Contraindications	• Unfavorable anatomy of the sella (small or asymmetric sella) • Unfavorable tumor characteristics (firm consistency, anterior/posterior/lateral extension) • Prolactinomas responding to medication • Sphenoid sinusitis • Ectatic midline ICA
Alternative approaches for above contraindications	• Expanded endonasal • Transcranial approaches (pterional, supraorbital)

Positioning/ Preparation	• **Patient position:** supine
	• **Mayfield clamp**
	• **Head (aim:** align midline axis with surgeon's angle of view, bridge of nose parallel to floor)
	  – **Elevation:** above heart
	  – **Rotation:** 5–15 degree to the right
	  – **Lateral flexion:** to the left
	  – **Sniffing position**
	• **Navigational systems ± C-arm**
	• **Antibiotics**
	• **100 mg hydrocortisone iv** (not for Cushing pts)

Surgical field preparation	• Face + nose preparation • Nostrils preparation (with iodine-soaked cottonoids) • Face is completely draped except for the nostrils • Pack nose with cottonoids soaked with oxymetazoline • Infiltrate nasal mucosa (septum, turbinates) with lidocaine–epinephrine solution • Put Kerlix gauze in oropharynx (prevents blood drainage into esophagus) • Preparation of right lower abdominal quadrant/right thigh (for fat ± fascia graft harvesting)

10.8.2 Key Procedural Steps (Table 10.8b)

1. Endonasal stage	• Endoscope into right nostril • Identify floor, inferior turbinate, choana • Identify middle turbinate • Direct endoscope superiorly and posteriorly and identify the superior turbinate • Identify the sphenoid ostium posteriorly to superior turbinate
2. Posterior septum removal	• Cauterize mucosa of posterior septum and surrounding sphenoid ostium • Detach septum from sphenoid rostrum and displace contralaterally • Remove posterior septum (keep vomer pieces) → two nostrils should communicate

3. Orientation		• Sagittal plane: confirm with navi ± C-arm • Midline: use landmarks (middle turbinate, sphenoid ostia, keel of rostrum)
4. Entry into sphenoid sinus (sphenoidotomy)		• Locate ostia (posterior to superior turbinate, two-third up the anterior wall of sphenoid sinus) • Drill through rostrum • Consider bilateral approach for wider view • Remove sphenoid sinus septae and mucosa
5. Entry into sella		• Identify landmarks in posterior wall of sphenoid sinus (optic and carotid protuberances, opticocarotid recess, see also ▶ Fig. 9.7) • Drill sella (if bone not thinned by tumor) • Expand opening of sella with Kerisson rongeur (up to cavernous sinuses) • Expose dura of floor of sella
6. Dura opening		Cruciate incision (incise dura from midline to lateral) → cauterization of dural leaves !! Open from medial to lateral to decrease risk of carotid injury
7. Adenoma removal	Microadenoma	• After dura opening, we encounter the pituitary gland • Initial small incision in the gland • Blunt dissection through gland • Tumor removal with a small curette
	Macroadenoma	• After dura opening, we encounter the tumor • Piecemeal tumor removal from its inferior margin • Dissection proceeds superiorly – laterally until diaphragm sella prolapses • Use 30 degree endoscope for lateral tumor removal
8. Sella floor repair	MicroadenomasW/O CSF leak	• Dura graft + vomer pieces • Fibrin glue
	Macroadenomas + intra-op CSF leak	• Fat graft into tumor bed • Repair anterior sellar wall with dura graft + vomer pieces • Pack sinus with sandwich layers with rectus abdominus fascia + fat + Gelfoam® • LD
9. Closure		• Septum returned to place • Pack nose

10.8.3 Pearls for Each Procedural Step (Table 10.8c)

Pre-op preparation	Pre-op W/U	• Endocrine evaluation (hormone levels, hormone replacement PRN) • **Neuro-ophthalmological evaluation:** visual acuity, visual fields	
	Planning based on pre-op imaging studies	MRI	• Lesion relations to chiasm, ICA, cavernous sinus • Distance between cavernous internal carotid arteries • In case of not very obvious microadenomas, look for pituitary stalk deviation away from the side of lesion !! **Caution** for cases of aneurysms resembling adenomas
		CT	• Sphenoid sinus septae • Sellar bony anatomy
	Intra-op navigation (MRI ± CT) ± C-arm	• Ideally always OR at least in cases of distorted anatomy • Always confirm registration with patient's surface anatomical landmarks	
Endonasal stage	Keep vomer pieces	Keep pieces of the removed vomer and use them in order to reconstruct sellar floor	
	Do not cauterize mucosa over ostium	In order to reveal sphenoid ostium, do not cauterize mucosa overlying it, but rather preserve vascular nasal mucosal flap for closure, in order to reduce risk for CSF leak	
Sphenoidal stage	Do not place tips of nasal speculum inside the sphenoid sinus	If the tips of the nasal speculum are placed into the sphenoid sinus, opening the speculum can cause fracture to the optic strut (optic nerve injury) or carotid prominence (ICA injury)	
	Sphenoid sinus ostium localization	Sphenoid sinus ostium is usually located two-third up on the face the sphenoid sinus	
	Always be oriented	**Horizontal orientation**	• Use navi + anatomical landmarks (opticocarotid recess, no further lateral than ICA groove) • Risk in case of disorientation: injury of ICA, cavernous sinus, optic canal

		Vertical orientation	• Use navigation or intra-op C-arm • Risk in case of disorientation: entry into cribriform plate →brain injury, CSF leak
Sphenoidal stage	Identify opticocarotid recess		Prior to removing sellar floor bone, always identify opticocarotid recess to better understand location of ICA
	ICA localization		Intraoperative micro-Doppler can be used for ICA identification
Intradural stage	Dura opening		Always open dura from midline to lateral, in order to decrease the risk of puncturing ICA
	Techniques for tumor delivery in case of suprasellar extension		• Valsalva maneuver • Wait until CSF pulsations deliver tumor • Expanded exposure (remove bone superiorly) • Use 30-degree endoscope
	Do not overpack tumor bed with fat graft		• Overpacking can cause chiasm compression • Brain pulsations should be transmitted by the fat graft packed in the tumor bed

10.8.4 Complications: Avoidance + Mx (Table 10.8d)

Complications	Consequences	Avoidance/Mx
ICA injury	Massive arterial bleeding	• Avoid by staying midline • Avoid with navi use • Avoid with identification of ICA with micro-Doppler • Mx with packing + DSA (Dx + coiling)
Cavernous sinus injury	• Venous bleeding • Injury of CN III (diplopia, mydriasis, ptosis) • Injury of CN IV, VI (diplopia)	• Avoid by staying midline • Avoid with navigation • Mx with packing and Floseal
Optic nerve/chiasm injury	Visual impairment	• Avoid with navigation • Do not drill optic protuberances • Do not overpack sella after tumor removal • Preserve arteries supplying optic nerve/chiasm

(Continued) ▶

CSF rhinorrhea	Infection	• Avoid with gentle dissection of tissue off diaphragma • Avoid by not extending too superiorly (entry into cribriform plate) • Mx with fat graft + anterior sellar wall repair + LD • See Chapter 11, Table 11.1g
Diabetes insipidus	Hypernatremia Severe dehydration	• Try not to pull or manipulate stalk during tumor removal • Avoid with close monitoring (serum Na+, urine specific gravity, hormones) • **Mx:** ADH replacement
Hormone deficiency (TSH, cortizole, sex hormones)		• Avoid by identifying and preserving normal pituitary gland • Mx with hormone replacement
Hydrocephalus	Neurologic deterioration (even coma)	Tx with emergent EVD placement

Other: infections, anterior nasal perforation

10.9 Unilateral Decompressive Hemicraniectomy

10.9.1 Basic Information (Table 10.9a)

Indications	• Medically refractory ↑ intracranial pressure (ICP) in TBI or ischemic stroke[8,9] • Malignant middle cerebral artery infarct (primarily nondominant hemisphere) • Similar flap can be used for the treatment of ICH or acute subdural hematoma

Positioning	• **Patient position:**
	  – Supine
	  – Small roll under ipsilateral shoulder
	• **Foam headrest** (do not use Mayfield head holder in case of trauma)
	• **Head:**
	  – Rotation: to contralateral side (take C-spine injury precautions in case of trauma)
	  – Elevation: just above heart level

Incision	Always large reverse question mark • **Starts:** 1 cm anterior to tragus (root of zygoma) • Curves posteriorly just above pinna • Courses far behind ear in parietal area (≈ 4–5 cm) • Curves medially toward sagittal suture • Curves anteriorly around 1–2 cm lateral to sagittal suture • Courses parasagittally • **End:** just before the end in the frontal area, the incision crosses over to contralateral frontal area along the hairline ! **Depth:** down to the bone (incl. temporalis muscle) !! Preserve STA (if possible)

10.9.2 Key Procedural Steps (Table 10.9b)

1. Musculotaneous flap elevation	• Subperiosteal dissection and anterior reflection
	• **Extents of temporalis dissection to facilitate max temporal craniectomy:**
	   – Zygoma root
	   – Pterior (as far below keyhole as possible)
	! **Caution:** emergently use Raney clips to expedite opening without significant blood loss

2. Craniotomy	• Several burr holes (≥ 3) (place of them at root of zygoma)
	• **Size:** 10 × 15 cm (AP extent from keyhole = 15 cm)
	• **Extents:**
	   – **Anteriorly:** as low to the anterior cranial fossa floor as possible (‼ beware of frontal sinus)
	   – **Posteriorly:** ≈ 1–2 cm from transverse sinus
	   – **Medially:** ≈ 1.5 cm from superior sagittal sinus
	   – **Laterally:** as low to the middle cranial fossa floor as possible

3. Additional craniectomy	• **Craniectomy:**
	   – Remove temporal bone with Leksell rongeurs down to middle fossa floor (‼ beware of mastoid air cells)
	   – Remove sphenoid wing with Leksell rongeurs/drills
	• **Aim:** maximum decompression of lateral brain stem

4. Dura opening	In stellate fashion (‼ beware of location of venous sinuses)
5. Associated hematomas evacuation + hemostasis	
6. Bone flap placement in abdomen	Prep abdomen and surgically create SQ pocket to store craniotomy flap
7. Closure	• Place dural substitute over dural leaves • Galea closure • Skin closure (running suture)

10.9.3 Pearls for Each Procedural Step (Table 10.9c)

Pre-op preparation	Study pre-op imaging studies	Look for: • Location, size of hematoma • Fracture over major sinus • Possible vascular lesion responsible for hematoma (ask for CTA) • Hydrocephalus
	Mayfield use	• **In trauma:** do not use due to possible skull fracture • **ICH due to possible aneurysm:** use Mayfield
	Check jugular vein	Check jugular vein for compression → venous outflow compression

(Continued) ▶

Craniotomy	Avoid midline	Always avoid midline during craniotomy (!! mark midline before incision)
	Mastoid air cells	Push wax into air cells rather than swiping wax across air cells
Dura opening	Slow dura opening	Open dura slowly !! Caution: sudden ICP reversal can cause cardiovascular collapse and hypotension
	Dural tack up sutures	Always place large number of peripheral tack-up sutures
	Epidural sinus bleeding control	• Pack epidural space with Gelfoam® soaked in thrombin • Place tack-up sutures
Closure	Dura expansion	• In case of craniotomy due to high ICP, always expand dura by patch *(continued)* ▶ • Leave dura open and overlay dural substitute
	Anterior tip lobectomy	Indication: in case of severe brain herniation due to ↑ ICP
	Difficulty closing galea	Consider: • Releasing cuts under the flap may help • Anterior tip lobectomy
	Sudden intra-op ICP increase	Consider intra-op U/S or CT to R/O new hemorrhage
	EVD placemenet	Place EVD for additional relaxation or better medical/anesthetic management of ICP

10.9.4 Complications: Avoidance + Mx (Table 10.9d)

Complications			Consequences	Avoidance/Mx
Wound complications			• Skin necrosis • CSF leak • Infection	Avoid with: • Multiple closely spaced galeal stitches • Skin closure with running suture
Frontal sinus violation			CSF rhinorhea	Avoid by: • Studying pre-op CT • Covering frontal sinus with pericranial flap (see Table 10.4c)
Hematoma	Epidural	Ipsilateral (under skin flap)	Life-threatening	• Avoid with meticulous hemostasis • Hematoma evacuation if increased ICP or midline shift > 5 mm associated to hematoma
		Contralateral (under bone fracture)	Life-threatening	• **Dx** with STAT post-op CT (OR) • **Suspect** with intra-op sudden external brain herniation after ipsilateral decompression in the presence of contralateral skull fracture/small EDH • **Mx** with craniotomy – EDH evacuation

Complications			Consequences	Avoidance/Mx	
	Intracerebral		↑ ICP, life-threatening	Avoidance	• Blood pressure monitoring – control • Checking and correcting coagulation status
				Mx	• Conservative measures for lowering ICP (hyperventilation, mannitol, narcotic analgesics, etc.) (see Chapter 5, Table 5.8b) • Hematoma evacuation for ICP > 22 mm Hg, midline shift > 5 mm Hg
Infection			• Drainage from wound • Nonhealing wound • Fever, malaise, nightsweating • Meningitis • Lab tests findings (↑ CRP, leukocytosis)		• Antibiotics (6 weeks iv + 6 weeks po) • Wash-out and debridement in OR (if not responding well to antibiotics or if empyema) (see also Table 11.3c)
Acute brain swelling		Avoidance	• External herniation of brain matter through craniotomy		• Head should be elevated • Internal jugular vein should not be compressed (no neck flexion, no ties around neck)
		Mx	• Difficulty closing surgical wound		• Head elevation • Verify good venous outflow • Mannitol (1 g/kg iv) • Hyperventilation • EVD • Check for new hemorrhage w/ intra-op U/S • Lobectomy (see Chapter 11, Table 11.1a)
Venous sinus injury	• Air embolism • Hemorrhage • Infarction			Avoidance	• Mark midline on scalp before incision • Study pre-op CT for fractures over sinuses
				Mx	• Notify anesthesia to be ready with IV fluids and blood • Irrigate field continuously to avoid air embolism • Gentle tamponade w/ Gelfoam • Repair if bigger hole (see also Chapter 11: Surgical Complications)

10.10 Far Lateral Suboccipital Approach

10.10.1 Basic Information (Table 10.10a)

Indications	Exposure	270 degree around medulla oblongata (including lateral aspect of ventromedial p-fossa) in the following areas: • Inferior clivus, inferior petroclival junction • Anterior/anterolateral foramen magnum • Occipital condyle • Posterior aspect of jugular foramen • Cervicomedullary junction

	Lesions	• **Tumors**
		  – Extra-axial (extradural/intradural)
		    ◦ Chordoma, chordosarcoma
		    ◦ Metastasis
		    ◦ Glomus jugulare
		    ◦ Meningioma
		    ◦ Schwannoma
		  – Intra-axial tumors with extension to the anterolateral surface of medulla oblongata and lower pons
		• **Vascular lesions**
		  – Aneurysms (VA, PICA, vertebrobasilar junction)
		  – AVMs

Contraindications		• Lesions located in ventral brain stem above pontomedullary junction • Lesions located in the upper acoustic meatus and tentorium (prefer retrosigmoid) • Ventromedial compartment of lower p-fossa (petroclival region, lateral aspect of lower two-third of clivus) (the endonasal transclival approach is an option for this area) • P-fossa lesions with supratentorial extension (require combined approaches)

Positioning/ preparation		• **Patient position:**
		  – Three-quarter prone (park bench)
		  – Contralateral shoulder: down
		  – Contralateral arm: in a shoulder sling off the edge of the bed
		  – Ipsilateral shoulder: up in mild flexion on arm rest, pulled away from head
		• **Mayfield clamp:**
		  – Posterior paired pins → contralateral occipital bone (equator)
		  – Anterior single pin → ipsilateral frontal bone above superior temporal line
		• **Head (aim:** posteromedial portion of ipsilateral occipital condyle at highest point)
		  – Slight flexion
		  – Slight lateral flexion toward floor
		  – Slight elevation
		  – Rotation: 45 degree away from lesion (toward contralateral shoulder)
		• **Intra-op neuromonitoring:** MEPs, SSEPs, brainstem auditory evoked potentials, EMG (facial muscles, tongue, soft palate), endotracheal tube electrodes, nerve stimulator

Incision	Hockey-stick shaped
	• **Midline vertical incision:** from C7 spinous process → to just above inion
	• **Horizontal incision:** from just above inion → along superior nuchal line (transverse sinus) → to just above mastoid tip
	• **Small vertical incision:** along posterior edge of mastoid process (from just above→ to just below)

10.10.2 Key Procedural Steps (Table 10.10b)

1. Soft tissue elevation	• **Subperiosteal muscle elevation – exposure of bony landmarks:**
	– Exposure of all hemiocciput down to foramen magnum
	– Exposure of medial surface of mastoid process down to its tip
	– Exposure of C1 laterally up to the tip of its transverse process
	• Reflect large musculocutaneous flap laterally – posteriorly by starting soft-tissue dissection from level of C6 spinous process
2. VA mobilization	• Use intra-op Doppler for localization of VA
	• Identify – cauterize – divide venous plexus around VA
	• Dissect VA off perivascular venous plexus
	• Remove posterior bony part of foramen transversarium
	• Untether VA by dividing several periosteal attachments
	• Mobilize VA inferomedially away from occipital condyle w/ vessel loop
3. Unilateral suboccipital craniotomy	**Craniotomy cuts**
	• **Medial vertical cut** (just lateral to midline): from foramen magnum → up to just before transverse sinus. (always cut away from sinus)
	• **Lateral vertical cut** (curvilinear): from just inferomedial to asterion → down to foramen magnum (as lateral as possible just posterior to condyle).
	• **Horizontal cut:** along inferior edge of transverse sinus (between superior extents of vertical cuts)
	!! Primary author uses high-speed drill to make all cuts for safer exposure of the edges of transverse and sigmoid sinuses
4. C1 hemilaminectomy	**Aims:** allows inferior extent of dural incision
5. Retrosigmoid mastoidectomy	**Aims:** exposure of jugular bulb
6. Bony skeletonization of venoussinuses	**Bony skeletonization of:**
	• Transverse sinus
	• Sigmoid sinus
	• Beginning of jugular bulb
7. Occipital condyle drilling[10] (transcondylar variation)	• **Extent of drilling:** ≤ half of condyle posteriorly (extra drilling requires occipitocervical fusion)
	• **Aim:** additional anterior visualization
	• Hypoglossal canal serves as the landmark for the anterior limit of condylar drilling (see Table 10.10c: Occipital condyle drilling)

(Continued) ▶

8. Dura opening	• **P-fossa dura (lazy J insicion):** from transverse–sigmoid junction → to foramen magnum (just posterior to the VA intradural entry)
	• **Cervical dura (linear paramedian incision):** from foramen magnum → down to upper edge of C2 lamina
	!! Beware of circular sinus (marginal sinus)
9. Intradural dissection (depending on pathology)	• Open cisterna magna → allow egress of CSF
	• Dissect arachnoid between tonsils–medulla → retract tonsils to allow exposure of deeper structures
	• Identify CN VI–XII, verterbral artery, vertebrobasilar junction, PICA
	• Divide dentate ligament for more ventral exposure
	• Dissection depending on lesion
10. Closure	• Watertight dura closure
	• Bone flap replacement
	• Muscle and galea closure by layers
	• Skin closure (prefer running nylon sutures – oversew)

10.10.3 Pearls for Each Procedural Step (Table 10.10c)

Pre-op preparation	Pre-op CTA and MRA/MRV	Study pre-op CTA and MRA to identify:
		• The exact course and the dominance of VA (also study PICA anatomy)
		• Anatomy and dominance of sinuses
	Pre-op Dandy burr hole for EVD	Main author leaves burr-hole ready pre-op for EVD placement
Soft tissue elevation	Always be oriented to spinal midline	Early identification of intramuscular septum → identification of spinal midline → exposure of C1–C3 hemilamina
	C1 dissection	Always dissect C1 on inferior laminar border in order to initially avoid sulcus arteriosus
VA dissection	VA localization	• Use Doppler to identify VA
		• VA is located in the floor of the suboccipital triangle (formed by superior oblique, the inferior oblique, and the rectus capitis major muscle) (see Chapter 9, Fig. 9.9)
		• Palpate the groove for VA on the lateral aspect of posterior arch of C1 with a Penfield No 4 to estimate location of VA (see also ▶ Fig. 9.2)
	VA venous plexus bleeding control	Control bleeding from venous plexus around VA with thrombin soaked morcelized Gelfoam

Extra bone removal	Additional C2, C3 hemilaminectomies	**Pros:** ↑ visualization (if req.)
	Bony skeletonization of transverse–sigmoid sinus	**Pros:** ↑ working angle → view parallel to petrosal cerebellar surface + ventral brain stem
	Mastoid air cells	Always wax mastoid air cells after sigmoid sinus exposure
Dura opening	Be aware of the circular sinus	**For dura incision:** ligate circular sinus with clips → divide sinus → oversew
Occipital condyle drilling	**Tips to avoid hypoglossal canal violation during occipital condyle drilling**	Drill occipital condyle from po*(Continued)* ▶ anterior (cortical bone and then cancellous bone) → while drilling cancellous bone beware of change in bone constistency (cortical bone surrounding hypoglossal canal) and color (bluish color due to hypoglossal venous plexus)
	Preserve atlanto-occipital joint	During occipital condyle drilling (transcondylar variation), preserve the atlanto-occipital joint in order to prevent instability
Intradural stage	**Tips to avoid use of retractors**	• Opening of cisterna magna → allow CSF drainage • Park-bench position allows natural cerebellum retraction from gravity • Mannitol • Tumor debulking – pull tumor into surgical field instead of retracting neurovascular structures

10.10.4 Complications: Avoidance + Mx (Table 10.10d)

Complications	Consequences	Avoidance/Mx
Venous sinus injury		• Avoid by preferring to unroof sinuses with drill rather than craniotome • **Mx:** see Table 10.7d and Table 11.1d
CSF leak	• CSF otorrhea or rhinorrhea • CSF leak from wound • Subcutaneous CSF collection • Infection, meningitis	**Avoid by:** • Waxing mastoid air cells • Watertight dura closure • Meticulous layered closure (for Mx, see Table 11.1f)
Air embolism		See Table 10.7d
VA injury		• Avoid by being oriented to spinal midline • Always have a set of permanent and temporary aneurysm clips

(Continued) ▶

Complications	Consequences	Avoidance/Mx
Hypoglossal nerve injury	• Ipsilateral tongue deviation • Dysarthria • Swallowing difficulties	Avoid by preserving canal (see also Table 10.10c)
Lower CN injury	• Aspiration risk • Swallowing difficulties • Hoarseness	Avoid by sharp arachnoid dissection to minimize tension during manipulation

Craniocervical instability		• Avoid by:
		  – Preserve atlanto-occipital joint
		  – Drill < half of occipital condyle
		• **Tx:** occipitocervical fusion

10.11 Anterior Cervical Diskectomy and Fusion G

10.11.1 Basic Information (Table 10.11a)

Indications	• Radiculopathy due to cervical disk herniation causing:
	  – Persistent arm pain despite conservative measures
	  – Progressive neurologic deficit
	• Cervical myelopathy
	• Neoplasia
	• Infection (discitis/epidural empyema limited to one disk level)

Contraindications	• Posterior compression → prefer posterior approaches • Professions that depend on use of voice (e.g., singers) • Ossification of the posterior longitudinal ligament (relative contraindication)

Positioning	• **Patient position:**
	  – Supine
	  – Roll between scapulae
	  – Gentle caudal shoulder traction with tape
	• **Neck:** slight neck extension (in cervical myelopathy, be careful not to overextend and use fiberoptic intubation to avoid mechanical injury of spinal cord)
	• **Pre-op cervical level localization for skin incision:**
	  – **Use anatomical landmarks**
	    ○ Hyoid bone → C3 vertebra
	    ○ Thyroid cartilage → C4–5 disk space
	    ○ Carotid tubercle or cricoid ring → C6
	  – **Confirm w/ lateral x-ray**
	• Neurophyshiologic monitoring (EMG, MEPs, SSEPs)

Incision	Transverse skin incision (along skin crease if possible): • **Starts:** at medial border of sternocleidomastoid muscle • **Ends:** to just past midline

10.11.2 Key Procedural Steps (Table 10.11b)

1. Platysma incision	

2. Develop avascular plane to prevertebral fascia	• Use blunt dissection along medial border of sternocleidomastoid
	• Develop an avascular plane retracting:
	  – Sternocleidomastoid muscle and carotid laterally
	  – Trachea–esophagus medially

3. Longus coli detachment	Detach longus coli muscle laterally → expose vertebral bodies. Beware of location of sympathetic trunks (see ▶ Fig. 9.10)
4. Intra-op x-ray	Place a spine needle into disk space → confirm cervical level w/ x-ray
5. Place retractors underneath each longus colli muscle	• Expose vertebral bodies – disks • Retraction on the mediolateral axis
6. Place Caspar retractors	Place pins in the midportion of vertebral bodies → attach Caspar distractor → interbody distraction (in cephalocaudal axis) in the involved disk level
7. Diskectomy	• Incise disk annulus w/ scalpel (four separate cuts, create square) • Dissect disk material from end plate w/ curette • Remove anterior two-third of disk w/ curettes and pituitary rongeur • Remove posterior one-third of disk w/ drill up to posterior longitudinal ligament • Perform foraminotomies as needed
8. Remove cartilagenous end plates	Use high-speed drill
9. Divide posterior longitudinal ligament	Use careful sharp disection
10. Remove osteophytes	• Use high-speed drill • Confirm adequate decompression with blunt nerve hook ! Beware of the use of Kerisson punch → foot plate may lead to cord injury
11. Place graft in disk space	! Caution: • Release disk space distraction before graft measurement • Make sure graft does not overdistract disc space
12. Place metal plate	• Place shortest plate possible • Screw plate into vertebrae
13. Closure	• Meticulous hemostasis (drain placement is optional) • Confirm integrity of trachea/esophagus and vessels (carotid, internal jugular vein) • Platysma closure • Skin closure

(Continued) ▶

10.11.3 Pearls for Each Procedural Step (Table 10.11c)

Pre-op measures/ precautions	Pre-op study of MRI/CT	• Study thoroughly the pre-op MRI/CT images and correlate the sites of neural compression with the patient's symptoms • Ask for CT to look for osteophytes and calcified ligaments/disks
	Fiberoptic intubation	In pts with cervical myelopathy, ask for fiberoptic intubation to avoid neck extension, which can cause a mechanical spinal cord injury
	Key maneuvers to avoid recurrent laryngeal nerve palsy	• Once retractors open, deflate endotracheal cuff momentarily (until there is an air leak and then barely reinflate) → allows nerve to change position • Release Cloward retractors q 45 min (see also precautions in reop) ! Recurrent laryngeal nerve courses in a groove between esophagus – trachea
	Precautions in reop	• Ask for orogastric tube placement in order to identify easier esophagus • In case of reoperation, use ipsilateral side approach or if you will use contralateral side → always ruleout vocal cord paralysis with direct laryngoscopy on the side of the previous approach
Approach	Place incision inferior to involved diskspace	Place incision 1 cm below disk space → this allows visualization along the angle of disk space, which courses on a sagittal plane from anterior–caudal to posterior–cephalad
	Carotid protection	During the initial stage of developing a plane to the prevertebral fascia, always retract pulsatile carotid with a finger of the nondominant hand during dissection → this always allows to locate the carotid, thus avoiding its injury
	Place Cloward retractors underneathlongus colli	In this way, longus colli bear all the force from retraction → soft-tissue injury is prevented
	Disk space distraction in case of multilevel procedure	Distract only one disk space at a time
Diskectomy	Lateral margin of diskectomy	Identify uncal joints as lateral margin of disk resection
	Beware of VA	• Mean distance between the medial border of the uncinate process – foramen transversarium is approximately 5 mm (see also ▶ Fig. 9.10) • Always maintain midline orientation → prevents lateral deviation • Do not use Kerisson punch > 10 mm from midline

Graft instrumentation	Graft placement	• Release disk space distraction prior to estimating/measuring graft placement • Do not overdistract disk space with graft • Avoid or minimize bone wax use for bone bleeding control in the intervertebral space → it may interfere with fusion
	Plate placement	Remove anterior vertebral osteophytes with high-speed drill → to allow the plate to lie flat on vertebral bodies
	Screw placement	Screws should be convergent in order to increase pull-out strength

10.11.4 Complications: Avoidance + Mx (Table 10.11d)

Complications	Consequences/symptoms	Avoidance/Mx
Dysphagia (10%)		• R/O hematoma • Avoid excessive esophagus retraction • Typically transient
Post-op hematoma (6%)	• Breathing difficulties (stridor, respiratory distress) • Swallowing difficulties	• Avoid by using blunt retractors • STAT evacuation, when pt develops breathing OR swallowing difficulties (see Chapter 11, Table 11.2e)

Recurrent laryngeal nerve palsy (3%)	Hoarseness	• **Avoidance tips:**
		  – Once retractors open, deflate endotracheal cuff just before there is an air leak
		  – Release Cloward retractors q 45 min
		• Usually neuropraxic → transient (3–6 mos)

VA injury		• **Small injury:** packing → post-op DSA • **Significant injury:** may require expanding exposure for primary arterial control (see also Chapter 11: Surgical complications)
Carotid artery injury		primary repair
Dural perforation	CSF subdural collection or CSF leak	• Primary repair • LD always (see also Chapter 11: Surgical complications)

(Continued) ▶

Complications	Consequences/symptoms	Avoidance/Mx
Pharynx/esophageal perforation	• Dysphagia, fever • Subcutaneous emphysema • Mediastinitis	• In case of excessive retraction → check esophageal undersurface for small tears • Primary repair (see also Chapter 11: Surgical complications)
Tracheal perforation		Primary repair
Horner's syndrome	• Miosis • Enophthalmos, ptosis • Face anidrosis	Avoid by not excessively detaching the longus colli
Instrumentation failure: • Graft collapse OR shift OR nonunion • Instrumentation shift		• Revision surgery • Consider posterior approaches
Myelopathy worsening		• R/O graft migration with cord compression • R/O insufficient decompression → if present, decompress further posteriorly • Avoid neck hyperextension

Others: infection, adjacent level degeneration, nerve root injury, pneumothorax (for lower C-spine)

10.12 Lumbar Microdiskectomy G

10.21.1 Basic Information (Table 10.12a)

Indications	**Disc herniation causing:** • Radiculopathic pain failing to improve with conservative measures • Progressive severe weakness **! Caution:** make sure that both symptoms and clinical findings can be attributed to the imaging findings of disc herniation
Contraindications	• Large central disk herniation causing cauda equina syndrome) → perform full laminectomy • Mechanical back pain • Drop foot due to peroneal nerve compression at the head of fibula • Symptoms due to peripheral neuropathy (usually easily diagnosed due to bilateral extremities involvement and nonradicular distribution of pain/numbness) • Vascular claudication

Positioning	• **Patient position:**
	– Prone
	– Chest rolls, Wilson frame
	• **L-spine:** flexion
	• **Pre-op lumbar level localization:**
	– W/ x-ray
	– Imaginary line from anterior superior iliac crest to the L-spine crosses roughly L4–L5 interspace
Incision	Linear midline incision (based on the pre-op level localization with x-ray)

10.12.2 Key Procedural Steps (Table 10.12b)

1. Subcutaneous dissection	
2. Fascial incision	• Identify thoracolumbar fascia • Dissect subcutaneous fat off fascia w/ periosteal elevator • Paramedian fascial incision w/ monopolar electrocautery (allows fascial cuff for closure, incision may be extended under the skin incision)
3. Subperiosteal paravertebral muscle dissection	Detach paravertebral muscles subperiosteally from the spinous processes and laminae at the involved lumbar level unilaterally using monopolar electrocautery
4. Intra-op x-ray	**Always use the pedicle of the verterbra as a reference** for x-ray localization of disk fragment and for planning hemilaminectomy
5. Hemilaminectomy	• Find interspace of interest (expose lower margin of lamina above and upper margin of lamina below) • Perform a lateral laminectomy and medial facetectomy w/ drill – Kerrison punch
6. Removal of ligamentum flavum	• Split ligamentum flavum medially just under the spinous processes w/ a right-angled instrument until you identify the whitish thecal sac • Create a window through ligamentum flavum using Kerrison rongeurs • Remove ligamentum flavum window using pituitary rongeur • Extend window opening medially to laterally using Kerrison rongeurs

(Continued) ▶

7. Diskectomy	• Identify involved root coursing around the pedicle below
	• Retract gently nerve root–thecal sac to midline using a nerve root retractor
	• Make a small incision in the posterior longitudinal ligament w/ No. 11 blade (from medial to lateral directing the blade's sharp edge away from thecal sac)
	• Remove disk material w/ pituitary rongeur
	• Explore disk space by making a small linear incision in the disk annulus removing residual free disk material w/ pituitary rongeur
	• Explore foramina above and below the disk herniation for stenosis
	• Irrigate disk space under high pressure to remove free disk material
8. Closure	• Meticulous hemostasis
	• Meticulous fascial closure (w/ interrupted 2–0 sutures)
	• Subcutaneous layer closure
	• Skin closure

10.12.3 Pearls for Each Procedural Step (Table 10.12c)

Pre-op preparation	Complete pre-op and intra-op understanding of source of root compression	• Study carefully the pre-op MRI/CT to R/O facet hypertrophy causing lateral recess stenosis OR foraminal stenosis → if present, additional decompression and/or foraminotomy is required (apart from diskectomy) • Intraoperatively use probe to confirm adequate decompression in the canal and through the foramen
	Use of pedicle for localization	Always use pedicle for X-ray localization of disk fragment preoperatively and intraoperatively
	Positioning	• Place L-spine in slight flexion → this opens interlaminar space allowing entry into the canal with less bone removal • Frame should leave abdomen hanging → this reduces intra-abnominal pressure and thus epidural venous pressure leading to less bleeding in the operative field
Hemilaminectomy	Bone bleeding control	Control w/ wax on a Freer elevator → push w/ cottonoid – bayonet forceps
	Avoid destabilization of spine	• A medial facetectomy is quite often used to expose the lateral dura margin • Thus, always be aware of the lateral border of the pars interarticularis, so that during initial exposure, sufficient bone width in the pars area (from its lateral border) is left

| Diskectomy | Aggressive vs. conservative diskectomy (controversial)[11] | Definitions | • **Conservative:** removal of only the herniated disk fragment
• **Aggressive:** removal of herniated disk fragment + curettage of disk space |
| | | Comparison | • **Persistent back/leg pain:** ↑ w/ aggressive discectomy
• **Recurrent disk herniation:** non-significant ↑ w/ conservative discectomy |

10.12.4 Complications: Avoidance + Mx (Table 10.12d)

Complications	Consequences	Avoidance/Mx

Dura violation		• **Intra-op identification:** primary closure under microscope:
		  – Primary dura closure (6–0 nylon continuous suture, oversew, Castroviejo needle holder) + fibrin glue
		  – Watertight fascia closure
		• **Post-op CSF leak from wound:** oversewing of wound → if persistent, dura repair ± lumbar drainage at a superior point (if leak is from lower lumbar spine)
		(see also Chapter 11: Surgical complications)

Recurrent disc herniation		Treat like fresh disk. First conservatively and only if it fails proceed with reoperation
Injury of great abdomen vessels	• Unexplained hypotension • Unexplained blood in disk space • • life threatening	• Can be avoided by marking the allowed depth (≈ 35 mm) on the instruments (rongeurs, curettes) • See Chapter 11, Table 11.3c
Wrong level surgery		Avoid by using intraoperative x-ray localization and correlating intraoperative findings with pre-op imaging
Spine destabilization		**Avoid by:** • Not extending medial facetectomy > 50% of facet • Preserving pars interarticularis
Back pain		Avoid curettage of the end plates and overagressive removal of normal disk material

(Continued) ▶

Complications	Consequences	Avoidance/Mx
Nerve root injury		• Beware of conjoined nerve root • Mx: steroids + repair of dura (if violated)
Wound infection		See Chapter 11: Surgical complications
Discitis	• Severe post-op back pain few weeks post-op exacerbated by any movement • Fever w/ chills (not always) • Limitation of range of motion spine • **spine tenderness**	TLSO + antibiotics (6 weeks po + 6 months iv) + analgesics
Epidural hematoma		• Avoid w/ subfascial drains • Emergent reexploration to evacuate hematoma

10.13 Lumbar Laminectomy

10.13.1 Basic Information (Table 10.13a)

Indications	• Neurogenic claudication due to spinal stenosis confirmed by imaging • Large central disk herniation causing cauda equina syndrome • Initial step of exposure for decompression of spinal canal due to other pathologies (tumors, epidural hematoma/empyema) • Tethered spinal cord ! **Caution:** make sure that both symptoms and clinical findings can be attributed to the imaging findings (for degenerative spinal stenosis)
Contraindications	• Vascular claudication • Peripheral neuropathy • Mechanical back pain • Coexisting spine instability and/or deformity (may require additional instrumentation) • Medical comorbidities with increased surgical risk

Positioning	• **Patient position:**
	  – Prone
	  – Chest rolls, Wilson frame
	• **L- spine:** flexion (↑ interlaminar space)
	• **Pre-op lumbar level localization:**
	  – W/ x-ray
	  – Imaginary line from anterior superior iliac crest to the L-spine crosses roughly L4–L5 interspace

Incision	Linear midline incision (depending on pre-op imaging and pre-op X-ray localization)

10.13.2 Key Procedural Steps (Table 10.13b)

1. Subcutaneous dissection	
2. Fascial incision	• Identify thoracolumbar fascia • Dissect subcutaneous fat off fascia w/ periosteal elevator • Midline fascial incision
3. Subperiosteal paravertebral muscle dissection	• Dissect paravertebral muscles subperiosteally off the spinous processes and laminae at the involved lumbar levels bilaterally using Bovie electrocautery • Expose facet joints as well • If fusion is planned, also expose transverse processes
4. Intra-op x-ray	• Always use the pedicle of the verterbra as a reference for x-ray localization and for planning laminectomies • Ask for x-ray localization after exposing one level → then extend exposure as needed
5. Laminectomies	• Remove spinous processes w/ Leksell rongeurs • Remove laminae (from caudal → to cephalad) w/ Leksell rongeurs as much as possible • Thin laminae w/ drill • Complete laminectomies w/ Kerrison rongeurs (from caudal to cephalad) preserving initially the underlying ligamentum flavum and epidural fat, which serve to prevent inadvertent dura violation (cottonoids can also be used for dura protection during laminectomy)
6. Removal of ligamentum flavum	• Split ligamentum flavum w/ a right-angled instrument until you identify the whitish thecal sac • Remove ligamentum flavum and epidural fat until thecal sac is decompressed • Assistant may protect dura with Woodson dental instrument
7. Further widening of laminectomy (medial facetectomy)	• Partial removal of medial facet (allows lateral recess decompression) • Removal of ligamentum flavum and osteophytes from the medial surface of pedicle • Use probe to look for potential residual compression of thecal sac and especially nerve roots • If present, decompress further
8. Foraminotomies	• Identify corresponding pedicle • Identify root take-off from dural sac • Follow root from take-off to foramen and decompress along its course as needed • Remove dorsal compressive pathology in foramen w/ Kerisson punch • Place blunt probe in the foramen to confirm sufficient decompression
9. Closure	• Meticulous hemostasis (use of subfascial drains at surgeon's preference) • Muscle layer closure (controversial) • Meticulous fascial closure (w/ interrupted 2–0 sutures) • Subcutaneous layer closure • Skin closure

10.13.3 Pearls for Each Procedural Step (Table 10.13c)

Pre-op preparation	Complete pre-op and intra-op understanding of source of root compression	• Study carefully the pre-op MRI/CT to R/O foraminal stenosis → if present, foraminotomy is required • Intraoperatively use probe to confirm adequate decompression in the canal and through the foramen
	Positioning	• Place L-spine in slight flexion → this opens interlaminar space • Frame should leave abdomen hanging → this reduces intra-abnominal pressure and thus epidural venous pressure leading to less bleeding in the operative field
	Caution w/ reoperations	• Study pre-op CT • First expose "virgin" bone surfaces surrounding all previous surgical fields • Start laminectomies from there
Muscle dissection	Paravertebral muscle dissection	Dissect paravertebral muscles of the spinous processes/laminae using Bovie cautery from caudal to rostral: More efficient removal of muscle insertions Less blood loss
Laminectomy	Always keep bone removed during laminectomies	May be needed if a posterolateral fusion is later decided during case
	Bone bleeding control	Control w/ wax on a Freer elevator → push w/ cottonoid – bayonet forceps
	Preserve pars interarticularis	In lumbar laminectomy, always preserve pars interarticularis to avoid fracture and/or instability
Duralsac decompression	Tips to avoid dura violation	• **During removal of ligamentum flavum:** place a cottonoid between dura–ligament → advance Kerisson rongeur on cottonoid before each bite • **During laminectomy:** prefer overlapping Kerisson rongeur bites → no bony sharp spurs are formed, preserve ligamentum flavum/epidural fat initially
	Beware of midline raphe	In L5/S1 interspace, beware of midline raphe between dura and ligament flavum in order to avoid pulling on it and potentially causing an inadvertent midline durotomy
	Control of epidural venous plexus bleeding	• Place thrombin soaked Gelfoam over venous plexus • Push Gelfoam in place with cottonoid – bayonet forceps

| Foraminotomy | Foraminotomy indications | • Radiculopathic pain distribution attributed to specific nerve root (clinically ± EMG confirmation)
• Pre-op imaging findings of foraminal stenosis (CT, MRI)
• Intra-op nerve root compression at the foramen |

10.13.4 Complications: Avoidance + Mx (Table 10.13d)

Complications	Consequences	Avoidance/Mx

Dura violation		• Beware of spina bifida
		• Intra-op identification: primary closure under microscope:
		  – Primary dura closure (6–0 nylon continuous suture, oversew, Castroviejo needle holder) + fibrin glue
		  – Watertight fascia closure
		• Post-op CSF leak through wound: oversewing of wound → if persistent, dura repair ± LD at a superior point (if leak is from lower lumbar spine)
		
		(see also Chapter 11: Surgical complications)

Spinal destabilization/ spondylolisthesis		May require instrumentation
Inadequate decompression	Persistence of symptoms	Reimaging with MRI with contrast. If instrumentation has been placed then obtain CT myelogram
Wrong level surgery		Avoid by using intraoperative x-ray localization and corelating intraoperative findings with pre-op imaging
Nerve root injury		• Beware of conjoined nerve root • Mx: steroids + repair of dura (if violated)
Wound infection		See Chapter 11: Surgical complications
Epidural hematoma		• Avoid w/ subfascial drains • Emergent re-exploration to evacuate hematoma

References

[1] Coscarella E, Vishteh AG, Spetzler RF, Seoane E, Zabramski JM. Subfascial and submuscular methods of temporal muscle dissection and their relationship to the frontal branch of the facial nerve. Technical note. J Neurosurg. 2000; 92(5):877–880

[2] Babakurban ST, Cakmak O, Kendir S, Elhan A, Quatela VC. Temporal branch of the facial nerve and its relationship to fascial layers. Arch Facial Plast Surg. 2010; 12(1):16–23

[3] Aziz KMA, Froelich SC, Cohen PL, Sanan A, Keller JT, van Loveren HR. The one-piece orbitozygomatic approach: the MacCarty burr hole and the inferior orbital fissure as keys to technique and application. Acta Neurochir (Wien). 2002; 144(1):15–24

[4] Shimizu S, Tanriover N, Rhoton AL, Jr, Yoshioka N, Fujii K. MacCarty keyhole and inferior orbital fissure in orbitozygomatic craniotomy. Neurosurgery. 2005; 57(1, Suppl):152–159, discussion 152–159

[5] Jandial R, McCormick P, Black PML. Core Techniques in Operative Neurosurgery. Philadelphia, PA: Elsevier Saunders, 2011

[6] Rhoton AL. Cranial Anatomy and Surgical Approaches. Philadelphia, PA: Lippincott Williams & Wilkins, 2003

[7] Fossett DT, Caputy AJ. Operative Neurosurgical Anatomy. New York, NY: Thieme, 2002

[8] Hutchinson PJ, Kolias AG, Timofeev IS, et al; RESCUEicp Trial Collaborators. Trial of decompressive craniectomy for traumatic intracranial hypertension N Engl J Med. 2016; 375(12):1119–1130

[9] Cooper DJ, Rosenfeld JV, Murray L, et al; DECRA Trial Investigators. Australian and New Zealand Intensive Care Society Clinical Trials Group. Decompressive craniectomy in diffuse traumatic brain injury. N Engl J Med. 2011; 364(16):1493–1502

[10] Rhoton AL, Jr. The far-lateral approach and its transcondylar, supracondylar, and paracondylar extensions. Neurosurgery. 2000; 47(3, Suppl):S195–S209

[11] McGirt MJ, Ambrossi GLG, Datoo G, et al. Recurrent disc herniation and long-term back pain after primary lumbar discectomy: review of outcomes reported for limited versus aggressive disc removal. Neurosurgery. 2009; 64(2):338–344, discussion 344–345

Suggested Reading

Connolly ES, McKhann GM, Huang J. Fundamentals of Operative Techniques in Neurosurgery, 2nd edition. New York: Thieme, 2011

Fessler RG, Sekhar LN. Atlas of Neurosurgical Techniques: Spine and Peripheral Nerves. Thieme, 2016

Greenberg MS. Handbook of Neurosurgery, 8th ed. New York, NY: Thieme, 2016

Jandial R, McCormick P, Black PML. Core Techniques in Operative Neurosurgery. Philadelphia: Elsevier Saunders, 2011. • D. T. Fossett and A. J. Caputy, Operative Neurosurgical Anatomy. New York: Thieme, 2002

Lawton MT. Seven Aneurysms: Tenets and Techniques for Clipping. New York, NY: Thieme, 2011

Rhoton L. Cranial Anatomy and Surgical Approaches. Philadelphia: Lippincott Williams & Wilkins, 2003

Vaccaro R, Todd AJ. Spine Surgery: Tricks of the Trade. Thieme, 2016

11 Surgical Complications

11.1 Complications After Cranial Procedures

Acute brain swelling and herniation during craniotomy (Table 11.1a 🔊)

Presentation	• Acute brain swelling • External herniation of brain matter through craniotomy
Diagnostic studies	May consider intraoperative U/S to rule out intracranial hemorrhage
Treatment	• Elevate head-end of the bed (reversed trendelenburg) • Verify good venous outflow • Mannitol 1 g/kg intravenous (IV) • Hyperventilate • Emergent ventriculostomy for CSF drainage • Address parameters that could contribute (volatile anesthetics, high arterial blood pressure) • Increase narcotic analgesia • Lobectomy or hemicraniectomy • Barbiturates

Intraoperative seizure during craniotomy (Table 11.1b)

Presentation	• Sudden often violent shaking of patient • Unexplained rise in systolic blood pressure • Unexplained difficulty ventilating patient
Diagnostic studies	None
Treatment	• Irrigate brain with ice-cold ringer's solution • Discontinue inciting event (e.g., Intraoperative cortical stimulation, deep brain stimulation [DBS], etc.) • Administer IV anti-epileptic drug (midazolam, phenytoin, levetiracetam) • R/O acute cause, such as intracerebral hemorrhage (ICH), pin perforation, etc. • Beware of patient pulling out of pins • If persistent, consider barbiturates

Intraoperative acute hydrocephalus (Table 11.1c)

Presentation	Acute external herniation of brain matter during surgery, typically in posterior fossa surgery and surgeries within ventricles, due to obstruction from blood clot
Diagnostic studies	• Usually a clinical diagnosis • May consider use of intra-op U/S
Treatment	Emergent placement of ventriculostomy **Remember: to prep for emergent EVD placement before surgery or place drain before even starting craniotomy (safest)**

Venous sinus laceration (Table 11.1d)

Presentation	Sudden massive dark venous bleeding
Diagnostic studies	Pre-op magnetic resonance venography (MRV): preoperatively assess sinus dominance, patency, and proximity to surgical site
Treatment	• Notify anesthesia to be ready with IV fluids and blood • Irrigate field continuously to avoid air embolism • Hold gentle tamponade with gelfoam or muscle patch or "sinus patty" (patty + surgicel + floseal/surgiflo) • Consider collagen powder (avitene), fibrin glue, and other hemostyptic agents. Beware not to inadvertently pack them within Lumen of critical sinuses, since this may lead to sinus occlusion • If necessary, attempt repair with direct suturing or with use of patch (i.e., Pericranial flap) • Do not attempt to use bipolar coagulation; this maneuver only enlarges the hole • If all else fails and not a critical/dominant sinus, then sacrifice **Remember: always notify anesthesiologist before operating near venous sinus**

Venous air embolism (Table 11.1e ◀))

Presentation	• Direct visualization of air being sucked into vein or venous sinus • Sudden and unexplained hypotension • Unexplained sudden drop in end-tidal Pco_2
Diagnostic studies	• Transesophageal echocardiography (has to be placed before surgery in cases with increased risk) • Precordial doppler U/S intraoperatively • Aspiration of blood foam through central venous catheter (has to be placed before surgery in cases with increased risk)
Treatment	• Lower the head end of the bed immediately (Trendelenburg) • Flood operative field with copious irrigation • Repeated aspiration of blood foam via central venous catheter until foam clears • If source of embolism is apparent (i.e., venous sinus), attempt repair • Place patient in left lateral decubitus position, so that the air bubble moves to the right atrium • Start patient on 100% oxygen **Remember: always notify anesthesiologist before operating near venous sinus**

CSF leak after craniotomy (Table 11.1f)

Presentation	• Common after certain surgeries (up to 30% of skull base surgeries have CSF leaks)
	• May present as:
	  a. External leakage of clear or nearly clear fluid leaking from wound, ear, nose, or into mouth
	  b. Subgaleal CSF collection (internal leakage; wound closed but CSF collection apparent)

Diagnostic studies	Studies to identify source of leakage: a. Often not needed as source is apparent b. If site is not apparent, consider thin-cut CT or cisternogram. Usually, there are air bubbles intracranially or opacified air sinus near leakage site

Treatment	1. Always R/O hydrocephalus
	2. Basics:
	  • Head of bed up 15 degrees
	  • Avoid straining or blowing nose
	  • Stool softeners
	  • Consider short-term acetazolamide 250 mg orally every day (reduces CSF production)
	3. For external skin leak: oversew the leak (use running–locking sutures over the leaking part + 1 cm proximal and 1 cm distal → convert external drainage into internal CSF collection)
	4. CSF diversion for 3–7 d:
	  • Lumbar drain (remember: this is a volume-driven CSF diversion and not pressure driven)
	  • Start with 5 ml/h → increase daily as tolerated (headaches!!)
	Caution: pneumocephalus—if air is sucked in from negative CSF drainage pressure
	5. Apply external counter pressure for 3–14 d: tight head wrap with elastic bandage (ace bandage) ± tapping collection
	6. Repeat surgery for direct repair: consider use of duraplasty, dura tissue glue (fibrin or other)
	7. Lumboperitoneal (LP) shunt: if leak persists, some practitioners use LP shunt (communicating CSF spaces) or ventriculoperitoneal shunt. The primary author does not employ this because of high risk of pneumocephalus and infection

CSF leak after transsphenoidal surgery (Table 11.1g)

Presentation	• Usually, obvious clear-fluid drainage from nose or into pharynx • Positional headaches

Diagnostic studies	• Signs/studies indicating that rhinorrhea is due to CSF:
	  – Reservoir sign
	  – CSF target/ring sign
	  – β_2-transferrin or beta trace-protein test
	• Studies to identify source of leakage in difficult cases:
	  – Intrathecal dye head CT study with thin-cut slices
	  – Intrathecal fluorescein, followed by nasal endoscopy (direct visualization of CSF leak)

Treatment	a. If CSF become apparent during surgery	1. Repair anterior sellar wall with dura graft + vomer pieces 2. Pack sinus with sandwich layers with rectus abdominis fascia + fat + gelfoam 3. Consider placement of lumbar drain after surgery (even prophylactically)
	b. If CSF in postop period	1. CSF diversion for 3–7 d: • Lumbar drain (remember: this is a volume-driven CSF diversion and not pressure driven) • Start with 5 ml/h, increase daily as tolerated (headaches!!) **Caution: pneumocephalus (if air is sucked in from negative CSF drainage pressure)** 2. If CSF leak persists after clamping of lumbar drain following drainage for 7 d: • Return to OR and attempt primary repair as described above (may use fluorescein to identify leakage site) • Post-op continue lumbar drainage for 3–7 d

Carotid injury during transsphenoidal surgery (Table 11.1h)

Presentation	Massive arterial bleeding often obscuring view
Diagnostic studies	Post-op intraoperative angiography is a must
Treatment	1. Apply occlusive pressure to carotid arteries in the neck to slow bleeding down 2. Obtain hemostasis with hemostatic agents and direct pressure. Pack area 3. If necessary, place foley catheter in sphenoid sinus and inflate balloon to tamponade 4. Proceed directly to angiography suite for endovascular repair 5. Monitor postoperatively for formation of pseudoaneurysm

Bleeding during stereotactic needle biopsy (Table11.1i)

Presentation	Blood dripping out of biopsy needle during surgery (hemorrhage is the most common complication of stereotactic biopsy occurring in > 5% of patients)
Diagnostic studies	• Usually a clinical diagnosis • May consider intra-op U/S • Obtain STAT postop head CT to determine extent of hemorrhage and need for further treatment
Treatment	• Leave biopsy needle in place and open: allow blood to drain until bleeding stops on its own • If bleeding does not stop after 5–10 min, consider injecting a small amount of hemostatic agent (surgiflo, floseal) and taking patient emergently to CT while informing OR to prepare for craniotomy

Inadvertent opening of air sinus (Table 11.1j)

Presentation	Following craniotomy, sinus mucosa or air cells become visible	
Diagnostic studies	None	
Treatment	**a. Frontal paranasal sinus**	1. If mucosa is intact, may just repair bony defect
		2. If mucosa is violated cranialize sinus:
		• Strip mucosa (study frontal sinus anatomy, beware of duplicate orbital roof)
		• Drill thin layer of bone from entire sinus wall (in order to ensure that all mucous secreting cells have been removed)
		• Plug nasofrontal duct with gelfoam soaked with bacitracin ointment followed by muscle plug
		• Apply vascularized pericranium graft
	b. Small air cells (mastoid cells)	Push wax into air cells rather than swipe wax across air cells

Pneumocephalus after craniotomy (Table 11.1k)

Presentation	• Unspecific headaches • Neurological compromise is possible **Caution: deteriorating neurological status indicates tension pneumocephalus**
Diagnostic studies	CT head
Treatment	• For routine cases: 100% O_2 via non-rebreather mask for 24 h • Tension pneumocephalus is an emergency!! → Emergently place needle into tension pneumocephalus for air aspiration (may be done under CT guidance). Occasionally, return to or for evacuation is required (see also Table 5.17)

Facial nerve palsy management (Table 11.1l)

Presentation	Postoperative CN VII palsy	
Diagnostic studies	Serial ENoG (electroneuronography) studies	
Treatment	• Besides cosmetic issues, the main concern is corneal abrasions, which may even lead to blindness • Unless nerve is clearly transected during surgery, watchful waiting for up to 6–12 mo is indicated	
	General measures	• Eye patch at night • Protective glasses • Lacri-Lube

Specific surgical treatments	• Primary nerve graft repair during initial surgery, if nerve transected
	• CNs VII to XII nerve anastomosis
	• Temporalis muscle transposition
	• Eyelid gold weight implant
	• Tarsal strip
Long-term outcome	• Depends on initial House–Brackmann grade
	• Synkinesis of facial branches is common
	• Crocodile tears

11.2 Spine Surgery $\boxed{\text{G}}$

Posterior lumbar spine surgery with retroperitoneal vessel injury (Table 11.2a)

Presentation	• Occurs typically during routine spine surgery, when entering the disc space too deeply and causing anterior disc perforation
	• In most cases, there is no visible severe bleeding in surgical field (due to bleeding into retroperitoneal space)
	• Venous injury more likely than arterial injury
	• First sign is precipitous blood pressure drop or drop in end-tidal P_{CO_2} reading
Diagnostic studies	Usually, a clinical diagnosis that can be verified with imaging:
	a. In unstable patient, proceed directly to laparotomy with assistance of vascular surgeon
	b. In stable patient, obtain CTA of abdomen and pelvis, intra-op U/S, conventional angiogram
Treatment	1. Pack disc space tightly with gelfoam or similar material
	2. Close wound immediately and fast
	3. Notify vascular surgery team and interventional vascular team
	4. Start immediate fluid/blood resuscitation:
	a. If patient is unstable, obtain STAT intraoperative imaging studies to confirm free retroperitoneal fluid and proceed with laparotomy with the assistance of vascular surgeon
	b. If patient is stable, proceed with CTA and plan for endovascular repair if possible

Vertebral artery injury during cervical surgery (Table 11.2b)

Presentation	Profuse arterial bleeding in field
Diagnostic studies	CTA, digital subtraction angiography (DSA)
Treatment	1. If possible, expose artery and attempt primary repair with 8–0 prolene 2. Tamponade/pack 3. If bleeding will not stop, sacrifice injured vertebral artery 4. Proceed directly to endovascular imaging and repair 5. Long-term imaging follow-up to R/O pseudoaneurysm formation

C5 palsy (Table 11.2c)

Presentation	• Presents with deltoid weakness and shoulder pain 1–3 d after C4/C5 surgery • Incidence: 5% • Higher incidence in: posterior approaches, male patients, ossification of the posterior longitudinal ligament (OPLL)
Diagnostic studies	MRI cervical spine to R/O hematoma or other compression
Treatment	• Physical therapy for up to 1 y • Consider short-term steroids • Consider pregabalin for pain • Usually self-resolving • If weakness persists for >3 mo, consider orthopedic consultation in order to avoid shoulder dislocation

Esophageal or pharyngeal tear in anterior spinal surgery (Table 11.2d)

Presentation	Intraoperatively	Air bubbles or gastric content visible in wound especially after placing retractors
	Postoperatively	Mediastinitis: • Difficulty swallowing • Choking • Aspiration • Fever, malaise
Diagnostic studies	Intraoperatively	Try to identify tear visually. May be helpful to have esophageal probe placed
	Postoperatively	• Gastrografin swallowing study • Noncontrast CT neck and chest (R/O pneumothorax) • Flexible endoscopy (pharynx, esophagus, bronchus)

Treatment	• Mediastinitis is a potentially life-threatening complication (mortality up to 10%) if not identified and treated properly
	• STAT surgery and ENT (ear, nose, and throat) consult. Intraoperative repair is best option!!
	• Multimodality approach necessary, including:
	  – Long-term nasogastric tube and nothing by mouth status often necessary for days or weeks
	  – If primary repair not possible, healing by secondary intention (esophageal–cutaneous fistula)
	  – Broad-spectrum IV antibiotics	

Wound hematoma after anterior cervical discectomy and fusion (ACDF) surgery (Table 11.2e)

Presentation	Immediately after anterior cervical surgery:	
	• Hoarseness, stridor	
	• Difficulty breathing after extubation	
	• Patient complains of severe swallowing difficulty	
	• Swelling in area of surgery, that is more pronounced than usual	
	• Obvious laryngeal or tracheal deviation	
Diagnostic studies	• X-ray to identify tracheal deviation and increased retropharyngeal/ retrotracheal space	
	• CT neck	
Treatment	a. Unstable patient	1. Open skin wound and platysma in postanesthesia care unit (PACU) and drain hematoma
		2. Then proceed to or for proper closure
		Antibiotic IV coverage
	b. Stable patient	1. Intubate and stabilize patient
		2. Return to or for adequate hemostasis, wound closure
		Antibiotic IV coverage

CSF leak after spine surgery (Table 11.2f)

Presentation	• Visible fluid egress from wound or moist dressing	
	• Positional headaches	
	• Significant palpable soft swelling in wound area	
Diagnostic studies	• Usually a clinical diagnosis	
	• CT/mri	
Treatment	a. Cervical area following ACDF surgery (significant subcutaneous CSF collection in anterior neck)	1. Difficult to repair directly. Place fibrin glue over tear intraoperatively, if leak identified during initial surgery
		2. If wound is leaking through skin, oversew entire wound with running-locking nylon
		3. CSF diversion via lumbar drain for 5–7 d
		4. Usually self-resolving
	b. Lumbar area	1. Key is to stop CSF from leaking through skin. Subcutaneous pocket usually only a cosmetic issue
		2. If wound is leaking through skin, oversew entire wound with running-locking nylon sutures
		3. Apply pressure corset for up to 3 mo
		4. If above do not suffice, return to OR for direct repair

Change in neuromonitoring during spine surgery (Table 11.2g)

Presentation	Decreased amplitude of somatosensory evoked potentials (SSEP) or motor evoked potentials (MEP) during spine surgery
Diagnostic studies	Verify that all electrode connections are intact
Treatment	• Increase systolic bp to 130–140 mm hg • Hydrate • Warm patient • Consider IV steroids • Reduce any traction on spinal cord and check for compressive spinal lesion • Consider changing patient positioning • Consider removing any placed instrumentation • Repeat SSEP and MEP readings • If amplitude drop is 50% or more, consider aborting procedure

11.3 Other Complications

Bowel perforation during shunt placement (Table 11.3a)

Presentation	Hollow viscus content visible during placement of peritoneal catheter
Diagnostic studies	None
Treatment	• Obtain immediate intraoperative general surgery consultation. Primary repair is preferred • Abort shunt implantation procedure • Place ventriculostomy, if patient shunt dependent • Obtain infectious disease consult and start appropriate antibiotics

Retained foreign objects (drains, catheters, electrodes, etc.) (Table 11.3b)

Presentation	May be incidental finding or suspected after incomplete removal	
Diagnostic studies	• X-rays • CT • C-arm fluoroscopy	
Treatment	No need for removal	Consider leaving the retained objects if sterile and educated patient
	Mandatory removal	Indications: • Infection • CSF leak • Patient preference
		Catheter localization: • Obtain preoperative (CT) and intraoperative imaging (C-arm fluoroscopy) • Locate object by means of triangulation (anteroposterior [AP], lateral, oblique views) • Consider intra-op U/S

Wound infection (Table 11.3c)

Presentation	• Drainage from wound • Nonhealing wound • Fever, malaise, night sweating • Meningitis

Diagnostic studies	• MRI with contrast, CT with contrast
	• Laboratory tests: complete blood count (CBC) with differential, erythrocyte sedimentation rate (ESR), C-reactive protein (CRP), procalcitonin
	• Wound drainage culture
	• Shunt tap for suspected shunt infection
	• Organisms:
	  • Common organisms include staphylococcus aureus, S. Epidermis, streptococcus viridans, gram-negative organisms
	  • Beware of indolent organisms such as propionibacterium, when infections appear late or indolent
	  • Do not forget about nonbacterial pathogens such as fungi, etc.
	• SOS: always try to obtain sample for cultures before starting antibiotics!!

Treatment	a. Craniotomy infection	1. Washout and debridement in OR: remove infected bone flap. Remove all old sutures 2. Obtain intra-op cultures 3. Close with single-layer nylon suture 4. Infectious diseases consult, consider peripherally inserted central catheter (PICC) line 5. Six weeks of IV followed by 6 wk of oral antibiotics 6. Follow with serial laboratory tests as above, serial contrast MRI scans 7. Cranioplasty once infection is cured
	b. Spinal infections	1. Superficial wound infections may be treated with antibiotics alone 2. Deep wound infections require surgical debridement. Remove all old sutures 3. Obtain intra-op cultures 4. If infection is clearly superficial to fascia, do not open fascia 5. Wash out with pulse irrigator 6. If possible, remove all foreign bodies, including instrumentation and bone graft 7. Minimize sutures used to close deep wound and if possible use antibiotic impregnated sutures. Close skin with single-layer nylon suture 8. Infectious diseases consult, consider PICC line 9. Six weeks of IV followed by 6 wk of oral antibiotics 10. Follow with serial laboratory tests as above, serial contrast MRI scans

c. DBS/vagus nerve stimulation (VNS)/ intrathecal pump infection	1. All foreign bodies and instruments must be removed, including batteries, pumps, catheters and electrodes. Remove all old sutures 2. Infectious diseases consult, consider PICC line 3. Six weeks of IV followed by 6 wk of oral antibiotics 4. Follow with serial laboratory tests as above 5. For intrathecal pump, treat patient with appropriate corresponding oral medications in order to avoid acute withdrawal
d. Shunt infection	1. Obtain CSF cultures 2. Check with CT for distal infection site in abdomen, including loculated CSF collection 3. Surgically remove the entire system. If the patient is shunt dependent, then place antibiotic covered EVD 4. Infectious diseases consult 5. After full course treatment with antibiotics, replace shunt system only after two consecutive CSF cultures have been finalized negative.

11.3.1 Baclofen, Opioid, and Ziconotide (Prialt) Withdrawal and Overdose (Related to Intrathecal Pumps) (Table 11.3d) [G]

		Baclofen	Opioid	Ziconotide (Prialt)
Presentation	Withdrawal	• Severe muscle spasms • Seizures • Respiratory difficulty • Delirium • Hyperthermia **Life-threatening**	• Jitteriness and tremors • Abdominal cramping pains • Nausea • Diarrhea **Not life-threatening**	None
	Overdose	• Decreased consciousness • Fixed pupils • Miosis or mydriasis • Respiratory difficulty • Hypotension • Seizures **Life-threatening**	• Decreased consciousness • Fixed pupils • Miosis • Respiratory difficulty **Life-threatening**	• Confusion, sedation, stupor • Ataxia, dizziness • Speech difficulty • Nausea, vomiting Not life-threatening
Diagnostic studies		AP and lateral X-rays abdomen, lumbar, and thoracic spine CT of abdominal wall is rarely needed (see Table 11.3e)		

Treatment	Withdrawal	• Benzodiazepines	IV opioid drip	
		• Tizanidine		
		• Propofol		
		• Intrathecal baclofen		
	Overdose	• CSF removal (side port, spinal tap) • Physostigmine	• CSF removal (side-port, spinal tap) • Naloxone	Symptomatic treatment

	For all patients (withdrawal/ overdose)	1. Admission to ICU
		 2. Interrogate intrathecal pump; stop delivery for overdose!!
		 3. Identify source of problem (programming error, refill error, dosing error, catheter problem)
		 4. Surgical catheter repair or replacement for catheter malfunction
		  • REMEMBER:
		   a. Withdrawal: most likely a catheter problem or programming error (pump ran empty)
		   b. Overdose: most likely a dosing error, refill error, or programming error		

Intrathecal pump and catheter complications (Table 11.3e)

Presentation	• Sudden return of symptoms, which were present before placement of pump or stimulator • Signs of intrathecal medication overdose or withdrawal (often medication mixture!) • Signs of infections at implanted hardware sites
Diagnosis	• Interrogation of intrathecal pump • X-rays of the entire implanted system • CT abdomen (rarely needed) • C-arm fluoroscopy study • MRI with contrast for intrathecal granuloma (**caution: device has to be MRI safe**)

Complications	Findings	Treatment

Withdrawal	• Pump is empty on interrogation
	 • X-ray shows:
	  – Catheter disconnection
	  – Catheter not in spinal canal
	  – Catheter kinked
	  – Catheter fractured
		1. Admission for treatment of withdrawal (consider ICU admission for baclofen withdrawal)
		 2. Administer supportive medical and medication support as per above chart
		 3. Diagnostic studies:
		  a. Catheter problems: surgical repair of disconnected, dislodged, kinked or broken catheter
		  b. Empty pump: refill and reprogramming of empty pump:
		   – If patient has been without medication for hours, restart pump at previous rate
		   – If patient has been without medication for days or more, restart pump at a rate appropriate for new implant (rate for "medication-naive" patient)

(Continued) ▶

Overdose	• Diagnostic studies usually normal
	• Check most recent refill or reprogramming records
	• Almost always:
	  – Programming error
	  – Dosing error
	  – Refill error:
	    ◦ Medication injected through side port
	    ◦ Medication not injected into reservoir
		1. Admission or ICU admission (baclofen or opioid overdose)
		2. Stop the pump and empty the reservoir (side-port aspiration of CSF if necessary)
		3. Once patient is stable and has recovered from overdose (this may take 1–2 wk), intrathecal pump therapy has to be restarted at a rate appropriate for new implant (rate for "medication-naive" patient)
		Caution: stopping the pump may destroy the pump mechanism; new pump implantation may be required
		Overdose of undetermined origin: patient IV self-injection of pump opioid medication has been reported (residual pump volume much lower than programmer indicates)

Audible alarm pump	• Alarm is audible (may take several minutes in a quiet room) • Pump interrogation shows alarm error	Always interrogate pump to visually verify the type of alarm: a. Low reservoir alarm: routine pump refill procedure, as long as patient is not at risk for withdrawal b. Low battery alarm: indicating imminent battery failure (usually within a few months). Schedule elective pump replacement surgery c. Critical alarm: indicates that medication is no longer flowing. Patient at high risk of withdrawal. Perform replacement of pump

Granuloma formation	• Patient may present with:
	a. Symptoms of compression: mass effect can cause either spinal cord compression or nerve root compression
	b. Symptoms of medication undertreatment: granuloma impedes medication flow
	• MRI lumbar and thoracic spine with contrast: shows catheter granuloma
		a. If spinal cord or nerve root compression: immediate surgery for removal of granuloma and placement of new catheter.
		b. If no neurological compromise:
		  1. Reduce intrathecal medication concentration (mostly morphine)
		  2. Switch to different medication if possible
		  3. If granuloma persists: remove catheter and implant new intrathecal catheter with the tip at different site (this may cause repeat granuloma formation)
		  4. If granuloma persists: granuloma resection, catheter removal, and discontinuation of intrathecal therapy

Abbreviations

- /: Or
- #: Fracture
- ACom: anterior communicating
- ant: anterior
- AP: anteroposterior
- ASDH: acute subdural hematoma
- BG: basal ganglia
- b/l: bilateral
- CC: corpus callosum
- CC axis: cephalocaudal axis
- CPA: cerebellopontine angle
- cons: disadvantages
- contra: contralateral
- crani: craniotomy
- CSF: cerebrospinal fluid
- C-spine: cervical spine
- CT: computed tomography
- CTA: computed tomography angiography
- Dx: diagnosis
- EAM: external acoustic meatus
- EDH: epidural hematoma
- esp.: Especially
- EVD: external ventricular drain
- F2: middle frontal gyrus
- FM: foramen magnum
- FMo: foramen of monro
- GCS: glasgow coma scale
- GSPN: greater superficial petrosal nerve
- HCP: hydrocephalus
- IAM: internal acoustic meatus
- ICA: internal carotid artery
- incl.: Including
- inf: inferior
- inj: injury
- ipsi: ipsilateral
- JF: jugular foramen
- LD: lumbar drain
- L-spine: lumbar spine
- max: maximum
- mb: morbidity
- meds: medications
- mid-fossa: middle cranial fossa
- ML axis: mediolateral axis
- MRI: magnetic resonance imaging
- Mx: management
- Na$^+$: sodium ion
- navi: navigation
- neuro: neurologic
- OR: operating room
- OZ: orbitozygomatic
- p-fossa: posterior cranial fossa
- post: posterior
- PRN: when necessary
- pros: advantages
- pt: patient
- req.: Require / requirement
- R/O: rule out
- SMA: supplementary motor area
- sol: solution
- SSS: superior sagittal sinus
- STA: superior temporal artery
- STAT: immediately
- sup: superior
- supratent.: Supratentorial
- T2: middle temporal gyrus
- T3: inferior temporal lobe
- TBI: traumatic brain injury
- traj: trajectory
- T-spine: thoracic spine
- Tx: treatment
- U/S: ultrasound
- Usu.: Usually
- VA: vertebral artery
- vis.: Visualization
- vs.: Versus
- W/O: without
- W/U: workup

12 Neurology for Neurosurgeons

12.1 Electromyography and Nerve Conduction Studies (Nerve Conduction Velocity) (Table 12.1) G

Electromyography (EMG)	
Normal	Abnormal
No electrical activity with muscle at rest	A. Muscle at rest: Spontaneous electrical activity with may be a sign of: • *Denervation:* fibrillation potentials and positive sharp waves (fibrillations may not be present in first 3 wk) • *Myotonic disorders:* waxing/waning frequency and amplitude and "dive bomber" sound on audio • *Amyotrophic lateral sclerosis and progressive motor neuron disorders:* fasciculations *Remember:* Complex repetitive discharges are nonspecific (seen in both neuropathic and myopathic disorders) B. **Muscle in minimal (to identify recruitment pattern) and maximal contraction (interference pattern analysis):** Motor unit action potentials reflect the number of motor units activated in contraction: a. *Myopathy* presents with decreased (amplitude/duration) motor unit action potential. Also, in myopathy, there is early/increased recruitment of motor units (the opposite happens in neurogenic conditions) b. *Lower motor neuron disorder* presents with increased (amplitude/duration) motor unit action potential

Nerve conduction velocity		
Nerve	Conduction velocity[1]	Distal latency
Median nerve	Sensory: ≥ 49 m/s Motor: ≥ 49 m/s	4.5 ms
Ulnar nerve	Sensory: ≥ 49m/s Motor: ≥ 43 m/s	3.7 ms
Peroneal nerve	Motor: ≥ 37 m/s	6.5 ms

NCV includes not only the study of the velocity of electrical stimulation but also the latency (time needed from stimulation to recording site in milliseconds) and the amplitude (the intensity of response measured in millivolts)

i. *EMG and nerve conduction studies facilitate differential diagnosis between nerve dysfunction, muscle dysfunction, or dysfunction of neuromuscular transmission.*
ii. *Preganglionic vs. postgaglionic brachial plexus lesions: Sensory nerve action potential is normal in preganglionic lesions and reduced in postganglionic lesions. Consequently, it helps in diagnosing plexus disorders (reduced sensory potential with no fibrillations in paraspinal muscles) and root avulsion (typically normal sensory potential)*
iii. *Cervical roots can ONLY be evaluated C5 and below*

12.2 Weakness (Table 12.2 ◀))) G

Disease	Presentation	Diagnostics	Treatment
Guillain–Barre[2]	• **Weakness** is: – symmetrical – primarily proximal • Usually occurs days weeks after respiratory/gastrointestinal infection (*Campylobacter jejuni*)	1. **Lumbar puncture:** increased protein in CSF 2. **NCV:** decreased	1. Plasmapheresis 2. Immunoglobulin therapy
Myasthenia	• **Weakness** is worse at the end of the day • **Commonly affects** eyes (ophthalmoplegia/ptosis/diplopia), face, and swallowing ability	1. **Chest X-ray:** rule out thymoma 2. **Tensilon test** (edrophonium: no longer popular as it may cause life-threatening bradycardia): positive if muscles get stronger with Tensilon 3. **Nerve conduction study/EMG**	1. Acetylcholinesterase inhibitors (pyridostigmine/neostigmine) 2. Immunosuppressants 3. Removal of thymus 4. Plasmapheresis 5. IV immunoglobulin (in crisis)
Lambert–Eaton	• **Weakness:** – improves with activity – primarily proximal • **Dysfunction of autonomic system** (dry mouth/constipation/blurred vision) • Usually occurs **in the setting of paraneoplastic syndrome** (frequently small cell lung cancer)[3]	1. **EMG/NCV** (compound motor action potentials and single-fiber examination) 2. **Antibodies** against pre-synaptic voltage-gated calcium channels 3. **CT** to find the cancer (small cell lung). If negative, it may have to be repeated within a few months. Consider bronchoscopy and PET	1. Treat cancer 2. Steroids 3. Immunosuppressants

Disease	Presentation	Diagnostics	Treatment
Polymyositis	• **Weakness** is primarily proximal (shoulders and hips usually affected first) • Spares eyes • Muscle pain • Dysphagia • Increased risk of malignancy, heart failure, interstitiallung disease	1. Increased **creatine phosphokinase** (CPK) 2. **EMG** 3. Positive **muscle biopsy**	1. Steroids 2. Immunosuppressants 3. Physical therapy
Steroid myopathy	1. **Weakness** is primarily proximal 2. **Associated with chronic use of steroids** (ICU/asthma/chronic obstructive pulmonary disease/connective tissue disorders) 3. In addition to chronic form, there is also an **acute form** (generalized weakness) associated with rhabdomyolysis	Vs **Epidural lipomatosis:** • commonly associated with: – long-term steroid use – endogenous overproduction – obesity • Treatment: – Discontinue steroids – Weight loss – Surgery	1. Discontinue or reduce steroids 2. Physical therapy (not high intensity)

Note: When myopathy is suspected, investigate ability to stand up from chair/climb stairs.

12.3 Parkinson's Disease and Parkinson Plus Syndromes (Table 12.3) G

Disease	Presentation	Diagnostic	Other	Treatment
	Symptoms common to all Parkinsonian syndromes: • Resting tremor • Rigidity (lead pipe or cogwheel) • Bradykinesia • Postural instability			1. **L-Dopa** (long-term use leads to dyskinesias) 2. **L-Dopa + Carbidopa** (Sinemet: peripheral dopa decarboxylase inhibitor with less side effects) used primarily for freezing episodes 3. **Dopamine agonists** (bromocriptine, pergolide, cabergoline): less effective than L-Dopa but with delayed risk of dyskinesias 4. **MAO-B inhibitors** (selegiline) 5. **Surgery (deep brain stimulation):** Patients with neuropsychiatric disorders are CONTRA-INDICATED **Prognosis:** Usually very good with treatment Often near-normal life expectancy
	Disease-specific symptoms			
Parkinson's disease	• Starts out asymmetrical • Progressively: – Hypophonia – Dementia – Depression – Frequently alteration of smell		Degeneration of compacta substantia nigra + Lewy bodies (alpha-synuclein)[4]	
Progressive supranuclear palsy (Steele–Richardson–Olszewski syndrome)	• Symmetrical • Reduced voluntary saccades (especially vertical and downward) • Poor response to L-DOPA	**"Hummingbird" sign** on MRI (atrophy of midbrain with preservation of pons)	Tauopathy	1. No treatment 2. **Prognosis:** death in 7 y (from pneumonia + swallowing difficulties)

Disease	Presentation	Diagnostic	Other	Treatment
Multiple system atrophy or Shy–Drager syndrome or olivopontocerebellar atrophy or striatonigral degeneration	• **Autonomic dysfunction** (orthostatic hypotension/sphincter disturbances/erectile dysfunction) • Ataxia • There are two types: Parkinsonian and cerebellar		Accumulation of alpha-synuclein in glial cells	1. **L-DOPA** typically does *not* work. (droxidopa/fludrocortisone) 2. **For systolic blood pressure:** increase salt intake/compression stockings 3. **For bladder dysfunction:** anticholinergics (oxybutynin/tolterodine) **Prognosis:** average survival 6 y
Corticobasal degeneration	1. Asymmetrical[5] 2. Alien hand syndrome 3. Apraxia/aphasia	Involves cerebral cortex and basal ganglia	Tauopathy	1. Poor response to L-DOPA 2. **Prognosis:** death within 8 y

Note: Parkinson plus syndromes: progressive supranuclear palsy, multiple system atrophy, corticobasal degeneration.

12.4 Side Effects of Antipsychotics (Table 12.4) G

Disease	Presentation	Treatment

Tardivedyskinesia	• **Stereotyped movements:**
	  – Face and tongue
	  – Lip smacking
	  – Extremities: chorea
	• **Caused by** postsynaptic dopamine hypersensitivity induced by medication
		1. Stop antipsychotics
		2. **Valbenazine** (reduces the available dopamine in synapses)
		3. **Benzodiazepines** (clonazepam): tolerance is progressively developed
		4. Symptoms may start after first dose and may be irreversible even with treatment

Drug-induced Parkinsonism	1. **History of antipsychotics use** (but may also be caused by antiemetics, antiepileptics, calcium-channel blockers)[6] 2. **Parkinson-like symptoms** (classically symmetric but not always)	1. Reduce dose or stop the responsible drug 2. Anticholinergics in the young 3. Amantadine in the elderly

Note: Antipsychotics are dopamine antagonists as is metoclopramide (antiemetic). Risk is less with atypical antipsychotics (olanzapine) than typical (haloperidol).

12.5 Various Movement Disorders (Table 12.5)

Disease	Presentation	Treatment
Essential tremor or familial tremor or idiopathic tremor[7]	• The **most common** movement disorder • Tremor **ONLY with movement** (usually action or postural) • Usually upper extremities/head/neck and oropharynx • Present **only when awake**	1. **Beta-blockers** (propranolol, nadolol, timolol) 2. **Antiepileptics** (topiramate, gabapentin, levetiracetam)/benzodiazepines, alcohol 3. Avoid stress/caffeine 4. **Deep brain stimulation** (ventral intermediate nucleus thalamus [VIM])
Dystonia	• Slow sustained repetitive posture • **Several forms** (generalized, focal, multifocal, segmental with involvement of adjacent body parts, hemidystonia) • Cervical dystonia (spasmodic torticollis) and blepharospasm are the most common forms of focal dystonia	1. **Botulinum injection**[8] (in affected muscles) with subsequent relief for 3–6 mo; then repeat 2. **Medications:** anticholinergics/benzodiazepines/carbidopa or levodopa 3. **Selective neurotomy** (sternocleidomastoid denervation for cervical dystonia) 4. **Deep brain stimulation:** globus pallidus for early/childhood-onset variant and generalized form

12.6 Dorsal Colum sfunction (Table 12.6)   G

Disease	Presentation	Other	Treatment

B12 deficiency (subacute combined degeneration of spinal cord)	• **Affects** dorsal column + corticospinal tract + peripheral nerves, causing significant ataxia along with upper and lower motor neuron weakness
	• Also **causes:**
	  – megaloblastic anemia
	  – gastrointestinal symptoms
	  – dementia
	  – depression
		High levels of methylmalonic acid (MMA) → damages myelin	B12 injections or oral administration

Friedreich's ataxia	• **Affects** dorsal column > cerebellar tract > corticospinal tract leading to:
	  • ataxia
	  • nystagmus
	  • speech disturbance
	  • minimal weakness
	• **Associated with** scoliosis, heart disease, diabetes
		Autosomal recessive (expansion of GAA triplet reduces expression of mitochondrial protein frataxin)[9]	1. No truly effective treatment
			2. Speech therapy/physical therapy
			3. Treat the associated symptoms and diseases

Tabes dorsalis or syphilitic myelopathy	• Dorsal column dysfunction (typical gait) + peripheral nerves • Weakness/paresthesias (often painful)/degeneration of the joints • Argyll Robertson pupil and visual disturbances • Personality changes/dementia/deafness/Loss of bladder control	• The **clinical manifestations** may be delayed for many years. • There is demyelination caused by untreated *Treponema pallidum* infection (tertiary syphilis)	1. IV penicillin 2. Treat the pain (opiates and carbamazepine) 3. Physical therapy

Note: Dorsal column: proprioception, vibration, discriminative touch.

12.7 Dementia (Table 12.7) G

Disease	Presentation	Diagnostics	Other	Treatment
Wernicke's encephalopathy	**Acute dementia** • Horizontal gaze palsy • Ataxia	**MRI fluid-attenuated inversion recovery (FLAIR):** signal is increased in: • Mammillary bodies • Dorsomedial thalamus • Tectal plate • Periaqueductal area in proximity of the 3rd ventricle	Deficiency of thiamine (vitamin B1)[10] as in: • chronic alcoholism • malnutrition • chemotherapy	100-mg thiamine (B1) IV + daily oral administration
Korsakoff's syndrome	**Chronic dementia** • Amnesia • Confabulation[11]			
Creutzfeldt–Jacob disease (CJD)	• Dementia • Myoclonus	1. **EEG:** periodic spikes (periodic sharp wave complexes [PSWC]) 2. **Lumbar puncture:** normal or maybe increased protein. 14-3-3 protein has highest sensitivity and specificity for CJD 3. **MRI (FLAIR and diffusion weighted imaging [DWI]):** abnormalities in cerebral cortex/striatum/thalamus		• **Treatment:** NONE • **Prognosis:** death in less than 1 y

Disease	Presentation	Diagnostics	Other	Treatment
Alzheimer's disease	The most common cause of dementia	**MRI:** temporal and parietal atrophy	**Neurofibrillary tangle** (abnormally phosphorylated tau protein; may also be present in other diseases) + **senile plaques** (β-amyloid)	1. **Cholinesterase inhibitors/ memantine** (for cognitive symptoms) 2. **Selective serotonin reuptake inhibitors** (for depression) 3. **Atypical antipsychotics** (for agitation). *CONCERNS:* use of these medications may increase risk of mortality, cerebrovascular events, cardiovascular and metabolic complications, infections, falls 4. Do not use benzodiazepines **Prognosis:** death in 5 y: 70%
Pick's disease	• Dementia • Changes in behavior • Progressive nonfluent aphasia	**MRI:** frontal+ temporal atrophy	Tau proteins in neurons (silver staining: Pick's bodies)	There is no therapy
Lewy body disease	• **Second most common** cause of dementia[11] • Sleep disturbance • May include Parkinsonian symptoms	**MRI:** temporal+ parietal + occipital atrophy	**Lewy bodies:** alpha-synuclein protein in neurons	1. **Cholinesterase inhibitors** (for cognitive symptoms) 2. **Levodopa** (in case of significant Parkinsonian symptoms) 3. **Melatonin and/or clonazepam** for sleep disorders 4. Use **atypical antipsychotics** if absolutely necessary. *Avoid the typical ones*

12.8 Multiple Sclerosis and Other Demyelinating Disorders (Table 12.8) G

Disease	Presentation	Diagnostics	Other	Treatment

Multiple sclerosis	• Optic neuritis/sensory motor symptoms/internuclear ophthalmoplegia
	• **Two attacks** in different places and different times
	• Females > males.
	• Three clinical types:
	  e. Relapsing remitting
	  – Primary progressive
	  – Secondary progressive (initially relapsing remitting)
	• **Clinical signs**
	  – *Uhthoff's sign* (symptoms worsen when temperature is higher)
	  – *Lhermitte's sign* (sense of current along the spine when bending the neck)
		1. **MRI:** white matter lesions:
		  • Acute lesion is enhancing
		  • Chronic lesion is a black hole in T2
		  • Spares basal ganglia and thalamus
		2. **CSF:** increased protein + oligoclonal bands
			Prevalence increases with distance from equator	1. **Acute phase:**
				  a. Steroids
				  b. Plasmapheresis (if no response to steroids)
				  c. IV immunoglobulins (if contraindication to steroids or plasmapheresis)
				2. **Preventative:**
				  a. Interferon beta (may produce flulike symptoms and liver dysfunction)
				  b. Daclizumab/ocrelizumab (for relapsing–remitting and primary progressive type)
				  c. Mitoxantrone (for secondary progressive type)

Disease	Presentation	Diagnostics	Other	Treatment
Devic's disease or neuromyelitis optica (NMO)	• Acute bilateral painful decrease of vision (optic neuritis) • Spinal injury symptoms (myelitis) • Females > males • Monophasic or recurrent	Antibodies against astrocyte's aquaporin-4 protein may be present (NMO-immunoglobulin G [IgG] test)[12]	Neurologic sequelae tend to be more severe and permanent than multiple sclerosis	Similar to acute multiple sclerosis: 1. IV steroids 2. Plasmapheresis
Balo's concentric sclerosis	• Headache • Impaired cognition • Seizures	MRI: T2 sequence presents concentric layers of demyelination[13]		• Treatment: similar to acute multiple sclerosis • Prognosis: generally fatal
ADEM (acute disseminated/ demyelinating encephalomyelitis)	• Presents 2 wk after infection or vaccination (usually against rabies) • Monophasic deterioration[14] with variable symptoms (among which are fever, seizures, confusion) • Usually children	1. MRI: lesions all over brain including basal ganglia and thalami 2. CSF: increased protein and lymphocytes		1. High-dose steroids 2. Plasmapheresis 3. IV IgG Prognosis: mortality of 20%

12.9 Vasculitis (Tabe 12.9) G

Disease	Presentation		Diagnostics	Other	Treatment
	Arteries involved	Symptoms			
Wegener's granulomatosis or granulomatosis with polyangiitis	Affects small and medium vessels	• **Head:** eyes, ears, sinuses, nasal or oral inflammation)/saddle nose deformity because of collapse of inflamed septum) • **Kidneys:** glomerulonephritis • **Respiratory:** hemoptysis due to lung lesion • **Skin:** palpable purpura • **Nervous system:** cranial and peripheral neuropathy	1. Increased erythrocyte sedimentation rate (ESR)/C-reactive protein (CRP; in active disease) 2. **ANCA** (antineutrophil cytoplasmic antibodies)[15] 3. **CT:** chest, sinuses 4. **Biopsy** (renal and lung are most specific)	Autoimmune	1. Steroids 2. Cyclophosphamide
Behcet's disease	Affects vessels of all sizes	• **Ocular** (anterior or posterior uveitis: can lead to blindness) • **Genital** (ulcers) • **Oral** (aphthous ulcers) • **Neurological** (white matter) lesions may be present (even meningitis)	1. **Oral ulcerations** are the most pathognomonic 2. Possibly positive pathergy test (not specific)	**Association with HLA-B51:** risk factor	1. Steroids 2. Immunosuppressants 3. Colchicine for mucosal involvement
Takayasu's arteritis	• Affects large and medium size vessels (aorta and its major branches typically) • Carotid and vertebral arteries	• Systemic arteritis • **Pulseless disease** (absent or weak pulse usually in upper extremities because of aorta involvement)	1. Increased ESR/CRP 2. Angiography/MRA/CTA (several stenotic areas) 3. Biopsy is not needed		1. Steroids 2. Endovascular treatment of aneurysms or stenosis)

Disease	Presentation		Diagnostics	Other	Treatment
	Arteries involved	Symptoms			
Polyarteritis nodosa or Kussmaul–Maier disease	1. Affects small and medium-sized arteries 2. Usually spares pulmonary arteries[16] 3. Possibly small aneurysms like **"beads of a rosary"**	• A multisystem disease that can affect almost any organ and even lead to polyvisceral failure. • Frequently testicular pain	1. Increased ESR/CRP 2. Hepatitis B surface antigen or antibody 3. **EMG** (peripheral neuropathy/mononeuritis multiplex is common and confirming it helps the diagnosis) 4. **Angiography** is not pathognomonic (aneurysms/stenoses of medium-sized vessels) 5. **Biopsy** (nerves with pathological NCV/muscle/skin)	Association with viral viral hepatitis (typically B and chronic)[16]	1. Steroids 2. Cyclophosphamide, if no response to steroids but not in viral hepatitis-related disease 3. Antiviral medication when indicated
Giant cell arteritis or temporal arteritis	Affects the cranial branches (mostly external carotid) of the arteries of the aortic arch	• Headache • Eye pain/visual symptoms. Can cause blindness • Tenderness over temporal artery/jaw pain after chewing • Aortic aneurysm (thoracic) or dissection • Stroke	1. Increased ESR/CRP 2. **Biopsy** (superficial temporal artery)	Often associated with polymyalgia rheumatica	Steroids (start immediately to prevent vision issues, even before biopsy when necessary, in case of strong suspicion)

12.10 Diseases Associated with Stroke (Table 12.10) G

Disease	Presentation	Diagnostics	Other	Treatment
Fibromuscular dysplasia (FMD)	• Transient ischemic attack (TIA) or stroke/headache/vertigo/pulsating tinnitus • Stenosis/aneurysm/dissection • Affects also renal artery (causing hypertension and bruits)	• "String of beads" appearance on angiogram • Irregularities in internal carotid artery (usually bilateral). Vertebral artery may also be affected		1. Anticoagulation (usually aspirin) 2. Angioplasty
CADASIL: Cerebral Autosomal Dominant *Arteriopathy* with Sub-cortical Infarcts and Leukoencephalopathy	• Migraine headaches often with auras/TIA or stroke[17] • **Progressively:** dementia/pseudobulbar palsy/incontinence	**Binswanger's like lacunae** but at an *early age* (lesions around basal ganglia, pons, periventricular white matter)	Familial. Chromosome 19 (*Notch 3* gene)	**Anticoagulants** (but they are associated with slight increased risk of microhemorrhages)
MELAS: Mitochondrial Encephalomyopathy, Lactic Acidosis, and Stroke-like episodes	• Stroke (frequently occipital) • **Multisystem disorder**[18] with usually childhood onset	1. Arterial lactate and pyruvate are elevated and possibly also CSF lactate 2. Analysis of mitochondrial DNA 3. **MRI:** high T2 signal (temporal/parietal/occipital) and cerebral atrophy 4. Muscle biopsy	Defective mitochondrial DNA (maternal inheritance)[18]	1. Coenzyme Q10/Idebenone has been tried 2. Avoid valproic acid (it has effect on mitochondria) as antiepileptic **Prognosis:** Progressive with poor prognosis

12.11 Anterior Circulation Vascular Occlusion (Table 12.11) G

Artery	Presentation	Other	Diagnostics	Treatment

Internal carotid	**Hemispheric infarction** unless collateral flow has developed		1. **CT:** to exclude hemorrhage (depending on timing may also define the infarct, which is typically identified after 24 h as low density area). Early signs are the loss of gray-white matter differentiation and the hyperdense artery (usually middle cerebral artery [MCA])
			2. **CT angiography:** Can also evaluate collateral circulation
			3. **MRI:**
			  a. Increased T2 signal and reduced T1 (obviously more sensitive than CT)
			  b. DWI (evaluates infarcted area but not penumbra) and perfusion weighted imaging (PWI; identifies viable areas)
			4. **Digital subtraction angiography** (DSA), if endovascular intervention or intra-arterial thrombolysis is planned)
				1. **Identify and when possible treat the cause:**
				  a. Cardiac disease
				  b. Atherosclerosis
				  c. Vasculopathy
				  d. Abnormal coagulation
				  e. Recent labor
				  f. Oral contraceptives
				  g. Cocaine/amphetamine
				Remember that trauma is the most common cause in patients <45 y.
				2. **Intravenous thrombolysis (t-PA)** in appropriate candidates within 3 h from neurologic deficit onset (recently extended to 4.5 h with some exceptions as age >80 y, history of stroke and diabetes, NIH stroke scale >25)
				  a. ***Dosage of t-PA:*** 0.09mg/kg IV in 1 min + infusion of 0.81 mg/kg in 1 h (max. dose 90 mg). No anticoagulants for 24 h
				  b. ***Candidates:***
				    • age > 18 y
				    • Systolic BP (SBP) < 180 mm Hg and diastolic BP (DBP) < 105 mm Hg
				    • No major surgery in last 2 wk

Ophthalmic	Involvement of central retinal artery will cause **monocular blindness**	Proximal occlusion may be asymptomatic because of collateral flow from external carotid that spares the central retinal artery		
Posterior communicating (PCom)	**Contralateral** • **Homonymous hemianopia** IF FETAL PCom • **Tremor/choreoathetosis** (involvement of anterior thalamoperforating artery)			

(Continued) ▲

Artery	Presentation	Other	Diagnostics	Treatment

Anterior choroidal	**Contralateral:**
	• Hemiparesis
	• Hemisensory deficit
	• Homonymous hemianopia
		Lesion in:
		• Posterior limb of internal capsule
		• Middle third of cerebral peduncle
		• Optic tract and lateral geniculate body
				• No trauma/no stroke in last 3 mo
				• No history of intracranial hemorrhage
				• No coagulation abnormality
				REMEMBER: there is a 6% risk of intracranial hemorrhage
				3. **Intra-arterial t-PA/mechanical embolectomy:**
				  a. Patients that present in <4.5 h from onset and do not respond to intravenous thrombolysis but are in good clinical condition
				  b. Patients that present between 4.5–6 h
				  c. Patients that present in 6–8 h after having done an MRI-DWI (contraindicated in infarcts greater than one-third of MCA distribution)
				4. **Endovascular thrombectomy:** patients who present 6–24 h after onset AND have mismatch between deficit (severe) and infarct size (small; on perfusion CT or DWI MRI)[19]

Anterior cerebral (A1)	• **Decreased motivation and memory disturbance** (orbital/frontopolar arteries) • **Dysarthria** (because Heubner's artery occlusion causes lesion to contralateral cranial nerves V, VII, XII nuclei) • **Ideomotor apraxia** (pericallosal artery involvement causes lesion to anterior corpus callosum) **PLUS** **Contralateral:** • Lower extremity weakness/hypesthesia • Pelvic floor weakness with subsequent incontinence • Mutism if left supplementary motor area is affected (callosomarginal artery)	Unilateral occlusion may be asymptomatic because of ACom (anterior communicating artery)		

Artery	Presentation	Other	Diagnostics	Treatment
Callosomarginal	**Mutism** if left supplementary motor area is affected			5. Urgent surgery: a. *Selected MCA infarcts:* decompressive craniectomy and dural opening. *Indications* include not otherwise controlled increased ICP, progressive clinical deterioration, nondominant hemisphere involvement b. *Posterior fossa infarcts:* decompressive craniectomy with dural opening or EVD
Pericallosal	• **Ideomotor apraxia** (lesion to anterior corpus callosum) • Leg Weakness			

Middle cerebral (M1)	**Contralateral:**
	• Hemiparesis (upper extremity more than lower)
	• Hemisensory loss
	• Homonymous hemianopia
	
	PLUS
	a. *Dominant hemisphere:*
	• Aphasia (Broca's and Wernicke's)
	• Agraphia
	• Acalculia
	• Apraxia
	• "Gerstmann's syndrome":
	  – Right to left confusion
	  – Finger agnosia
	  – Acalculia
	  – Agraphia
	b. *Nondominant hemisphere:*
	• Anosognosia
	• Constructional apraxia
	REMEMBER: The eyes look toward the infarct (ipsilateral deviation)			

(Continued) ▲

Artery	Presentation	Other	Diagnostics	Treatment
Lenticulostriate	Dysarthria and contralateral clumsy hand due to: • Hemiparesis (prominent in face and upper extremity) • Sensory loss (VP thalamic nucleus)			
Superior division of middle cerebral artery	Contralateral: • Weakness of lower face and upper extremity > lower • Hemisensory loss PLUS: a. *Dominant Hemisphere:* Broca's aphasia b. *Non-dominant Hemisphere:* Sensory neglect			
Inferior division of middle cerebral artery	• Contralateral homonymous hemianopia • Disorientation and agitation (limbic system) • Ideomotor apraxia PLUS *Dominant hemisphere:* Wernicke's aphasia			

Note: Risk factors: diabetes, hypertension, smoking, history of alcohol abuse. Time limit for posterior circulation strokes treatment is generally extended.

12.12 Brainstem Syndromes (Table 12.12)

Location	Medial		Lateral		Dorsal	
	Long tracts	Local structures	Long tracts	Local structures	Long tracts	Local structures
Midbrain	CST	CN3	Medial lemniscus	• CN3 • Red nucleus (Connections w/ dentate nucleus, thalamus)		Superior colliculus
Pons	• CST • Medial lemniscus	CN6	• Sympathetic • Spinothalamic tract	• CN5 • CN7 • CN8		MLF
Medulla	• CST • Medial lemniscus	CN12	• Sympathetic • Spinothalamic tract	• CN5 • CN7 • CN9/10/11		

Abbreviation: CST, corticospinal tract; MLF, medial longitudinal fasciculus

Location	Syndrome	Symptoms
Midbrain	Parinaud's or dorsal midbrain syndrome or pretectal syndrome	Dorsal midbrain lesion (*oculomotor nucleus, superior colliculus, Edinger–Westphal nucleus*): • Collier's sign (eyelid retraction) • Nystagmus retractorius (globe retracts when attempting to look upward) • "Setting sun" sign (conjugate down gaze in primary position[20]) • Difficulty regarding convergence/accommodation/upward gaze • Light/near dissociation (pupil constricts to object approaching but not to light)
	Weber's syndrome	• Cranial nerve III lesion • CONTRALATERAL hemiplegia (corticospinal tract lesion)
	Benedikt's or paramedian midbrain syndrome	• Weber's plus • CONTRALATERAL dyskinesia, tremor, ataxia (red nucleus lesion)
Pons	Millard–Gubler syndrome	• Cranial nerve VI lesion • Cranial nerve VII lesion • CONTRALATERAL hemiplegia (corticospinal tract lesion)
Medulla	Wallenberg's or lateral medullary syndrome	• Vertigo (vestibular nuclei lesion)[21] • Dysphagia (nucleus ambiguus lesion) • IPSILATERAL Horner's syndrome (descending sympathetic fibers lesion) • IPSILATERAL facial sensory issues (spinal trigeminal nucleus/tract lesion) • CONTRALATERAL impaired pain and temperature sensation (lateral spinothalamic tract lesion) • Ataxia (inferior cerebellar peduncle lesion) • Palatal myoclonus (central tegmental area lesion)

12.13 Migraine (Table 12.13)

Disease	Presentation	Treatment
Common migraine	• **NO AURA OR DEFICIT** • **Pain** > 4 h • Most common type	• Includes acute pain relief and prevention • Avoid triggers **Medications:** a. Paracetamol b. Anti-inflammatory c. Triptans[22] d. Ergotamine
Classic migraine	• **AURA LASTING** <24 h (transient focal neurological symptom, most common visual). *(if aura lasts for more than 24 h, exclude ischemic lesion)* Typical duration is <30 min • **Pain** >4 h	e. Antiepileptics (topiramate, valproate) and similar (gabapentin, pregabalin) f. Beta-blockers (propranolol, atenolol, timolol) g. Calcium channel blockers (verapamil) h. Antidepressants (amitriptyline) **Other treatments:** a. Alternative medicine (acupuncture, biofeedback, massage)
Acephalgic migraine. (may be called migraine equivalents)	• **AURA WITHOUT HEADACHE** (for example gastrointestinal symptoms, dysarthria etc.→ *(exclude TIA / seizures)* • Females, children and young adults	b. Cefaly (Food and Drug Administration [FDA] approved device causing transcutaneous supraorbital nerve stimulation)

Notes:
• Migraines are considered neurovascular disorders that may last up to 72 hours and may be accompanied by nausea, vomiting, irritability photophobia, or sensitivity to sound/smell.
• Possibly there are four stages of migraine: prodrome (hours to days before), aura (immediately before), headache, postdrome (after).
• Status migrainosus: pain >72 hours.

12.14 Other Headache Syndromes (Table 12.14)

Disease	Presentation	Diagnostics	Treatment
Cluster headache	• Very intense with rapid onset ("suicide headaches") • Unilateral pain around eye (usually with accompanying lacrimation/nasal congestion/sweating/pupil constriction on same side)[23] • **Pain** < 4 h. Each cluster of episodes usually lasts 6–12 wk	History and symptoms	a. Calcium channel blockers (verapamil is recommended preventive treatment) b. Oxygen c. Steroids (for a short period) d. Topiramate e. Triptans

(Continued) ▶

Disease	Presentation	Diagnostics	Treatment
Spontaneous intracerebral hypotension	Spontaneous positional orthostatic headache (no history of trauma or iatrogenic cause) **REMEMBER:** Subdural hemorrhage without trauma → search for spine leak	1. **Low CSF pressure** (< 6 cm H_2O)/not always 2. **MRI brain and spine**/coronal/ thin cuts (frequently not helpful) 3. **MRI brain imaging findings:** • pachymeningeal enhancement • sagging brain • pituitary hyperemia • subdural collections • engorged veins 4. **CT myelogram** (brain and spine) to identify the leak (images immediately after contrast- and in delayed fashion)	• **Delayed diagnosis** makes treatment more difficult • **Treat like post lumbar puncture headache:** 1. Bed rest 2. Hydration 3. Caffeine 4. Epidural blood patch[24] that can be repeated (10–20 mL of autologous blood in epidural space with patient placed in Trendelenburg after injection) 5. Surgical repair[24] (exact site of leak must be known)
Pseudotumor cerebri or benign (or idiopathic) intracranial hypertension	• Fat/fertile age/ female /forty years old • **Common symptoms:** – Headache – Papilledema/ enlarged blind spot/constricted visual field (this being the best test for following vision). Blindness may occur but is rare • **Uncommon symptoms:** – Cranial nerve VI palsy – tinnitus – nausea – stiffneck	1. **MRV:** Exclude sinus thrombosis 2. **MRI brain:** c. slit ventricles d. empty sella 3. **Lumbar puncture:** CSF pressure > 20 cm H_2O (REMEMBER: there are possible variations during day, so if there is strong suspicion repeat the test)	1. Weight loss (recent gain can worsen vision) 2. Salt restriction 3. **Diuretics** (acetazolamide, furosemide) 4. **Topiramate** 5. **Steroids** for a *short period* if no response to diuretics 6. **Serial lumbar punctures** (consider especially in pregnancy) 7. **Surgery:** a. *Headache ± visual disturbance:* • Ventricular peritoneal shunt • Lumbar peritoneal shunt (may cause tonsillar herniation, sciatica) b. *Visual disturbance with no headache:* – Shunt or – Optic fenestration **REMEMBER:** Spontaneous remission, but also relapse, is common. Close follow-up.

12.15 Other Cranial Nerves Issues (Table 12.15a) G

Disease	Presentation	Diagnostics	Other	Treatment pearls
Facial nerve palsy	1. **Central (supranuclear):** upper face is spared 2. **Nuclear:** paralysis is complete. (Upper and lower face.) 3. **Peripheral:** Symptoms depend on exact anatomic location of lesion along the nerve **Lesion proximal to:** 1. *Pterygopalatine ganglion-greater superficial petrosal nerve:* absence of lacrimation plus all of the below 2. *Nerve to stapedius muscle:* hyperacusis plus all of the below 3. *Chorda tympani nerve:* no taste in anterior 2/3 of tongue with reduced salivation plus all of the below 4. *Outside the stylomastoid foramen (usually at parotid gland):* temporal, zygomatic, buccal, mandibular, cervical branches with loss of associated facial motor function	A. Determine level of dysfunction through **neurologic examination** B. **Depending on history:** 1. *MRI* if mass lesion is suspected (intracranial, parotid, etc.) or if no response to treatment after 2 mo. 2. *CT* in cases of trauma 3. Consider *blood tests* to exclude: d. inflammation (complete blood count, ESR) e. diabetes (glucose level: hemoglobin A1c) 4. *EMG/NCV* may be used to monitor recovery	• **Frequent causes:** a. Idiopathic (Bell's palsy), the most common cause b. Herpes zoster oticus c. Skull base fracture d. Tumors (schwannomas and parotid gland) e. Sarcoidosis f. Diabetes g. Lyme's disease h. Traumatic labor and Möbius' syndrome • **House and Brackmann's scale determines severity (grade 1–6).** *1:* normal at rest and during movement *3:* normal at rest, disfiguring during movement *6:* disfiguring at rest, no movement	1. **Protect the eye:** (artificial tears, ointment, sunglasses). Tarsorrhaphy or eyelid gold weight may be needed 2. **Steroids for Bell's palsy**[25]: prednisone 30 mg twice a day for 1 wk and taper (total treatment duration of 10 d) starting as early as possible (within 72 h) 3. There is strong indication that the use of antivirals (acyclovir/valacyclovir) offers limited or no benefit in case of no obvious herpetic viral infection[25] 4. Treat **underlying systemic disorders** (sarcoidosis, etc.) 5. **Early physical therapy** 6. **Surgical treatment for anatomical disruption:** a. Direct anastomosis b. Use of jump graft (sural nerve) c. Anastomosis to hypoglossal or spinal accessory nerves **Prognosis for Bell's palsy** is excellent with most people recovering within 1 mo. About 10% of people have some residual findings such as synkinesis, etc.

12.15.1 Multiple Cranial Nerve Involvement (Table 12.15b)

Frequent causes to consider
1. **Brainstem syndromes**
2. **Meningitis:** neoplastic/infectious (Lyme disease, tuberculosis, herpes viruses)
3. **Skull base tumors** (metastases, schwannoma, meningioma, paraganglioma, multiple myeloma)
4. **Granulomatous** (Sarcoidosis) and **vasculitic** (Wegener's granulomatosis) **processes**
5. **Peripheral nerves involvement** (Guillain–Barre, *Myasthenia gravis*, diabetes)
6. **Trauma**

12.16 Seizures (Table 12.16a)

Type	Change in mental status	Motor/sensory symptoms	Treatment
Simple partial or focal onset aware seizure	No loss of consciousness	Focal motor or sensory symptoms (no tonic clonic activity)	**Medication options include** levetiracetam, oxcarbazepine, carbamazepine, lamotrigine, topiramate, valproic acid, and phenytoin, among others
Complex partial or focal onset impaired awareness seizure	Positive alteration of consciousness	Focal motor or sensory symptoms (no tonic clonic activity) Automatisms (lip smacking, chewing, tapping, etc.) Usually start in temporal/frontal lobe	Treatment practically as in simple partial
Generalized	Positive alteration of consciousness	Tonic clonic/nonfocal motor activity (except *absence*, which has alteration of consciousness with no motor or sensory component)	a. **Tonic clonic:** phenytoin, valproic acid, carbamazepine, topiramate, clonazepam b. **Absence:** valproic acid, ethosuximide
Status epilepticus[26]: duration of seizure > 5 min OR seizure persists after first- and second-line antiepileptics	Practically any type of seizure can present with status		"Status epilepticus" treatment algorithm

Note: For medical treatment prefer, when possible, monotherapy with best tolerated medication. For surgical treatment of epilepsy, see Chapter 7: Functional Neurosurgery.

12.16.1 Status Epilepticus (Treatment Algorithm) (Table 12.16b) G

Steps	Remember
1. Airway/breathing/circulation	
2. Assess vital signs and neurological condition	

2. (continued)
- Electrocardiogram
- Monitoring
- O_2 saturation

3. **Check labs including GLUCOSE level and establish satisfactory IV access**
- GLUCOSE and electrolytes (Na, Ca, Mg)
- CBC
- Antiepileptic levels
- LFTs
- ABG
- CRP

Remember (step 3):
- EEG monitor
- Consider need for CT

4. **Treat potential underlying causes:**
- *thiamine deficiency:* 100 mg thiamine IV
- *hypoglycemia:* 50 mL of 50% Dextrose IV
- *narcotic overdose:* 0.4mg naloxone

5. **First-line antiepileptic therapy:**
   Administer immediately:
   a. *Lorazepam* 0.1 mg/kg IV over 2 min (in adults: 4 mg in pediatric pts > 13 kg: 2 mg
      OR
   b. *Midazolam* 10 mg IM (in pediatric pts > 13 kg: 5 mg)
      OR
   c. *Diazepam* rectal is also an alternative (0.5mg/kg)

Remember (step 5):
- Repeat lorazepam every 5 minutes
- Beware of respiratory depression

6. **Second-line therapy:**
   Proceed to this step during the repeat dose of benzodiazepine
   a. *Fosphenytoin* 20 mg sodium phenytoin equivalents/kg IV (faster infusion than phenytoin at 150 mg/min)
      OR
   b. *Phenytoin* 20 mg/kg IV at 50 mg/min in adults and 1–3 mg/kg/min in pediatric pts
      OR
   c. *Phenobarbital* 20 mg/kg at 100 mg/min in adults and 1 mg/kg/min in pediatric pts
      OR
   d. *Valproate* 30 mg/kg at 100 mg/min
      OR
   e. *Levetiracetam* 20mg/kg over 15 min

Remember (step 6):
- Respect infusion rate because of risk of severe hypotension and cardiac arrhythmias
- If no response with loading dose of Fosphenytoin/phenytoin, repeat loading of 10 mg/kg after 20 min
- Each time you load, check levels 10 minutes after
- Phenobarbital 30 mg/kg can be repeated after 10 minutes

7. **Intubation in case of persistent seizure for > 30 min along with anesthetic dose medications**
   a. *Load with midazolam* 0.2 mg/kg and continue 0.5 mg/kg/h
      OR
   b. *Load with propofol* 2 mg/kg and continue 5 mg/kg/hr

Remember (step 7):
Paralytics may mask seizures

8. **If none of the above work, consider:**
   Pentobarbital 5 mg/kg and infuse at 2.5 mg/kg/hr

12.16.2 Specialized Epilepsy Syndromes (Table 12.16c)

Type	Presentation	Pathognomonic EEG	Treatment

Juvenile myoclonic epilepsy	• **Myoclonic jerks after waking.**
	  – Absence seizures may present years before the myoclonic jerks.
	  – Generalized tonic clonic seizures may present years after the myoclonic jerks
	• Usually presents in puberty and may be inherited
		EEG: Polyspike discharge (4–6 Hz) and slow waves	1. **Valproic acid** (risk of teratogenicity in pregnant women)
			2. **Alternatives** include levetiracetam, lamotrigine, topiramate

West syndrome or infantile spasms	• **Salaam seizures** are typical (rapid flexion of head, torso, limbs/less often extension) • Associated with cognitive impairment • Usually presents in first year of life • Must exclude tuberous sclerosis	**EEG:** Hypsarrhythmia (very disorganized background activity + high-amplitude irregular spikes waves)	1. **ACTH** (high levels of CRH are a possible cause of the disease with ACTH and steroids possibly suppressing them) 2. **Steroids**
Lennox–Gastaut syndrome	• Usually **atonic/drop attacks** but also tonic and other types • Cognitive impairment[28] • Children • Exclude tuberous sclerosis • Up to 50 seizures/d	**EEG:** Slow background rhythm + spike-wave bursts (frequency < 2.5 Hz)[28]	1. **Drug resistant** (try valproic acid, lamotrigine, topiramate) 2. **Vagus nerve stimulator** 3. **Callosotomy** (reduces drop attacks)
Rasmussen's syndrome	• Seizures + one enlarged hemisphere • Encephalitis (probably autoimmune) • Children	1. Various, nonspecific, findings related to clinical progression 2. **EEG:** Persistent high-amplitude delta activity in inflamed hemisphere	1. Frequently resistant to antiepileptics 2. Steroids 3. IV immunoglobulins/plasmapheresis 4. Hemispherectomy[29]

12.17 CSF Pathognomonic Findings in Disease (Table 12.17a ◀))

Disease	White blood cells	Protein	Glucose	Other
Multiple sclerosis	↑ (5–50/mm³) monocytes	Normal or ↑	Normal	Oligoclonal bands
Guillain–Barre	Normal	↑	Normal	Albuminocyto-logic dissociation (increased protein without increased cell count)
Bacterial meningitis	↑ (PMN's)	↑	↓	Turbid appearance
Viral meningitis	↑ (but usually not as much as in bacterial)/ Lymphocytes	↑ (but usually not as much as in bacterial)	Normal	Clear
Tuberculosis	↑ (lymphocytes then monocytes)	↑	↓	• Yellowish/fibrin clot • Positive acid-fast bacilli (AFB) culture/ Ziehl–Neelsen

Note: Normal CSF: clear, no polys, no red blood cells, 0–5 mononuclear cells, 15–45 mg/dL protein, glucose is 50–75% of serum value, and opening pressure is 7–18 cm H_2O measured in lateral decubitus.

12.17.1 CSF versus Other Liquid (Table 12.17b)

CSF   Glucose > 30 mg/dL
           REMEMBER: exclude coexisting cause for low CSF glucose such as bacterial meningitis

           β2-transferrin (protein electrophoresis)

           Halo sign (small ring of blood in center with clear fluid ring around it)

           Patient may describe **taste of salt** (in case of rhinorrhea)

12.18 Genetic Disorders (Table 12.18)

Disease	Presentation	Diagnostics	Other	Treatment
Huntington's disease	• **Chorea** worse with walking • Progressively dementia and inability to walk • Psychiatric disturbances • **Possible systemic abnormalities** such as cardiac failure, impaired glucose tolerance, osteoporosis	**MRI:** caudate atrophy, rounding of frontal horns	• Autosomal dominant chromo- some 4 • May present earlier in every subsequent generation[30]	1. **Tetrabenazine** (inhibitor of vesicular monoamine transporter 2. **Antipsychotics** **Prognosis:** death within 15–20 y
Wilson's disease	• Dysarthria/ataxia/Parkinsonism • Psychosis[31] • **Systemic:** eye deposits (brown Kayser–Fleischer ring at edge of cornea)/hepatitis portal hypertension/hemolytic anemia	• Low blood levels of ceruloplasmin • Low serum copper with elevated urine copper levels	• Autosomal recessive (chromosome 13) • Copper accumulates in brain, eyes, liver	1. Diet modification 2. Penicillamine (may worsen neurological symptoms)/trientine hydrochloride/zinc 3. Possibly liver transplant **Prognosis** is poor

12.19 Various (Table 12.19)

Disease	Presentation	Diagnostics	Other	Treatment

ALS (amyotrophic lateral sclerosis) or Lou Gehrig's disease	• **Upper and lower motor neuron findings/** muscle atrophy: weakness
	• Tongue fasciculations
	• Progressively:
	  – Dysphagia
	  – Dysarthria
	  – Respiratory difficulty
		EMG: fasciculations		1. No therapy
				2. **Riluzole** (decreases glutamate, may prolong survival)[32]
				3. **Edaravone** (initially developed for stroke treatment)
				4. **Noninvasive ventilation** improves quality of life
				Prognosis: death within 3 y

Disease	Presentation	Diagnostics	Other	Treatment
Transverse myelitis	Acute spinal cord deficit that peaks within 2 d	1. **MRI:** ↑ T2 signal 2. **Lumbar puncture:** may show elevated protein or increased lymphocytes/PMNs 3. May follow viral/bacterial infection or vaccination	If accompanied by optic neuritis: **Devic's disease**	1. **Steroids** in high doses 2. **Plasmapheresis** is an option in case of bad response to steroids **Prognosis:** usually there is at least partial recovery but it takes months. If no improvement in 3–6 mo: bad prognosis

Sarcoidosis	• **Cranial neuropathy** (possibly multiple). Most commonly:
	  – optic neuropathy
	  – peripheral facial nerve palsy (this can be bilateral)
	• ±hydrocephalus/seizures/meningitis/hypothalamus–pituitary dysfunction/peripheral neuropathy
		1. Elevated **serum ACE** (angiotensin converting enzyme)
		2. Hypercalcemia
		3. Usually requires **biopsy** for definitive diagnosis
			1. Formation of **granulomas** (initially *lungs*, lymph nodes, skin)
			2. 5–10% of sarcoidosis patients suffer from neurosarcoidosis
				1. Steroids
				2. Immunosuppressants (for example cyclosporine)

Malignant neuroleptic syndrome	1. Stupor 2. Hyperthermia 3. Rigidity 4. Hypotension		Associated with medications that block central dopaminergic transmission (haloperidol, chlorpromazine, prochlorperazine)[33]	1. Discontinue responsible medication 2. Hydration/cooling/bicarbonate 3. Bromocriptine
Malignant hyperthermia	Similar to malignant neuroleptic syndrome		Associated with halogenated inhalational anesthetics/succinylcholine. Secondary to calcium not re-entering sarcoplasmic reticulum	1. Discontinue responsible medication 2. Hydration/cooling/bicarbonate 3. **Dantrolene** (inhibits calcium release from sarcoplasmic reticulum)

12.20 Case

12.20.1 Status Epilepticus

Chief complaint/History of present illness	A 40 y/o man was recently diagnosed with low grade glioma located in the right temporal lobe after presenting with a generalized tonic-clonic seizure. He underwent a right temporal craniotomy and gross total resection of the tumor was achieved. Patient is prescribed levetiracetam 1000 mg bid. It's the third postoperative day and you are on call for the ward, when you are asked to treat this patient, who is already having a generalized tonic-clonic seizure for 7 minutes.
Physical examination	• Patient is having a generalized seizure. • Afebrile. • Shallow respirations, oxygen saturation is 89%. • Pupils: normal size, symmetric, reactive.

1. **What are the main types of seizures? How does mental status differ in each type? What is the presentation and what are the treatment options for each one?**
   Simple partial, complex partial, generalized. (See Table 12.16a).

2. **What is the definition of status epilepticus?**
   Duration of seizure for more than 5 minutes OR seizure persists after first- and second-line antiepileptics. (See Table 12.16a).

3. **What might cause status epilepticus in a patient operated for brain tumor?**
   The differential diagnosis is postoperative hemorrhage, infection (meningitis, abscess, subdural empyema), abnormal electrolytes, hypoglycemia, inadequate antiepileptic treatment. After stabilizing the patient, a head CT scan should be performed immediately to rule out hematoma.

4. **What would be the differential diagnosis in an adult patient with their first seizure?**
   Main causes for a first seizure are TBI, stroke (ischemic/hemorrhagic), CNS infection, inflammatory/autoimmune diseases, alcohol or drug use/withdrawal, medications, metabolic causes (glucose and electrolyte abnormalities, liver/kidney failure etc.), tumor.

5. **What are the first management measures of status epilepticus?**
   Stabilization (ABC), monitoring of vital signs, finger stick blood glucose, labs and head CT. (See Table 12.16b).

6. **What is the first-line antiepileptic therapy?**
   Choose one from the following: Lorazepam IV, midazolam intramuscular (IM), diazepam per rectum. (See Table 12.16b).

7. **What is the second-line antiepileptic therapy?**
   (See Table 12.16b).

8. **What is the third-line antiepileptic therapy?**
   Anesthetic doses of midazolam or propofol or pentobarbital. (See Table 12.16b).

References

[1] Chen S, Andary M, Buschbacher R, et al. Electrodiagnostic reference values for upper and lower limb nerve conduction studies in adult populations. Muscle Nerve 2016;54(3):371–377

[2] van den Berg B, Walgaard C, Drenthen J, Fokke C, Jacobs BC, van Doorn PA. Guillain-Barré syndrome: pathogenesis, diagnosis, treatment and prognosis. Nat Rev Neurol 2014;10(8):469–482

[3] Titulaer MJ, Lang B, Verschuuren JJ. Lambert-Eaton myasthenic syndrome: from clinical characteristics to therapeutic strategies. Lancet Neurol 2011;10(12):1098–1107

[4] Poewe W, Seppi K, Tanner CM, et al. Parkinson disease. Nat Rev Dis Primers 2017;3:17013

[5] Mahapatra RK, Edwards MJ, Schott JM, Bhatia KP. Corticobasal degeneration. Lancet Neurol 2004;3(12):736–743

[6] Shin HW, Chung SJ. Drug-induced parkinsonism. J Clin Neurol 2012;8(1):15–21

[7] Louis ED. Clinical practice. Essential tremor. N Engl J Med 2001;345(12):887–891

[8] Jankovic J. Treatment of dystonia. Lancet Neurol 2006;5(10):864–872

[9] Delatycki MB, Williamson R, Forrest SM. Friedreich ataxia: an overview. J Med Genet 2000;37(1):1–8

[10] Sechi G, Serra A. Wernicke's encephalopathy: new clinical settings and recent advances in diagnosis and management. Lancet Neurol 2007;6(5):442–455

[11] Zupancic M, Mahajan A, Handa K. Dementia with Lewy bodies: diagnosis and management for primary care providers. Prim Care Companion CNC Disord 2011;13(5):pii:PCC.11r01190

[12] Lana-Peixoto MA. Devic's neuromyelitis optica: a critical review. Arq Neuropsiquiatr 2008;66(1):120–138

[13] Hardy TA, Miller DH. Baló's concentric sclerosis. Lancet Neurol 2014;13(7):740–746

[14] Pohl D, Alper G, Van Haren K, et al. Acute disseminated encephalomyelitis: updates on an inflammatory CNS syndrome. Neurology 2016;87(9, Suppl 2):S38–S45

[15] Lutalo PM, D'Cruz DP. Diagnosis and classification of granulomatosis with polyangiitis (aka Wegener's granulomatosis). J Autoimmun 2014;48–49:94–98

[16] De Virgilio A, Greco A, Magliulo G, et al. Polyarteritis nodosa: a contemporary overview. Autoimmun Rev 2016;15(6):564–570

[17] Chabriat H, Joutel A, Dichgans M, Tournier-Lasserve E, Bousser MG. Cadasil. Lancet Neurol 2009;8(7):643–653

[18] El-Hattab AW, Adesina AM, Jones J, Scaglia F. MELAS syndrome: clinical manifestations, pathogenesis, and treatment options. Mol Genet Metab 2015;116(1–2):4–12

[19] Nogueira RG, Jadhav AP, Haussen DC, et al; DAWN Trial Investigators. Thrombectomy 6 to 24 hours after stroke with a mismatch between deficit and infarct. N Engl J Med 2018;378(1):11–21

[20] Baloh RW, Furman JM, Yee RD. Dorsal midbrain syndrome: clinical and oculographic findings. Neurology 1985;35(1):54–60

[21] Pearce JM. Wallenberg's syndrome. J Neurol Neurosurg Psychiatry 2000;68(5):570

[22] Perry CM, Markham A. Sumatriptan. An updated review of its use in migraine. Drugs 1998;55(6):889–922

[23] May A. Cluster headache: pathogenesis, diagnosis, and management. Lancet 2005;366(9488):843–855

[24] Davidson B, Nassiri F, Mansouri A, et al. Spontaneous intracranial hypotension: a review and introduction of an algorithm for management. World Neurosurg 2017;101:343–349

[25] Hazin R, Azizzadeh B, Bhatti MT. Medical and surgical management of facial nerve palsy. Curr Opin Ophthalmol 2009;20(6):440–450

[26] Glauser T, Shinnar S, Gloss D, et al. Evidence-based guideline: treatment of convulsive status epilepticus in children and adults: report of the Guideline Committee of the American Epilepsy Society. Epilepsy Curr 2016;16(1):48–61

[27] Genton P, Thomas P, Kasteleijn-Nolst Trenité DG, Medina MT, Salas-Puig J. Clinical aspects of juvenile myoclonic epilepsy. Epilepsy Behav 2013;28(Suppl 1):S8–S14

[28] Arzimanoglou A, French J, Blume WT, et al. Lennox-Gastaut syndrome: a consensus approach on diagnosis, assessment, management, and trial methodology. Lancet Neurol 2009;8(1):82–93

[29] Varadkar S, Bien CG, Kruse CA, et al. Rasmussen's encephalitis: clinical features, pathobiology, and treatment advances. Lancet Neurol 2014;13(2):195–205

[30] Roos RA. Huntington's disease: a clinical review. Orphanet J Rare Dis 2010;5:40

[31] Bandmann O, Weiss KH, Kaler SG. Wilson's disease and other neurological copper disorders. Lancet Neurol 2015;14(1):103–113

[32] Salameh JS, Brown RH Jr, Berry JD. Amyotrophic lateral sclerosis: review. Semin Neurol 2015;35(4):469–476

[33] Tse L, Barr AM, Scarapicchia V, Vila-Rodriguez F. Neuroleptic malignant syndrome: a review from a clinically oriented perspective. Curr Neuropharmacol 2015;13(3):395–406

Index